Childhood Rhinitis and Sinusitis

ALLERGIC DISEASE AND THERAPY

Series Editor

David G. Tinkelman

Medical College of Georgia,
Augusta, Georgia, and
Atlanta Allergy Clinic,
Atlanta, Georgia

Volume 1 Histamine and H_2 Antagonists in Inflammation and Immunodeficiency, *edited by Ross E. Rocklin*

Volume 2 Asthma as an Inflammatory Disease, *edited by Paul M. O'Byrne*

Volume 3 Childhood Rhinitis and Sinusitis: Pathophysiology and Treatment, *edited by Charles K. Naspitz and David G. Tinkelman*

Additional Volumes in Preparation

Childhood Rhinitis and Sinusitis

Pathophysiology and Treatment

edited by

Charles K. Naspitz

Escola Paulista de Medicina
São Paulo, Brazil

David G. Tinkelman

Medical College of Georgia,
Augusta, Georgia, and
Atlanta Allergy Clinic,
Atlanta, Georgia

MARCEL DEKKER, INC. New York and Basel

Library of Congress Cataloging-in-Publication Data

Childhood rhinitis and sinusitis

(Allergic disease therapy ; v. 2)
Includes bibliographical references.
1. Hay-fever in children. 2. Sinusitis in children.
I. Naspitz, Charles K. II. Tinkelman, David G.
III. Series. [DNLM: 1. Rhinitis, Allergic, Perennial--
in infancy & childhood. 2. Rhinitis, Allergic, Perennial--
physiopathology. 3. Rhinitis, Allergic, Perennial--
therapy. 4. Sinusitis--in infancy & childhood.
5.Sinusitis--physiopathology. 6. Sinusitis--therapy
WV 335 C536]
RJ386.3.C47 1990 618.92'202 90-2861
ISBN 0-8247-8228-3 (alk paper)

This book is printed on acid-free paper.

MARCEL DEKKER, INC.
270 Madison Avenue, New York, New York 10016

Current printing (last digit):
10 9 8 7 6 5 4 3 2 1

PRINTED IN THE UNITED STATES OF AMERICA

Series Introduction

Allergic disease and its therapy has long been a topic of discussion. The development of theories on the cause of allergic symptoms has consumed volumes of medical literature dealing with virtually all organ systems. From these postulations have come practical approaches to the diagnosis and management of allergic disorders. Despite the continuum of medical "breakthroughs," the answers to many of the questions relating to allergy remain unknown.

In this series, Allergic Disease and Therapy, the authors will attempt to concisely put forth reviews of past approaches as well as the most up-to-date information relating to a variety of different allergic states. Basic scientists, clinical researchers, and experts will combine their efforts to establish rational approaches to the diagnosis and management of the complex allergic problems of today. This will be a multidisciplinary approach by individuals spanning the globe in an effort to cover these topics from many different perspectives. From the genetics laboratories where complex questions concerning the role of certain gene pools in the develop of immunologic competence are being studied to the research facilities of pharmaceutical companies where new therapeutic products are being tested, this series will address many unanswered questions in the rapidly growing field of allergy and immunology. The goal of the series is to provide the practitioner with the background knowledge and tools with which to approach the allergic problems that are so common in today's society.

David G. Tinkelman

Foreword

Rhinitis is one of the most common disorders of children and may cause a varied spectrum of problems for the child and his family. Chronic rhinitis may cause sleep disturbances, interfere with normal psychosocial development, result in school absenteeism, and/or induce orthodontic problems. Sinusitis, a common complication of rhinitis, has been overlooked by pediatricians for almost two generations since it was declared a "nondisease" by a leading pediatric radiology textbook in the 1940s. Only recently have physicians caring for children recognized that childen do indeed develop acute and chronic infections of their sinuses with signs and symptoms that may be quite different from those of adults. For example, sinusitis in children can result in such diffuse symptoms as chronic fatigue and persistent coughing or may even increase the severity of asthma.

Though rhinitis and sinusitis represent a common problem in pediatric practice, very little attention is devoted to it in medical school or residency training. This is unfortunate since the complex interaction of the child with his environment, the interplay of allergens, irritants, and infectious agents, is so clearly seen in childhood sinusitis and rhinitis. Although many children with these disorders may be allergic, allergy is misunderstood by many physicians. On one hand, some physicians consider "allergy" to be the cause of all chronic rhinitis; on the other, allergic factors may not be recognized, and even when recognized may be managed inappropriately.

Drs. Naspitz and Tinkelman have assembled a distinguished group of authorities from the United States and England. Each, an expert in his or her own field, discusses pathogenesis, pathophysiology, diagnosis, and/or treatment of sinusitis or rhinitis in children. The focus is on the child and on the successful resolution of his or her problem. This book is for practicing physicians who care for children and should be of particular value to pediatricians, family physicians, and pediatric allergists. It should aid them in better controlling the morbidity from diseases of the nose and sinuses in children.

Warren Bierman, M.D., Clinical Professor, Department of Pediatrics, School of Medicine, University of Washington, Seattle, Washington; Visiting Professor, Paediatrics, United Medical and Dental School of Guy's and St. Thomas Hospital, University of London, London, England

Preface

Without question, symptoms related to the upper respiratory tract are the most frequent ones affecting children. Children all over the world experience the "common cold," allergy, and infection of the ears, nose, throat, or sinuses and regularly seek medical attention. In most cases the symptoms are treated without firm determination of the etiology of the problem. In the chronic or recurrent state more attention is given to making the diagnosis with respect to the causative agent so that more effective and, hopefully, long-lasting results can be attained. The approach to the diagnosis and management of the child with involvement of the upper respiratory tract is the emphasis of this book.

The influence of the developing child on the pathophysiology of the upper airway has more than simply academic interest. It is the essence of establishing a patient-specific diagnostic and management plan for a variety of disorders that affect children. In order to gain a better perspective on the interaction of the dynamics of a growing child and the presentation of many of these disorders, the approach of this book is to clearly establish the growth and development patterns of the anatomy and physiology of the normal child and, from there, to delve into the questions of the pathophysiological state.

As the subject of disorders of the nose and sinuses is varied and complex, we have joined the efforts of both otolaryngologists and allergists to create not only a comprehensive reference book, but also a practical guide for physicians who treat children. From the embryo to adolescence, these chapters deal with the latest theories of allergy, inflammation, diagnostic techniques, and treatment modalities. Both medical and surgical points of view are presented on how to approach acute and chronic nasal and sinus disorders. Experts from around the world have shared their knowledge, experience, and therapeutic strategies in their individual chapters. Their approach to similar problems may vary in some instances. However, in many of these problems there is no one "correct" way to proceed. We hope you will find it useful to read these differing opinions and will use them as guidelines for developing your own approach in each individual case. It is our intention that these scientifically stimulating and practical chapters will be a source of constant information regarding the latest theories on pathogenesis and diagnostic procedures and a guide to the preferred and alternative approaches for management of children with rhinitis and sinusitis.

We, as editors, would like to acknowledge the efforts and cooperation of the contributing authors. We value not only their expertise, but also their cooperation in meeting deadlines, which has put significant time demands on their already busy schedules. Without this effort this book would never have come to publication.

Charles K. Naspitz
David G. Tinkelman

Contributors

Martin D. Chapman, Ph.D. Assistant Professor of Medicine and Microbiology, Division of Allergy and Clinical Immunology, Department of Medicine, University of Virginia Health Sciences Center, Charlottesville, Virginia

Philip Fireman, M.D. Professor, Department of Pediatrics, University of Pittsburgh School of Medicine, and Director, Division of Allergy, Immunology, and Rheumatology, Children's Hospital of Pittsburgh, Pittsburgh, Pennsylvania

Brian K. Flowers, M.D. Department of Medicine, The Johns Hopkins University School of Medicine, Baltimore, Maryland

Gilbert A. Friday, Jr., M.D. Professor, Department of Pediatrics, University of Pittsburgh School of Medicine, and Chief, Clinical Services, Asthma and Allergic Disease Center, Children's Hospital of Pittsburgh, Pittsburgh, Pennsylvania

John W. Georgitis, M.D. Associate Professor, Department of Pediatrics, Bowman Gray School of Medicine of Wake Forest University, Winston-Salem, North Carolina

Peter W. Heymann, M.D. Assistant Professor, Department of Pediatrics, University of Virginia Health Sciences Center, Charlottesville, Virginia

Stephen T. Holgate, M.D., F.R.C.P. MRC Clinical Professor of Immunopharmacology, Medicine I, Southampton General Hospital and University of Southampton, Southampton, England

Peter H. Howarth, M.D. Senior Lecturer in Medicine, Medicine I, Southampton General Hospital and University of Southampton, Southampton, England

Eli O. Meltzer, M.D. Clinical Professor, Department of Pediatrics, Division of Allergy and Immunology, University of California—San Diego, and Allergy and Asthma Medical Group and Research Center, San Diego, California

Henry Milgrom, M.D. Associate Professor, Department of Pediatrics, University of Colorado Health Sciences Center, and Department of Pediatrics, National Jewish Center for Immunology and Respiratory Medicine, Denver, Colorado

Ahmed A. Mohiuddin, M.D. Department of Pediatrics, National Jewish Center for Immunology and Respiratory Medicine, Denver, Colorado

Robert M. Naclerio, M.D. Associate Professor of Otolaryngology and Pediatrics and Medicine, Department of Otolaryngology—Head and Neck Surgery, The Johns Hopkins University School of Medicine, Baltimore, Maryland

Charles K. Naspitz, M.D. Professor, Department of Pediatrics, Escola Paulista de Medicina, São Paulo, Brazil

Susan M. Pollart, M.D. Assistant Professor, Departments of Internal Medicine and Family Medicine, University of Virginia Health Sciences Center, Charlottesville, Virginia

Gail G. Shapiro, M.D. Clinical Professor, Department of Pediatrics, School of Medicine, University of Washington, and Division of Allergy, Children's Hospital and Medical Center, Seattle, Washington

Peter A. Shapiro, D.D.S., M.S.D. Professor and Chairman, Department of Orthodontics, University of Washington School of Dentistry, Seattle, Washington

Michael L. Steinberg, M.D. Fellow, Department of Allergy and Immunology, Children's Hospital of Pittsburgh, Pittsburgh, Pennsylvania

Aurapin Sukanich, M.D. Fellow, Department of Allergy and Immunology, Children's Hospital of Pittsburgh, Pittsburgh, Pennsylvania

David G. Tinkelman, M.D. Associate Clinical Professor, Division of Allergy, Department of Pediatrics, Medical College of Georgia, Augusta, Georgia, and Atlanta Allergy Clinic, Atlanta, Georgia

Gina M. Trask, D.D.S., M.S.D. Clinical Assistant Professor, Department of Orthodontics, University of Washington School of Dentistry, Seattle, Washington

Contents

1

Basic Aspects of Allergic Reactions

Peter H. Howarth and Stephen T. Holgate
Southampton General Hospital and University of Southampton, Southampton, England

I. INTRODUCTION

Rhinitis describes an inflammatory condition of the nasal mucosa associated with the symptoms of sneezing, nasal discharge, nasal blockage and nasal itching. In children with an atopic diathesis, rhinitis is the most common manifestation of allergic disease. Cumulative figures from questionnaire studies identify the prevalence of allergic rhinitis in westernized populations increasing from 1% in 4–6 year olds through 5–7% in 7 year olds, to 12–28% in university students (Table 1; 1–17). The comparative figures are higher in boys than girls (4,8). Few serial investigations have been undertaken to identify whether or not prevalences have changed with time, but studies from Switzerland (1,2,11) and Finland (10,8) suggest that allergic rhinitis has become more prevalent in the last two decades. Consistent with this, the National Morbidity surveys from The Royal College of General Practitioners research unit in Birmingham, England, have identified a quadrupling in the number of annual consultations for grass pollen seasonal allergic rhinitis between the years 1955/1956 and 1981/1982 (18,19). In three separate annual surveys (1955/1956, 1970/1971, 1981/1982), that are based on nationwide population surveys of about 300,000 individuals in England and Wales, there has been a progressive doubling of annual consultations for hay fever (Fig. 1). In these surveys, the consultations for hay fever in males was maximum in the aged group 5–15 and in females in the aged group 15–24. Although a number of factors could contribute to the increasing prevalence of consultations for hay fever treatment, it is likely that this represents a true increase in the prevalence of this condition, for a diagnostic change is unlikely because of the seasonal characteristic and nature of the symptoms and because no major therapeutic advance became available in the interval between the first two surveys.

II. ATOPY

Atopy describes a state of heightened sensitivity in which there is an exaggerated response to foreign protein. This exaggerated response can be demonstrated locally within the skin by the development of a wheal-and-flare response following intracutaneous inoculation of specific protein. An individual demonstrating such a response is termed *atopic*, and the protein to which they respond is called an *allergen*. The heightened sensitivity to allergens in atopic children is due to the presence in the tissue of excess immunoglobulin E (IgE), which is cell bound and allergen-specific. The skin wheal response in an individual correlates closely with the measurement of the circulating specific IgE level. The presence of atopy, thus, is detectable by skin-prick testing with specific allergens.

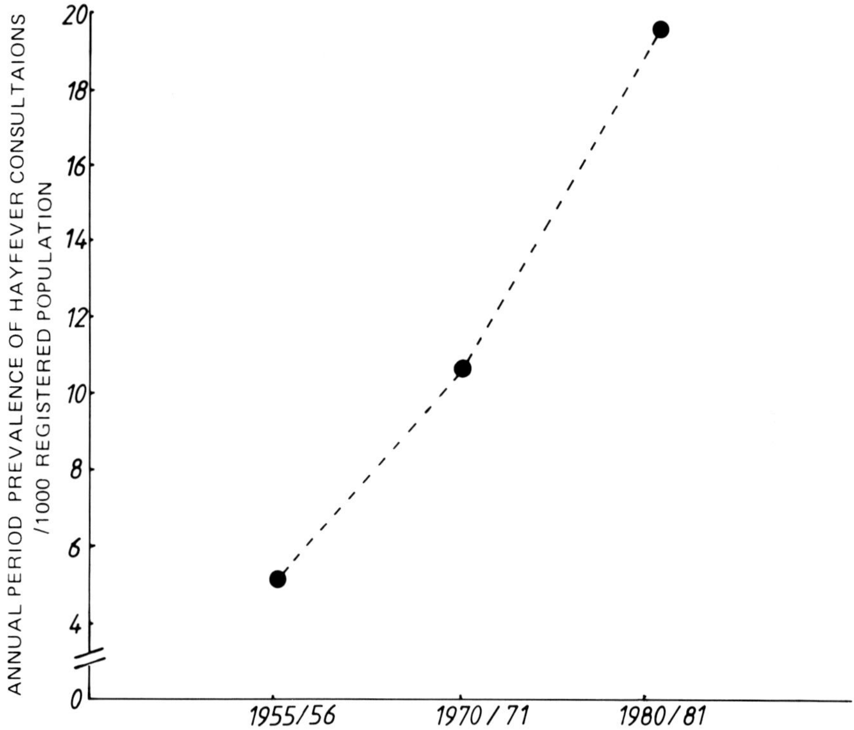

Figure 1 Annual period prevalence of hay fever consultations in general practice in the United Kingdom per 1000 of the registered population. (From Refs. 18 and 19.)

Not all children who exhibit a positive response on skin-prick testing have clinical symptoms related to that allergen, but the larger the wheal response, the greater the likelihood that they have, or will subsequently develop, rhinitic symptoms on specific allergen exposure. A serial study in university students identified that 71.4% of students with a 4+ skin wheal response to pollen had developed seasonal rhinitic symptoms within a 7-year follow-up period, compared with 7.7% of those with an initial negative response and 23.3% of those with a 1+ response (16). Concordant with this, a recent population survey reports a close positive correlation between the presence of allergic rhinitis and the positivity of the skin wheal response to common airborne allergens and, hence, the level of specific IgE (20).

Table 1 Prevalence of Allergic Rhinitis from Epidemiological Studies

Ref.	Author(s)	Date	Country	Age (yr)	Number studied	Prevalence (%)	Method
1	Varonier	1970	Switzerland	5–6	4781	0.5	1 + E
2	Varonier	1984	Switzerland	4–6	3270	1.1	Q + E
3	Giles	1968		7	8410	6.8	Q
4	Kjellman	1977	Sweden	7	1325	7.4	Q
5	Waite	1980	Tokelau	0–14	706	14	1 + E
	Waite	1980	New Zealand	0–14	1160	28	1 + E
6	Skerpaas and Gulsvik	1985	Norway	8–14	1772	5.4	Q
1	Varonier	1970	Switzerland	15	2451	4.4	1 + E
2	Varonier	1984	Switzerland	15	3500	6.1	Q + E
7	Wolstenholme	1979	Maldives	0–15	2903	20.4	1
8	Haahtela	1980	Finland	15–17	708	22	1 + E
9	Freeman and Johnson	1964		14–18	2235	19	Q + E
10	Alanko	1970	Finland	10–19	5287	2.7	1 + E
11	Wuthrich	1986	Switzerland	15–24		16	1
12	Tips	1954	USA	U.S.		16.2	
13	Van Arsdel and Motulsky	1959	USA	U.S.		12	
14	Maternowski and Mathews	1962	USA	U.S.		5.7	
15	Sherry and Scott	1968	USA	U.S.		13.9	
16	Hagy and Settipane	1969	USA	U.S.		19.7	
17	Malmberg	1979	Sweden	U.S.	315	28	

III. IMMUNOGLOBULIN E

Following its isolation in 1966 from the sera of ragweed-sensitive subjects, immunoglobulin E was identified as being the agent responsible for the transmission of the immediate hypersensitivity response (21), an action previously attributed to an unidentified "reaginic antibody." Immunoglobulin E is a tetrameric compound, composed of two light and two heavy chains, with a combined molecular mass of 190,000 Da (22). Papain digestion splits the molecule into two (Fab) fragments carrying the antibody-combining sites and an Fc section, which binds to specific receptors on cell surfaces (23). Immunoglobulin E directed to specific epitopes is synthesized by primed B lymphocytes and committed plasma cells in response to low levels of antigenic stimulation on mucosal surfaces. The differentiation of precursor B cells to IgE plasma cells is a complex process that has been investigated in rodents. In this species it involves immunoglobulin, isotype-specific, regulatory T-"helper" cells, which express Fc receptor (24) and secrete IgE-binding regulatory factors (IgE-BFs) under the further regulation of "suppressor" T lymphocytes. The influence of IgE-BFs on IgE production depends upon their degree of glycosylation, also under T-cell control (25). Glycosylated IgE-BF potentiates IgE synthesis, whereas unglycosylated IgE-BF suppresses IgE synthesis. Whether such a regulatory system also pertains to humans is still under investigation, and the basis for the enhanced IgE production characteristic of the atopic state is not fully clarified. Several proposals have been considered, including (1) a failure to exclude foreign protein at mucosal surfaces and (2) a failure of T-cell "suppressor" function that would normally regulate or terminate IgE production. Although elevated IgE levels can be found in some patients with IgA deficiency (26), direct evidence for the first hypothesis is deficient because no difference exists between atopic and nonatopic individuals in their nasal absorption of foreign protein (27). In mice, IgE antibody production is T-cell dependent and highly susceptible to suppression by both T cells and T-cell factors (25). Thus, it is possible that enhanced IgE synthesis in humans could be related to impaired T-cell "suppressor" function or exaggerated T-cell "helper" activity. Consistent with this hypothesis are the increased IgE levels that are a feature of states in which there is deficient T-cell suppressive function, as in congenital T-cell immunodeficiency disorders (Wiskott–Aldrich syndrome, ataxia telangectasia) and acquired T-cell immunodeficiency disorders (transient hypo-α-globulinemia, Hodgkin's disease) (28,29). In addition, diminished OKT8-lymphocyte levels and impaired T-cell function have been reported in hyper-IgE states and in atopic patients (30). Although it is not known whether these abnormalities represent a primary or a secondary defect, the finding that a reduction in T-cell suppressor function at 1 month precedes and increases the risk of atopy (31) suggests that it may be a primary abnormality in some infants. This interpretation is not exclusive and may not be the only imbalance between T-cell subsets, as there is also evidence in some instances of excess T-cell enhancing activity in the atopic state.

In the normal population, total serum IgE levels increase from birth, reaching the adult range at approximately 6 years of age (32). The mean total serum levels of IgE levels peak during the second decade of life and then decline with increasing age. Because IgE is predominantly cell bound, its serum concentration in normal subjects is low (0.1–0.7 μg/ml) in normal subjects, in comparison with the other immunoglobulins. The development of specific IgE to inhalant allergens is unusual before the age of 2 years, but may become apparent thereafter. In one serial study of 92 children of atopic parents, 20% had developed specific responses to inhalant allergens by the age of 5 years (33). In contrast to inhalant allergen sensitivity, the prevalence of egg-specific IgE approached 30% in these children within their first 2 years, with skin test positivity being maximum at 1 year and radioallergosorbent test (RAST) positivity maximal at 2 years. A number of other studies have also identified positive skin-prick tests to food allergens within the first year of life, ranging from 25–60% of populations of atopic-prone infants (34–36). Although these positive food allergen responses are not associated with rhinitis, it has been suggested that a positive skin-prick test response to a food allergen within the first year of life is a predictor of subsequent inhalant atopy and that skin test-positive infants will have a higher prevalence of allergic rhinitis than skin test-negative infants (37).

Several factors predispose to the development of atopy, of which the most powerful is genetic with 0–20%, 30–50%, and 60–100% being the reported occurrence of atopy in children with none, one, or two parents, respectively, with atopic disease (13,38–40). Expression of the atopic state is influenced by maternal smoking (41), month of birth (in relationship to seasonal inhalant allergens) (42,43), and possibly, also by respiratory infection (44). A temporal relationship has been observed in children between viral infection and the onset of sensitization to allergens. This relationship has recently been explored further in animal studies, and an enhanced IgE response to ragweed antigen is reported in mice infected intranasally with respiratory syncitial virus (45). No such response occurs in sham-infected mice, despite a comparable antigen exposure. This suggests that a mucosally restricted viral infection may enhance the development of sensitization and influence the magnitude of the antibody response to an inhalant allergen in susceptible individuals. An effect possibly related to either viral-induced epithelial disruption, permitting an increase in antigen uptake, or an alteration in antigen processing.

IV. IMMUNOGLOBULIN E RECEPTORS

The enhanced IgE response in atopy leads to symptom generation through the interaction of allergen with cell-bound IgE. Following the discovery of IgE, autoradiographic studies identified that IgE is preferentially bound to mast cells and basophils (46,47). This binding, mediated by the Fc portion of the IgE molecule, is to high-affinity Fc receptors (48), now designated Fc_ϵ RI (Table 2). This receptor class designation has arisen with the discovery that lower-affinity Fc receptors (Fc_ϵ RII) are present on other cell types (see Table 2). These receptors were not identified in the early autoradiographic studies because the procedures employed selectively discerned the high-affinity receptors. The low-affinity Fc_ϵ RII has now been described on lymphocytes, eosinophils, platelets, and cells of the monocyte–macrophage series (49).

V. MECHANISMS OF ALLERGIC RHINITIS

Until relatively recently, the main effector cells considered to be involved in the initiation of IgE-mediated allergic reactions have been tissue mast cells and circulating basophils, because both these cells possess high-affinity IgE_ϵ Fc receptors in high density. As rhinitis is a result of allergen–antibody interaction at a tissue mucosal surface, the mast cell has been considered the prime orchestrator of symptom generation at this site. An understanding of the mechanisms of allergic rhinitis has come from laboratory experiments investigating the immediate and late nasal responses to allergen challenge, from the investigation of the effects of mediators considered to be important in the nasal response to allergen and from investigations of the nasal cellular events in naturally occurring disease.

Table 2 Receptors for IgE

	Fc_ϵ RI	Fc_ϵ RII
Cells	Mast cell Basophil	Macrophage Monocyte Lymphocyte: B, T Eosinophil Platelet
Affinity	10^9–10^{12} mol/L	10^6–10^8 mol/L
Number/cell	10^4–10^6	10^3–10^5
Structure	Tetramer	Single polypeptide chain

A. Immediate Nasal Response

In atopic subjects nasal insufflation with an allergen to which they are sensitive induces immediate itching, sneezing, and rhinorrhea, with nasal blockage developing over 30 to 40 mins after challenge and persisting for up to 2 hr, depending on the strength of immunological challenge. During this immediate nasal response, lavage of the nasal cavity has identified increased local concentrations of histamine; kinins; prostaglandin D_2 (PGD_2); leukotrienes (LTs) C_4; D_4 and E_4; and tryptase, an enzyme that hydrolyzes the artificial substrate tosyl arginine methyl ester (TAME esterase) (50–52). The finding of increased levels of both PGD_2 and tryptase in lavage suggests a mast cell origin for these findings. Direct evidence of mast cell degranulation in the nose immediately after allergen challenge has been obtained by nasal biopsy (53).

1. *The Mast Cell*

The mast cell was first described in 1877 by Paul Erhlich, when investigating the histochemical-staining characteristics of some synthetic basic aniline dyes. He identified the presence of a connective tissue cell the granules of which exhibited a metachromatic property (alteration of the color of the dye). Because these cells were numerous in tissues that were "well nourished" he named them "mastzellen" (well-nourished cells). Human mast cells are 9–12 μm in size, contain a round to oval eccentrically placed nucleus, and their cytoplasm is occupied by granules and cytoplasmic filaments (54). The cytoplasmic granules contain a number of preformed mediators.

Preformed Mediators. The metachromatic-staining property of the mast cell was subsequently identified as being due to the presence within the cytoplasmic granules of the highly acidic proteoglycan heparin (55,56). In human mast cells this is a 60-kDa species of herapin, in contrast with the 750-kDa heparin associated with rodent mast cells (57). The metachromatic property of heparin resides in its unique carbohydrate structure. It consists of a central peptide core, comprising alternating glycine and serine residues, to which are attached sulfated chains of amino sugars called glycosaminoglycans (GAGs) (58). The GAG side chains are attached to every second or third serine residue of the peptide core and are made up of a series of disaccharide units composed of either glucuronic or iduronic acid linked to glucosamine (59). The complexity of the disaccharide subunit is increased further by the insertion of one carboxyl group and sulfate groups varying in number from one to four. This complex structure of heparin and its highly acidic and hydrophilic properties permit it to store other pre-formed mediators in an inactivated form (60,61). The other major preformed mediators of the mast cell are the amine—histamine—and the proteases—tryptase, carboxypeptidase B, and chymase (Table 3).

Table 3 Preformed Human Mast Cell Mediators

Mediator class	Mediator	Physiochemical characteristics (M_r)	Function
Biogenic amine	Histamine	2–5 pg/cell	H_1- and H_2-mediated effects on vascular endothelium, nerve endings, and cell function
Neutral protease	Tryptase	Tetramer ($\alpha_2\beta_2$, 37,000 and β-35,000)	Cleavage of C3 and C3a, fibrinogen, and fibronectin
	Chymase	CTMC[a] only (30,000)	Cleavage of type IV collagen, glucagon, fibronectin
	Carboxypeptidase	Isoenzyme-B	Acts in concert with other proteolytic enzymes
Acid hydrolases	β-Hexosaminidase	Isoenzyme-B-β_4 (108,000)	Cleavage of β-linked hexosaminidases
	β-Glucuronidase	Tetramer (75,000)	Cleaves β-linked glucuronic acid
	β-Galactosidase	Type A (72,000)	Hydrolyzes β-linked galactose
	Arylsulfatase	Isoenzyme B	Hydrolyzes aromatic sulfate esters
Oxidative enzymes	Superoxide dismutase	?	Converts O_2 to H_2O_2
	Peroxidase		Converts H_2O_2 to H_2O
			Inactivates leukotrienes
Chemotactic factors	Eosinophil oligopeptides	ECF-A	Eosinophil chemotaxis
	Neutrophil chemotactic activity (NCA)	High M_r NCA (600–700,000)	Neutrophil chemotaxis
Proteoglycan	Heparin	Heparin (60,000)	Anticoagulant
			Anticomplementary
	Chondroitin sulfate	Chondroitin 4+6 sulfate	

[a]CTMC, connective tissue mast cell.

Histamine is bound to the carboxyl groups of the glucuronic and iduronic acid. Neutral proteases in being highly cationic, bind to the anionic carboxyl and sulfate groups of the GAGs. This structure of the GAGs and their intracellular binding give rise to an orderly crystalline pattern, discernible within the granules on transmission electron microscopy (62). Four structures of intragranular crystals have been described: scrolls, lattices, gratings, and a serpertinelike structure, all of which have a common repeating periodicity of 7.5 A or multiples thereof, suggesting a similar basic chemical structure. In addition to heparin, histamine, and the neutral proteases, the mast cell granules contain smaller quantities of acid hydrolases (β-hexosaminidase, β-glucuronidase, β-galactosidase, and arylsulfatase), chemotactic factors [eosinophil chemotactic factors of anaphylaxis (ECF-A), high-molecular-weight neutrophil chemotactic activity (NCA)], superoxide dismutase, and a kininogenase (63).

Immunological Mast Cell Activation. In an atopic individual, specific IgE is bound by the Fc fragment to the Fc receptors on the mast cell surface (Fig. 2). The binding of antigen to the cell surface-bound IgE initiates the process of mast cell activation and secretion. Although 10^4–10^6 high-affinity IgE receptors exist per cell (49,64), it is probably that aggregation of only 1–2% of surface-bound IgE is required to initiate substantial histamine release, and that occupancy of only 10–15% of the antigen-binding capacity is necessary for optimal mediator secretion. The cross-linking of IgE by antigen brings the cell surface receptors into apposition and reveals a membrane serine esterase. Within 30 sec of mast cell activation substantial amounts of 1,2-diacylglycerol (DAG) are generated, either through cleavage of membrane-bound phosphatidylinositol (PI) by phospholipase C, or related enzymes (65), or through sequential phosphorylation of PI and cleavage by a phosphodiesterase (66). The subsequent metabolism of DAG by the calcium-dependent enzyme, diglyceride lipase, leads to the production of L-monoacylglycerol (MAG) and arachidonic acid (Fig. 3). In addition to providing arachidonic acid for further metabolism, the products of this pathway may contribute to the intracellular events that precede preformed mast cell secretion. These events include hydrolysis and swelling of the secretory granules, their transfer by cytoskeletal proteins to regions adjacent to the plasma membrane, fusion of the perigranular and cytoplasmic membranes, and liberation of the preformed mediators into the extracellular environment. First, inositol triphosphate, formed during the generation of DAG, can mobilize calcium from intracellular stores in the presence of ATP, making it available for Ca^{2+}-dependent enzymes; second, DAG activates the Ca^{2+}-dependent enzyme, protein kinase C, which is responsible for the conversion of myosin to its active phosphorylated form and, thereby, induces contraction of smooth muscle (in this instance the

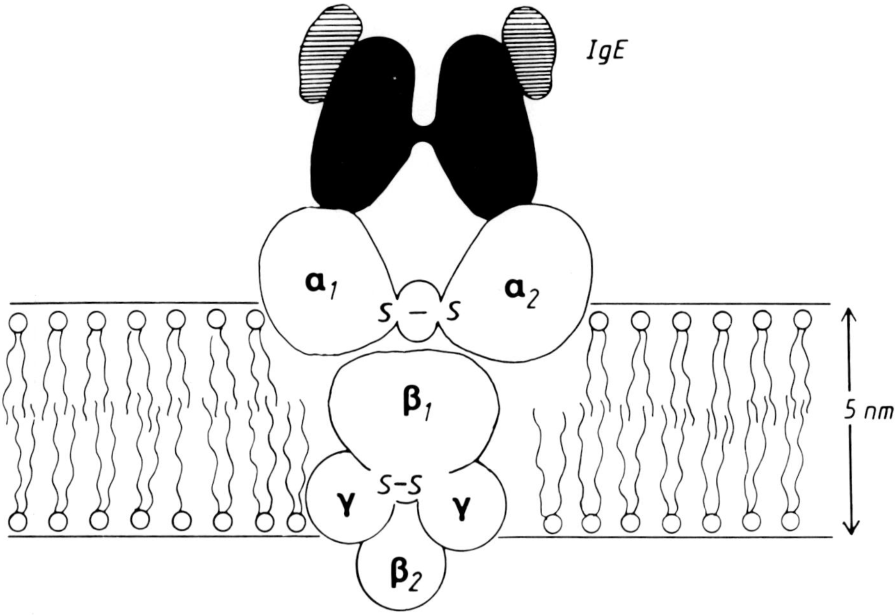

Figure 2 Schematic diagram of the cell-membrane-located, high-affinity IgE receptor plus associated IgE molecule. Receptor composed of two α and γ subunits linked by disulfide bonds and two β subunits.

cytoskeletal thin filaments) leading to the movement of the granule toward the mast cell plasma membrane; and third, both MAG and DAG are potent membrane fusagens. In addition, the change in membane PI levels may influence the membrane calcium pump to modify the intracellular/extracellular calcium balance in favor of an intracellular flux (67,68). Elevations in intracellular calcium also activate the membrane-bound phospholipase A_2 to amplify the arachidonic acid cleavage. The intracellular calcium influx is terminated by a rise in PI, generated from the conversion of DAG to phosphatidic acid and, hence, to PE by an energy-dependent process.

In addition to stimulation of these intracellular pathways, immunological activation of human mast cells has been shown to be accompanied by a transient increase in the cellular levels as a classic second messenger, cyclicAMP, which precedes mediator secretion (69).

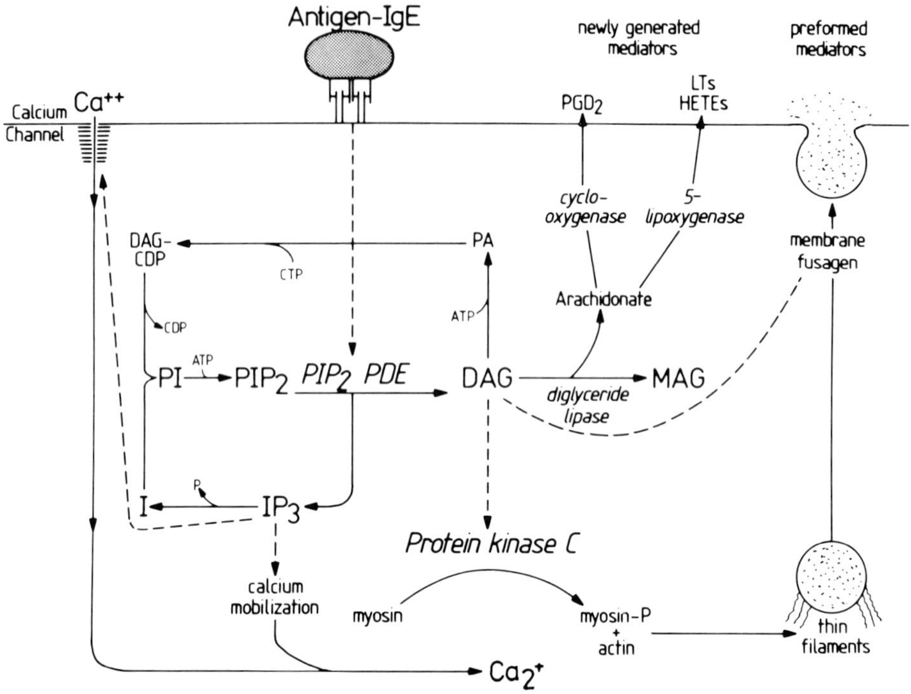

Figure 3 Proposed sequence of intracellular biochemical events following mast cell activation-secretion coupling.

Newly Generated Mediators. The arachidonic acid cleaved from the phospholipid membrane can be metabolized by either cyclooxygenase enzymes (Fig. 4) to produce prostaglandins (PGs) and thromboxanes (TXs) or lipoxygenase enzymes (Fig. 5) to produce hydroxyeicosatetraenoic acids (HETEs) or leukotrienes (LTs). Cyclooxygenase is a membrane-associated enzyme that catalyzes the incorporation of molecular oxygen into the arachidonic acid molecule, followed by ring closure, to yield the unstable endoperoxidase, PGG_2 and PGH_2 (70). These intermediates may then be converted enzymatically or nonenzymatically to yield PGD_2, PGE_2, $PGF_{2\alpha}$, PGI_2, and TXA_2 (71–73).

In isolated human mast cells dispersed from the lung by proteolytic enzymes and then purified by countercurrent centrifugal elutriation and density flotation (74,75), the most abundant cyclooxygenase product generated by immunological activation is PGD_2 (74,76), with only small quantities of PGE_2,

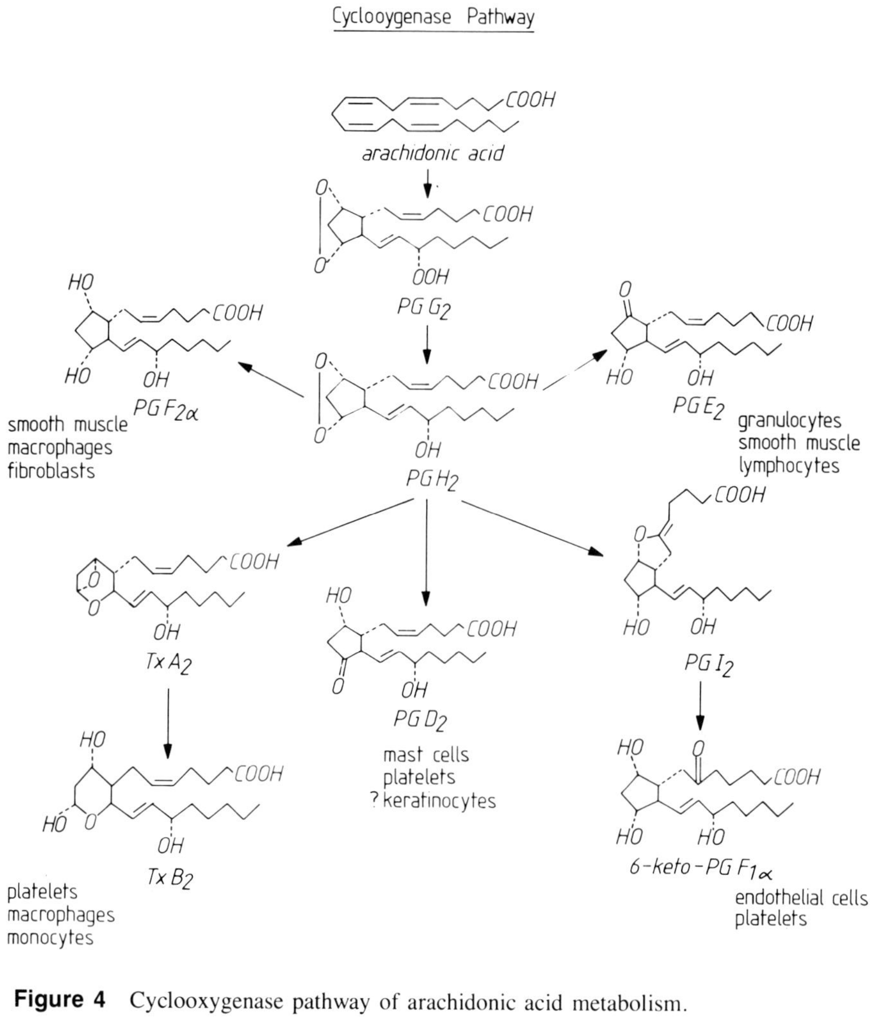

Figure 4 Cyclooxygenase pathway of arachidonic acid metabolism.

$PGF_{2\alpha}$, and the PGI_2 and TXA_2 metabolites, 6-keto-$PGF_{1\alpha}$ and TXB_2, being detectable (74). Prostaglandin D_2 is also the major prostanoid recovered after immunological activation of airway lavage mast cells (77). Arachidonic acid may also be metabolized by lipoxygenase enzymes to form, initially, an unstable acyclic hydroperoxyeicosatetranoeic acid (HPETE) (78). In the presence of

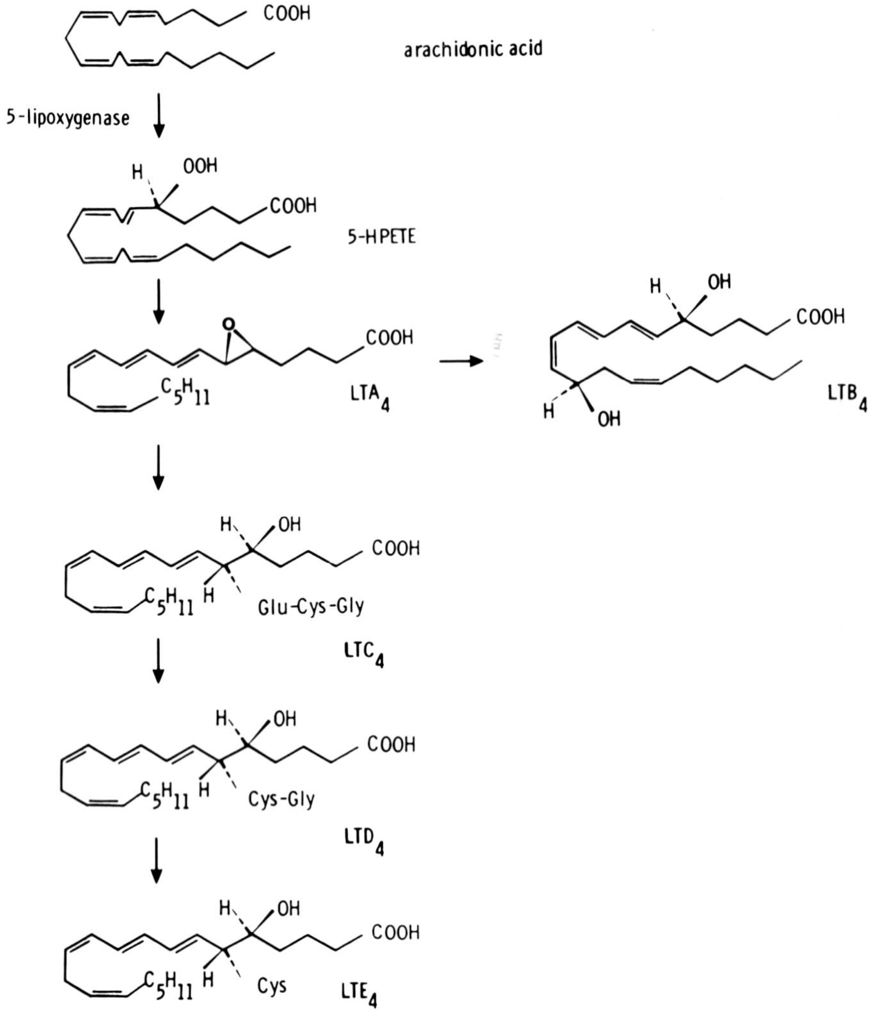

Figure 5 5-Lipoxygenase pathway of arachidonic acid metabolism.

the 5-lipoxygenase enzyme, this converts to LTA_4, which rapidly converts to LTC_4 in the presence of leukotriene C synthetase (79). Leukotriene C_4 is the only LT produced in experiments with immunological stimulation of highly purified human lung mast cells (80). In unpurified human lung cell preparations there is also generation of LTD_4 and LTE_4 (81), the enzymatic conversion products of LTC_4. Thus, LTC_4 released by mast cells may be converted to LTD_4 and LTE_4 by other cells in a local environment.

In contrast with the eicosanoids, less is known about the release of the other newly generated mediator, platelet-activating factor (PAF)-acether, from human mast cells. To date, the evidence suggests that human mast cells are not a major source of extracellular PAF-acether after immunological stimulation, despite a rapid intracellular synthesis (Fig. 6; 82). The synthesized PAF—acether remains cell bound.

Mast Cell Heterogeneity. It has been realized since the early 1900s that mast cells are not homogeneous among species and, indeed, among tissues in the same species. Considerable work has been undertaken in rodent species in this report, but only relatively recently has it been possible to isolate human mast cells and focus on their heterogeneity. Most of this work has been undertaken on human lung and skin mast cells (Table 4); with less functional work on the nasal mast cell, although morphological work is detailed in section VI.

In the rodent, there is a consistent relationship between morphological, physicochemical, and functional characteristics of mast cells derived from connective tissue and from mucosal sites. This division is not so clear in humans, but a major advance in the study of human mast cell heterogeneity has been

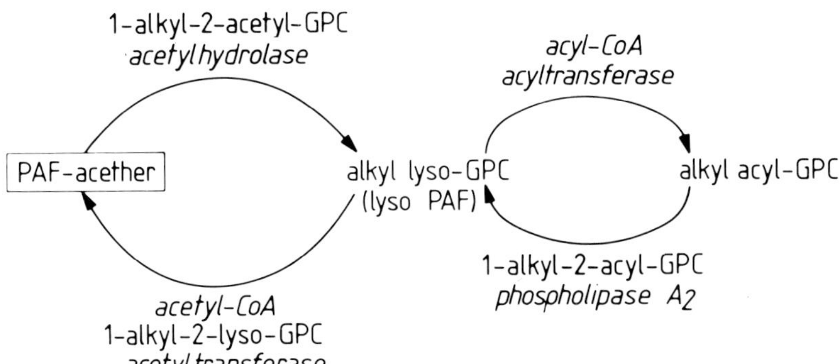

Figure 6 Biosynthesis of PAF-acether.

Table 4 Comparison of Human Mast Cell Subtypes

Variable	Mast cell source	
	Lung	Skin
Size	5–18 μm	5–18 μm
Formaldehyde fixation	Mainly sensitive	Mainly insensitive
Staining	Mainly alcian blue	Mainly safranin 0
MC^{TC}	<5%	<95%
Proteoglycans		
Heparin	65%	+
Chondroitin sulfate E	9%	?
Histamine	5 pg/cell	4 pg/cell
Prostaglandin D_2	++	++
Leukotriene C_4	+++	+
Activated by:		
IgE-dependent	Yes	Yes
Compound 48/80	No	Yes
Substance P	No	Yes
Effect of cromolyn	Yes	No

related to the development of specific antibodies against the proteases: tryptase and chymase. The use of double immunostaining techniques has shown that some mast cells contain only tryptase (designated MC^{T}), whereas others contain both tryptase and chymase (designated MC^{TC}). There is a preferential distribution of MC^{TC} in the connective tissue of skin and submucosal tissues of the small and large intestine, whereas MC^{T} are identified predominantly in lung tissue and the mucosal surfaces of the small and large intestine. A parallel between MC^{T} and the T-lymphocyte-dependent formaldehyde-sensitive mast cell of the rat intestinal mucosa is suggested by a marked reduction in numbers of MC^{T}, but not MC^{TC}, in the mucosa in patients with hereditary T-cell immunodeficiency disorders and acquired immunodeficiency syndrome. In addition to protease heterogeneity, there are dye-staining differences in relation to the proteoglycan content, differences in activation stimuli, and quantitative differences in the mediator elaboration (see Table 4).

B. Late Nasal Response

Allergen nasal challenge in children with symptomatic allergic rhinitis is also reported to be associated with late nasal reactions (83). Although this is a less consistent finding in the nose than in the lower airways after allergen challenge, it has been well characterized by the Baltimore group (84). The late nasal response is associated with increased lavage recovery of histamine, kinins, LTC_4, and TAME esterase. There is no elevation in PGD_2 in the late nasal response. Short-term treatment with glucocorticoids inhibits the mediator release occurring during the late nasal response to allergen challenge and has no effect on the immediate response (85). As glucocorticoids inhibit basophil, but not mast cell, degranulation in vitro (75,86), and PGD_2 is mast cell- and not basophil-derived (87), this has led to the suggestion that it is the basophil, and not the mast cell, that is important in the mediator elaboration associated with the late nasal response to allergen. Consistent with this is the finding of increased recovery of eosinophils and basophils, but not mast cells, in nasal lavage fluid during the late nasal response (88).

1. *The Basophil*

The basophil can be considered the circulating equivalent of the tissue mast cell, although it differs from the mast cell in its developmental origins, ultrastructure, and pharmacologic modulation. Basophils comprise 0.3% of nucleated cells in the bone marrow and 0.5–1.0% of the circulating leukocytes. They are considered to be derived from a myeloid bone marrow progenitor common to eosinophils and neutrophils (89). Circulating basophils are "end-cells," incapable of mitosis and division, having a life span of 8–12 days (90). Morphologically, basophils are best distinguished from mast cells by electron microscopy. In general, basophils are smaller, have a segmented nucleus, contain fewer and larger granules, possess fewer cytoplasmic filaments, and are characterized by the presence of glycogen particles and aggregates within the cytoplasm (91). The basophil differs from the mast cell in not generating PGD_2 on immunological stimulation (87,92,93), although producing comparable quantities of LTC_4. Differences also exist between the basophil and the mast cell relative to the preformed mediators. The basophil possesses less histamine; contains different proportions of proteoglycan, with predominantly chondroitin sulfate A and E and only a little heparin; has only 1–3% of the mast cell tryptase content; and contains small quantities of major basic protein (94,95). Pharmacologically, immunological mast cell degranulation is sensitive to the influence of β_2-adrenoceptor agonists and cromolyn (disodium cromoglycate), but it is insensitive to glucocorticoids (96). In contrast, cromolyn-like drugs and β_2-adrenoceptor agonists have little effect on immunologically stimulated basophil degranulation, whereas glucocorticoids inhibit immunologically stimulated histamine and LTC_4 release from human basophils. This may suggest the importance of the phospholipase A_2 pathway for arachidonic acid production in basophils, as this enzyme is steroid-sensitive and the phospholipase A_2 inhibitors, bromophenacyl bromide and 1-phenyl-3-pyrazolindinone (Phenidone), inhibit immunological basophil degranulation in vitro (97). The specificity of these compounds, however, has been questioned.

The appearance of the basophil within the nasal lavage in association with the late nasal response (88) might indicate a directed accumulation and migration from vascular compartments (see Sect. VI). Although little is known of those stimuli that initiate this event, the tissue migration of basophils that occurs in cutaneous basophil hypersensitivity is dependent on a combination of T-cell factors, homocytotropic antibodies, and vasoactive amines (98,99). Because T cells possess low-affinity IgE receptors, it is possible that they are activated at the initial allergen exposure and initiate the related cellular infiltration with both the basophil and the eosinophil.

2. *The Eosinophil*

The eosinophil is so named because of its characteristic pink staining with acid–aniline dyes, such as eosin, a feature described by Paul Erhlich in 1879. This property was subsequently identified as being due to the presence of highly basic proteins stored in secretory granules within the cytoplasm of this cell (Fig. 7). The eosinophil contains four major granule proteins: major basic protein (MBP), eosinophil cationic protein (ECO), eosinophil-derived neurotoxin (EDN), and eosinophil peroxidase (EPO). Of these MBP is the predominant preformed protein secreted in IgE-mediated reactions.

Major basic protein is localized to the crystalloid core of the eosinophil granules (100) and comprises approximately 55% of the granular protein content. It is a highly cationic protein, with an M_r of 10,000 Da (101), being composed of 117 amino acids. Because of a large number of sulfhydryl groups within the molecule, MBP tends to stick to surfaces (102) and may contribute to its toxicity toward parasites (103). Also, MBP is toxic toward ciliated epithelial cells (104), is a secretagogue for human basophils (105), and can inhibit whole blood clotting through an interaction with the coagulation pathway (106). Because of these properties, MBP has been implicated in the epithelial disruption apparent in allergic sinusitis (107).

Similar to the basophil, the eosinophil is marrow-derived. Its maturation is influenced by cytokines, including interleukin (IL)-2 (108), IL-3 (109), IL-5 (110), and granulocyte–macrophase colony-stimulating factor (GM-CSF) (111). Eosinophils bear receptors for IgG(Fc), IgE(Fc), and for activated complement fragments (CR1 and CR3) (112). The expression of complement receptors is enhanced by exposure of the eosinophil to histamine and eosinophil chemotactic factor of anaphylaxis (113). Immunological activation of the

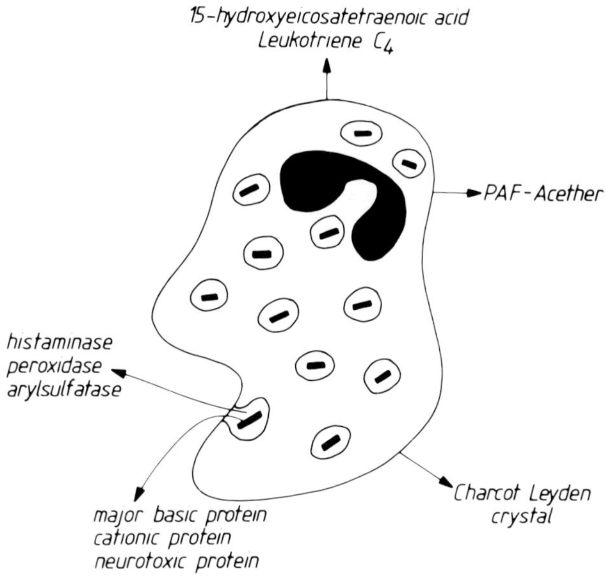

Figure 7 Eosinophil leukocyte, illustrating the granule and membrane-derived products following activation.

eosinophil, in addition to releasing the basic granule proteins, is associated with release of other granule-associated mediators, such as a collagenase, acetylcholinesterase, catalase, histaminase, arylsulfatase, alkaline phosphatase, cathepsin G, phospholipases B and D (114), and the generation of new mediators from the phospholipid membane.

Human eosinophils contain cyclooxygenase enzymes and produce PGE_2 and PGI_2 (prostacyclin) on their major prostanoids. Human eosinophils also possess 5- and 15-lipoxygenase activity (115,116), with LTC_4 being the major 5-lipoxygenase product (117). The ability of eosinophils to release LTC_4 is greatly enhanced if the cells have had prior exposure to a chemotactic stimulus such as LTB_4 or platelet-activating factor (PAF), or are preactivated by cytokines such as IL-3, IL-5, or GM-CSF (117). Interestingly, although human eosinophils can synthesize PAF, having the necessary acetyltransferase enzyme, most of this remains cell bound, with only 5–10% of that synthesized on immunological activation being released.

C. Mediator Relevance In Vivo

Allergen nasal insuflation produces immediate sneezing, itching, running, and nasal blockage. These symptoms are mimicked by histamine insuflation, implicating this mediator in their pathogenesis (Fig. 8). Consistent with this, H_1-antihistamines inhibit the immediate nasal symptoms induced by allergen. The effects of histamine are predominantly mediated by H_1-receptors, with only a small contribution to nasal blockage being related to vascular H_2-receptors (118). The hypersecretion is bilateral, after unilateral nasal challenge, whereas blockage is on only the challenge side. The bilateral hypersecretion is secondary to stimulation of afferent sensory nerves and reflex parasympathetic activity to the contralateral nasal glands. Despite these laboratory findings, antihistamines, although limiting itching, sneezing, and rhinorrhea, have little clinical effect on naturally developing nasal blockage in seasonal allergic rhinitis (119). Nasal blockage is mainly due to the local effects of mediators on the nasal vasculature, leading to engorgement of the nasal venous erectile

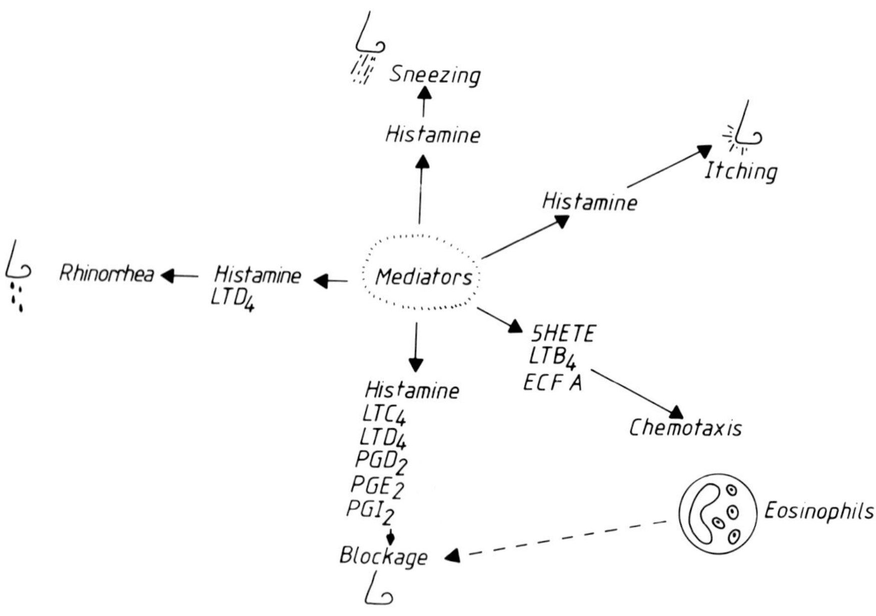

Figure 8 Nasal effects of inflammatory mediators associated with rhinitis. LT, Leukotriene; PG, prostaglandin; ECF-A, eosinophil chemotactic factor of anaphylaxis.

tissue. Thus, the lack of benefit of H_1-antihistamines in seasonal allergic blockage is due to the elaboration of other inflammatory mediators with more potent effects on the nasal vasculature. The effects of such mediators on the vasculature may be complex, depending on their site of release and site of action, as illustrated by PGE_2. Prostaglandin E_2 has been shown to be synthesized and metabolized by the normal nasal mucosa (120) as well as by the eosinophil. It is ten times as potent a constrictor of nasal venous erectile tissue as epinephrine (121) and, therefore, would be expected to reduce nasal resistance. However, PGE_2, is also a potent vasodilator of nasal resistance vessels and increases nasal blood flow (122), an action likely to increase nasal congestion and increase nasal resistance. In humans, PGD_2, LTC_4, and LTD_4, all produce sustained nasal blockage in the absence of itching or sneezing (123–125). These effects could be antagonized physiologically by PAF, because this lipid mediator reduces nasal resistance by decreasing mucosal blood flow and constricting venous capacitance vessels (126). In addition to these considerations, the interaction between the vasodilator properties of histamine, PGD_2, PGE_2, LTC_4, LTD_4, and histamine, LTC_4, and LTD_4, which all enhance vascular permeability, will lead to fluid extravasation and tissue edema, further compromising airflow through the nose. Mast cell-derived tryptase and kininogenase, acting on plasma precursors in the extravasated fluid, produce kinins, which stimulate afferent sensory nerves to produce sneezing and itch (127). Stimulation of sensory nerves by both kinins and histamine may amplify the response through activation of the nonadrenergic, noncholinergic nervous system. Substance P-containing nerves are present in the nasal mucosa in a perivascular, periglandular, and epithelial distribution. Nasal insuflation with substance P in humans causes nasal blockage (128) that may be a direct effect on the nasal vasculature, or, it may be secondary to substance P-induced mast cell degranulation, which causes histamine release in the absence of PGD_2 or LTC_4 generation (125).

VI. CELLULAR EVENTS AND CLINICAL DISEASE

Nasal cytology has been used to investigate cellular events within the nose in relationship to clinical disease. In infants and children, the normal nasal mucosal cytology consists of numerous epithelial cells, including ciliated and nonciliated columnar, goblet, and basal cells. There are normally no eosinophilic or basophilic cells and only a few neutrophils (130,131).

In allergic rhinitis, there is an increase in nasal mucosal eosinophils, with the diagnostic accuracy depending on the site and method of sampling (132). In one study of 60 schoolchildren with seasonal allergic rhinitis, 69% had a nasal eosinophilia, compared with only 7% of children (n = 70) without seasonal nasal symptoms (133). In general, the degree of nasal eosinophilia correlates well with active allergic disease in children, as indicated by both symptoms (17) and signs (134). A recent study, involving serial sampling in adults, identified a significant increase in nasal eosinophils in seasonal allergic rhinitis that correlated closely with pollen counts and symptoms (135), suggesting a relationship between eosinophils and allergic rhinitis. Consistent with this, corticosteroids, which improve nasal symptoms, also resolve nasal eosinophilia (136).

In the seasonal allergic rhinitis study (135), increases were also identified in mucosal mast cells and histamine-containing cells in nasal lavage. The identification of an increase in mucosal mast cells in seasonal allergic rhinitis confirms several previous studies (137,138) that have identified both a migration of mast cells from the lamina propria to the mucosa and an increase in total mast cell numbers. Consistent with this effect of allergen exposure, the numbers of mast cells in the nasal mucosa are higher in perennial allergic rhinitis than in nonrhinitic subjects (53). A significant correlation has been identified between nasal mucosal mast cells and symptoms of allergic rhinitis (139). These nasal mucosal mast cells differ from those at other sites, such as the skin and lung, in that they exhibit different staining characteristics and do not degranulate when challenged with the polyamine, 48/80 (140). These mucosal mast cells also differ from the metachromatic-staining cells recovered in nasal lavage fluid, which have been termed basophilic cells because they most closely resemble the circulating basophil (141). Whether these cells all represent differing lineages and, thus, reflect true heterogenicity, or represent differing stages of activation and development of the same progenitor in response to the local environment, is undetermined, but indirect evidence would favor the latter. In the rat, two populations of mast cells exist: a connective tissue mast cell and an inducible mast cell associated with mucosal surfaces, which increases in numbers during allergen or parasite exposure. This proliferation is cytokine-dependent, including T-cell-derived IL-3 (142,143) and is steroid-sensitive. Topical glucocorticoid therapy in the nose leads to a reduction in the formalin-sensitive mast cells (mucosal mast cells) and basophils (14), and regular corticosteroid therapy throughout seasonal allergen exposure limits their appearance (145). This evidence, plus the failure to identify any basophiloidlike cells in the lamina propria on electron microscopy (137), suggests that the characteristics of the metachromatic-staining cells in differing sites are likely to be related to growth and differentiation of a common progenitor, rather than to entirely separate populations.

VII. THERAPEUTIC IMPLICATIONS

From an understanding of the mechanisms of allergic rhinitis, it is possible to have a rational approach to therapy. This section will not deal with the prevention of atopy or avoidance of allergen exposure, but will concentrate on pharmacologic and immunotherapeutic intervention (Fig. 9).

A. Pharmacotherapy

It is apparent that histamine is involved in the allergic response in both the immediate and late nasal responses to allergen and will participate whether mast cell or basophil derived. As such H_1-antihistamines are the major oral therapy, a role enhanced by the advent of the newer nonsedating H_1-receptor antagonists (119). Because kinin generation will contribute to itch and sneeze, and LTC_4, which has been identified in association with clinical disease in children (146), and LTD_4 and PGD_2 will contribute to nasal blockage, treatment with H_1-antihistamines alone will not be fully effective treatment, unless an individual has mild intermittent symptoms confined to sneezing, itching, and rhinorrhea.

Corticosteroids exert a more fundamental effect on the disease process because they (1) inhibit the migration of mast cells into the nasal mucosa and the appearance of the basophiloid cell in nasal secretions (144), (2) induce a nasal eosinopenia (136), (3) inhibit basophil histamine release (86), and (4) modulate arachidonic acid metabolism in basophils and eosinophils through the induction of lipomodulin, an intracellular inhibitor of phospholipase A_2 activity (147). These effects will be maximized with regular treatment initiated before the pollen season in seasonal allergic rhinitis.

Other topical therapy includes β_2-adrenocepter agonists, cromolyn-like drugs, and sympathomimetic agents. Since the nasal blockage is vascular, sympathomimetic agents are effective in relieving this symptom, but they will have no effect on other aspects of rhinitis. Although β_2-adrenocepter agonists are potent inhibitors of immunological mast cell degranulation (148,149), their use in allergic rhinitis is disappointing. This may be related to nasal vasodilatation limiting their symptomatic efficacy or, more likely related to the heterogeneity of nasal metachromatic cells; β-agonists do not influence immunological basophil degranulation (96). Similarly, cromolyn has no effect on basophil degranulation (96), but some of its clinical benefit may derive from inhibition of immunological eosinophil activation (150), in addition to an effect on the mucosal mast cell.

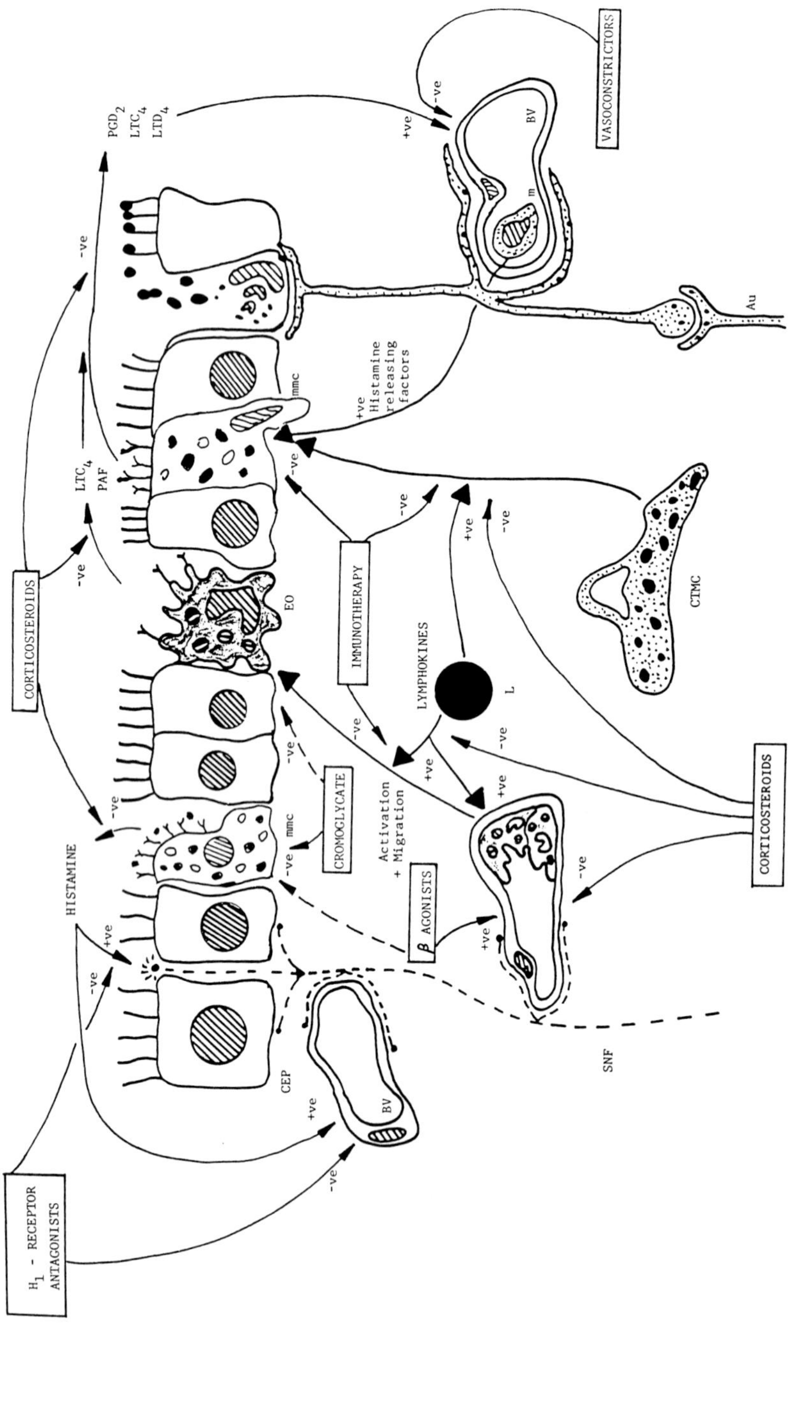

Figure 9 Schematic illustration of cellular events within the nose in allergic rhinitis and potential sites of therapeutic intervention. BV, blood vessel; CEP, ciliated epithelial cell; MMC, metachromatic mucosal cell; CTMC, connective tissue mast cell; EO, eosinophil; M, monocyte; L, lympocyte; AN, autonomic nerve; SNF, sensory nerve fiber.

B. Immunotherapy

Immunotherapy, similar to corticosteroids, can exert fundamental effects on disease activity. In allergic rhinitis, immunotherapy has been shown to reduce the number of metachromatic-staining cells (mast cells and basophils) and eosinophils in the nasal mucosa (151,152), possibly through regulation of T-lymphocyte function. This is reflected by a reduction in mediator secretion during the immediate nasal response to allergen (153), an effect correlating with individual efficacy of treatment. In addition, in vitro studies have identified that basophils are less responsive to allergen after immunotherapy (154). This may be due to an effect on cytokine–basophil interaction, because during immunotherapy, mononuclear cells synthesize less histamine-releasing factors (154).

VIII. CONCLUSIONS

Evidence suggests that allergic rhinitis is becoming more prevalent and that a number of environmental factors, including maternal smoking and childhood viral upper respiratory tract infections, may exaggerate the tendency to atopy and, hence, the likelihood of allergic nasal disease.

In the last decade there has been a considerable advance in the understanding of the mechanisms of allergic rhinitis, identifying the selective recruitment and accumulation of inflammatory cells in the nasal mucosa in association with active disease. Significant correlations have been identified between clinical symptoms and signs and the number of mast cells in the mucosa and eosinophils in secretions. The mediators released by both these cells on immunological activation can account for the symptoms of itching, sneezing, nasal discharge, and nasal blockage encountered in clinical practice. On the basis of this information, it is possible to identify stages for appropriate therapeutic intervention. A failure of classic "mast cell stabilizers" to have a major impact on disease expression may be related to the identification of metachromatic cell heterogeneity within the nose. Those cells recovered in nasal lavage having characteristics more suggestive of basophils than mast cells and, thus, having a different pharmacologic regulatory profile.

Future research directed at mechanisms of cell accumulation and cell activation within the nose may open additional avenues for successful symptom control. In addition, a broader awareness of environmental factors influencing the expression of atopy in children may lead to a reduction in the present progressive trend of an increasing prevalence of allergic rhinitis.

ACKNOWLEDGMENTS

The authors are most grateful to Mrs. Eileen Panks for typing this manuscript.

REFERENCES

1. Varonier HS. Prevalence of allergy among children and adolescents in Geneva, Switzerland. Respiration 1970; 27(suppl):115–120.
2. Varonier HS, De Haller J, Schopfer C. Prevalence de l'allergie chez les enfants et les adolescents. Helv Paediatr Acta 1984; 39:129–134.
3. Giles GG, Gibson HB, Lickiss N, Shaw K. Respiratory symptoms in Tasmanian adolescents: a follow up of the 1961 birth cohort. Aust NZ J Med 1984; 14: 631–637.
4. Kjellman NIM. Atopic disease in seven-year-old children: incidence to relation to family history. Acta Paediatr Scan 1977; 66:465–471.
5. Waite DA, Eyles EF, Tonkin SL, O'Donnell TV. Asthma prevalence in Tokelauan children in two environments. Clin Allergy 1980; 10:71–75.
6. Skarpaas IJK, Gulsvik A. Prevalence of bronchial asthma and respiratory symptoms in schoolchildren in Oslo. Allergy 1985; 40:295–299.
7. Wolstenholme RJ. Bronchial asthma in the Southern Maldives. Clin Allergy 1979; 9:325–332.
8. Haahtela T, Heiskala M, Suoniemi I. Allergic disorders and immediate skin test reactivity in Finnish adolescents. Allergy 1980; 35:433–441.
9. Freeman GL, Johnson S. Allergic diseases in adolescents. I. Description of survey: prevalence of asthma. Am J Dis Child 1964; 107:549–559.
10. Alanko K. Prevalence of asthma in a Finnish population: a study of symptomatic subjects tested for bronchial hyperreactivity. Scand J Respir Dis Suppl 1970; 1–64.
11. Wuthrich B, Schnyder VW, Henauer SA, Heller A. Epidemiology of pollinosis in Switzerland. In: Proceedings of the 13th Congress of EAACI 1986:656.
12. Tips RL. A study of the inheritance of atopic hypersensitivity in man. Am J Hum Genet 1954; 6:328–343.
13. Van Arsdel P, Motulsky AG. Frequency and heritability of asthma and allergic rhinitis in college students. Acta Genet 1959; 9:101–111.
14. Maternowski CJ, Mathews KP. The prevalence of ragweed pollinosis in foreign and native students at a midwestern university and its implications concerning methods for determining the inheritance of atopy. J Allergy 1962; 33:130–140.
15. Sherry MN, Scott RB. Prevalence of allergic diseases in freshman college students: a survey based on a predominantly Negro population. An Allergy 1968; 26: 335–338.
16. Hagy GW, Settipane GA. Bronchial asthma, allergic rhinitis and allergy skin tests among college students. J Allergy 1969; 445:323–332.
17. Malmberg H. Symptoms of chronic and allergic rhinitis and occurrence of nasal secretion granulocytes in university students, school children and infants. Allergy 1979; 34:389–394.

18. Logan WDP, Cushion AA. Morbidity statistics from general practice. Studies on medical and population subjects No 14. London: HMSO, 1958.
19. Fleming DM, Crombie DL. Prevalence of asthma and hay fever in England and Wales. Br Med J 1987; 294:279–283.
20. Burrows B, Fernando D, Martinez MD, Halonen M, Barbee RA, Cline MG. Association of asthma with serum IgE levels and skin-test reactivity to allergens. N Engl J Med 1989; 320:271–277.
21. Ishizaka K, Ishizaka T, Hornbrook MM. Physicochemical properties of human reaginic antibody. IV. Presence of a unique immunoglobulin as a carrier of reaginic activity. J Immunol 1966; 97:75–85.
22. Johansson SGO, Bennich H. Immunological studies of an atypical (myeloma) immunoglobulin. Immunology 1967; 13:381–394.
23. Ishizaka K, Ishizaka T, Lee EH. Biologic function of Fc fragments of E myeloma proteins. Immunochemistry 1970; 7:687–702.
24. Ishizaka K, Huff TF, Jardieu P, Moore KW, Martens CL. IgE-binding factors. Selective regulation of the IgE response by T cell factors. Int Arch Allergy Appl Immunol 1985; 77:13–18.
25. Ishizaka K. Regulation of IgE synthesis. Annu Rev Immunol 1984; 2:159–182.
26. Taylor R, Norman AR, Orgel MA, Stokes CR, Turner MW, Soothill JF. Transient IgA deficiency and pathogenesis of infantile atopy. Lancet 1973; 2:111–113.
27. Kontou-Karakitsos K, Salvaggio JE, Mathews KP. Comparative nasal absorption of allergens in atopic and non-atopic subjects. J Allergy Clin Immunol 1975; 55:241–248.
28. Berghind G, Finnstrom O, Johansson SGO, Moller KL. Wiskott-Aldrich syndrome. Acta Paediatr Scand 1968; 57:89–97.
29. Gajl-Peczalska KJ, Ballow M, Hansen JA, Good RA. IgE-bearing lymphocytes and atopy in a patient with X-linked infantile agammaglobulinaemia. Lancet 1973; 1:1254.
30. Geha RS, Reinherz E, Leung D, McKee KJ, Schlossman S, Rosen FS. Deficiency of suppressor T cells in the hyperimmunoglobulin E syndrome. J Clin Invest 1981; 68:783–781.
31. Chandra RK, Baker M. Numerical and functional deficiency of suppressor T cells precedes development of atopic eczema. Lancet 1983; 2:1393–1394.
32. Kjellman NIM, Johansson SGO, Roth A. Serum IgE levels in healthy children quantified by a sandwich technique (PRIST). Clin Allergy 1976; 6:51–59.
33. Rowntree S, Cogswell JJ, Platts-Mills TAE, Mitchell EB. Develoment of IgE and IgG antibodies to foods and inhalant allergens in children at risk of allergic disease. Arch Dis Child 1985; 60:727–735.
34. Cogswell JJ, Halliday DF, Alexander JR. Respiratory infections in the first year of life in children at risk of developing atopy. Br Med J 1982; 284:1011–1013.
35. Van Asperen PP, Kemp AS, Mellis CM. Skin test reactivity and clinical allergen sensitivity in infancy. J Allergy Clin Immunol 1984; 73:381–386.
36. Mathews DJ, Taylor B. Norman AP. Prevention of eczema. Lancet 1977; 1: 321–324.

37. Langeland T. A clinical and immunological study of allergy to hen's egg white. Clin Allergy 1983; 13:371–382.
38. Smith JM, Knowler LA. Epidemiology of asthma and allergic rhinitis. I. In a rural area. II. In a university-centered community. Am Rev Respir Dis 1965; 92:16–30; 31–38.
39. Kaufman HS, Frick OL. The development of allergy in infants of allergic parents: a prospective study concerning the role of heredity. Ann Allergy 1976; 37:410–415.
40. Orgel HA, Hamburger RN, Bazaral M. Development of IgE and allergy in infancy. J Allergy Clin Immunol 1975; 56:293–307.
41. Magnusson CGM. Maternal smoking influences cord serum IgE and IgD levels and increases the risk of subsequent infant allergy. J Allergy Clin Immunol 1986; 78:898–904.
42. Bjorksten F, Suoniemi I. Dependence of immediate hypersensitivity on the month of birth. Clin Allergy 1976; 6:165–171.
43. Bjorksten F, Sunoniemi I, Koski V. Neonatal birch pollen contact and subsequent allergy to birch pollen. Clin Allergy 1980; 10:585–591.
44. Frick OL, German DF, Mills J. Development of allergy in children. I. Association with virus infections. J Allergy Clin Immunol 1979; 63:228–241.
45. Leibovitz E, Freihorst J, Piedra PA, Ogra PL. Modulation of systemic and mucosal immune responses to inhaled ragweed antigen in experimentally induced infection with respiratory syncitial virus implication in virally induced allergy. Int Arch Allergy Appl Immunol 1988; 86:112–116.
46. Ishizaka K, Tomioka H, Ishizaka T. Mechanisms of passive sensitisation. I. Presence of IgE and IgG molecules on human leucocytes. J Immunol 1970; 105:1459–1467.
47. Tomioka H, Ishizaka K. Mechanisms of passive sensitization II. Presence of receptors for IgE on monkey mast cells. J Immunol 1971; 107:971–978.
48. Metzger H, Kinet J-P, Perez-Montfort R, Rivnay B, Wank SA. A tetrameric model for the structure of the mast cell receptor with high affinity for IgE. Prog Immunol 1983; 5:493–501.
49. Conrad DH. The receptor for immunoglobulin E. In: Holgate ST, ed. Mast Cells, Mediators and Disease. Kluwer Academic Publishers, 1988:99–127.
50. Naclerio RM, Meier HL, Kagey-Sobotka A, Adkinson NF, Meyers DA, Norman PS, Lichtenstein LM. Mediator release after nasal airway challenge with allergen. Am Rev Respir Dis 1983; 128:597–602.
51. Creticos PS, Adkinson NF, Kagey-Sobotka A, Proud D, Meier HL, Naclerio RM, Lichtenstein LM, Norman PS. Nasal challenge with ragweed pollen in hay fever patients. J Clin Invest 1985; 76:2247–2253.
52. Castells M, Schwartz LB. Tryptase levels in nasal-lavage fluid as an indicator of the immediate allergic response. J Allergy Clin Immunol 1988; 82:348–355.
53. Gomez E, Corrado OJ, Baldwin DL, Swanston AR, Davies RJ. Direct in vivo evidence for mast cell degranulation during allergen induced reactions in man. J Allergy Clin Immunol 1986; 78:637–645.

54. Dvorak AM. The fine structure of human basophils and mast cells. In: Holgate ST, ed. Mast cells, mediators and disease. Kluwer Academic Publishers, 1988:29–97.
55. Holmgren H, Willander O. Beitrag zur kenntnis der chemia und funktion der chrlichschen mastzellen. Z. Mikrosk Anat Forsch 1937; 42:242–278.
56. Schiller S, Dorfman A. The isolation of heparin from mast cells of the normal rat. Biochim Biophys Acta 1959; 31:278–283.
57. Metcalfe DD, Lewis RA, Silbert JG, Rosenberg RD, Wasserman SI, Austen KF. Isolation and characterisation of heparin from human lung. J Clin Invest 1979; 64:1537–1543.
58. Metcalfe DD, Smith JA, Austen KF, Gilbert JG. Polydispersity of rat mast cell heparin: implications for proteoglycan assembly. J Bio Chem 1980; 25: 11753–11758.
59. Hook M, Lindahl U, Hallen A, Backstromg X. Biosynthesis of heparin: studies on the microsomal sulfation process. J Biol Chem 1975; 250:6065–6068.
60. Uvnas B, Aborg C-H, Bergendorff A. Storage of histamine in mast cells. Evidence for ionic binding of histamine to protein carboxyls in the granule heparin protein complex. Acta Physiol Scand Suppl 1907; 336:1–14.
61. Schwartz LB, Riedel C, Caulfield JP, Wasserman SI, Austen KF. Cell association of complexes of chymase, heparin proteoglycan, and protein after degranulation by rat mast cells. J Immunol 1981; 126:2071–2078.
62. Caulfield JP, Lewis RA, Hein A, Austen KF. Secretion of dissociated human pulmonary mast cells. Evidence for solubulisation of granule contents before discharge. J Cell Biol 1980; 85:299–311.
63. Holgate ST, Kay AB. Mast cells, mediators and asthma. Clin Allergy 1985; 15:221–233.
64. Kulczycki A, Isersky C, Metzger H. The interaction of IgE with rat basophilic leukemia cells. I Evidence for specific binding of IgE. J Exp Med 1974; 139:600–616.
65. Sullivan TJ. Diacylglycerol metabolism and the release of mediators from mast cells. In: Becker EL, Simon AS, Austen KF, eds. Biochemistry of the acute allergic reactions. New York: Alan R Liss, 1981:229–238.
66. Berridge MJ, Irvine RF. Inositol triphosphate, a novel second messenger in cellular signal transduction. Nature 1984; 312:315–321.
67. Hawthorne JN. Polyphosphoinositide metabolism in excitable membranes. Biosci Res 1983; 3:887–904.
68. Lin SH, Wallace MA, Fain JN. Regulation of Ca^{2+}, Mg^{2+}, ATPase activity in hepatocyte plasma membranes by vasopresin and phenylephrine. Endocrinology 183; 113:2268–2275.
69. Ishizaka T, Conrad DH, Schulman ES, Sterk AR, Ishizaka K. Biochemical analysis of initial triggering events of IgE mediated histamine release from human lung mast cells. J Immunol 1983; 130:2357–2362.
70. Hamberg M, Svensson J, Samuelsson B. Novel transformations of prostaglandin

endoperoxidases: formation of thromboxanes. Adv Prostaglandin Thromboxane Res 1976; 1:19–27.

71. Hamberg M, Svensson J, Samuelsson B. Prostaglandin endoperoxidases: a new concept concerning the mode of action and release of protaglandins. Proc Natl Acad Sci USA 1976; 71:3824–3828.
72. Moncada S, Gryglewski RJ, Bunting S, Vane JR. An enzyme isolated from arteries transforms prostaglandin endoperoxidases to an unstable substance that inhibits platelet aggregation. Nature 1976; 262:663–665.
73. Hamberg M, Svensson J, Samuelsson B. Thromboxanes a new group of biologically active compounds derived from prostaglandin endoperoxidases. Proc Natl Acad Sci USA 1975; 72:2994–2998.
74. Lewis RA, Soter NA, Diamond PT, Austen KF, Oates JA, Roberts LJ. Prostaglandin D_2 generation after activation of rat and human mast cells with anti-IgE. J Immunol 1982; 129:1627–1631.
75. Schleimer RP, Schulman ES, MacGlashan DW, Peters SP, Hayes EC, Adams GK, Lichtenstein LM, Adkinson NF. Effects of dexamethasone on mediator release from human lung fragments and purified human lung mast cells. J Clin Invest 1983; 71:1830–1835.
76. Holgate ST, Burns GB, Robinson C, Church MK. Anaphylactic and calcium dependent generation of prostaglandin D_2 (PGD_2), thromboxane B_2 and other cyclooxygenase products of arachidonic acid by dispersed human lung cells and relationship to histamine release. J Immunol 1984; 133:2138–2144.
77. Agius RM, Howard PH, Robinson C, Holgate ST. Human bronchoalveolar mast cells and their mediators. In: Kay AB, ed. Asthma: clinical pharmacology and therapeutic progress. Oxford: Blackwell Scientific, 1986:274–285.
78. Hammarstrom S. Leukotrienes. Annu Rev Biochem 1983; 52:355–377.
79. Bach MK, Brashler JR, Murphy RC. Solubilization and characterization of the leukotriene C_4 synthetase of rat basophil leukemic cells: a novel, particulate glutathione-S-transferase. Arch Biochem Biophys 1984; 230:455–465.
80. Peters SP, MacGlashan DW, Schulman ES, Schleimer RP, Hayes EC, Rokach J, Adkinson NF, Lichtenstein LM. Arachidonic acid metabolism in purified human lung mast cells. J Immunol 1984; 132:1972–1979.
81. Dahlen SE, Hansson G, Hedquist P, Bjorck T, Granstrom E, Dahlen B. Allergen challenge of lung tissue from asthmatics elicits bronchial contraction that correlates with the release of leukotrienes C_4, D_4, and E_4. Proc Natl Acad Sci USA 1983; 80:1712–1716.
82. Schleimer RP, MacGlashan DW, Peters SP, Pinckard RN, Adkinson NF, Lichtenstein LM. Characterisation of inflammatory mediator release from purified human lung mast cells. Am Rev Respir Dis 1986; 133:614–617.
83. Price JF, Hey EN, Soothill JF. Antigen provocation to the skin, nose and lung in children with asthma; immediate and dual hypersensitivity reactions. Clin Exp Immunol 1982; 47:587–594.
84. Naclerio RM, Proud D, Togias AG, Adkinson NF, Meyers DA, Kagey-Sobotka

A, Plaut M, Norman PS, Lichtenstein LM. Inflammatory mediators in late antigen-induced rhinitis. N Engl J Med 1985; 313:65–70.
85. Pipkorn U, Proud D, Schleimer RP, Peters SP, Adkinson NF, Kagey-Sobotka A, Norman PS, Lichtenstein LM, Naclerio RM. Effects of short-term systemic glucocorticoid treatment on human nasal mediator release after antigen challenge. J Clin Invest 1987; 80:957–961.
86. Schleimer RP, Lichtenstein LM, Gillespie E. Inhibition of basophil histamine release by anti-inflammatory steroids. Nature 1981; 292:454–455.
87. MacGlashan DW, Schleimer RP, Peters SP, Schulman ES, Adams GK, Kagey-Sobotka A, Newball HH, Lichtenstein LM. Comparative studies of human basophils and mast cells. Fed Proc 1983; 42:2504–2509.
88. Bascom R, Wachs M, Naclerio RM, Pipkorn U, Galli SJ, Lichtenstein LM. Basophil influx occurs after nasal challenge: effects of topical corticosteroid pretreatment. J Allergy Clin Immunol 1988; 81:580–589.
89. Parwaresh MR. The human blood basophil. New York: Springer-Verlag, 1970.
90. Murakami I, Ogawa M, Amo H, Ota K. Studies on kinetics of human leukocytes in vivo with ^{3}H-thymidine autoradiogrpahy. II. Eosinophils and basophils. Acta Haematol Jpn 1969; 32:384–389.
91. Dvorak AM. The fine structure of human basophils and mast cells. In: Holgate ST, ed. Mast cells, mediators and disease. Kluwer Academic Publishers, 1988:29–97.
92. Findlay SR, Lichtenstein LM, Grant JA. Generation of slow reacting substance by human leucocytes. II. Comparison of stimulation by antigen, anti-IgE, calcium ionophore and C5-peptide. J Immunol 1980; 124:238–242.
93. MacGlashan DW, Peters SP, Warner JA, Lichtenstein LM. Characteristics of human basophil sulfidopeptide leukotriene release: releasability defined as the ability of the basophil to respond to dimeric cross-links. J Immunol 1986; 136;2231–2239.
94. Metcalfe DD, Bland CE, Wasserman SI. Biochemical and functional characterizaton of proteoglycans isolated from basophils of patients with chronic myelogenous leukemia. J Immunol 1984; 132:1943–1950.
95. Castells MC, Irani AM, Schwartz LB. Evaluation of human peripheral blood leucocytes for mast cell tryptase. J Immunol 1987, 138:2184–2189.
96. Church MK. Modulation of mast cell mediator secretion by drugs used in the treatment of allergic disease. In: Holgate ST, ed. Mast cells, mediators and disease. Kluwer Academic Publishers, 1988:259–279.
97. Warner JA, MacGlashan DW, Peters SP, Kagey-Sobotka A, Lichtenstein LM. The pharmacologic modulation of mediator release from human basophils. J Allergy Clin Immunol 1988; 82:432–438.
98. Askenase PW. Role of basophils, mast cells and vasoamines in hypersensitivity reactions with a delayed time course. Prog Allergy 1977; 23:199–320.
99. Dvorak HF. Cutaneous basophil hypersensitivity. J Allergy Clin Immunol 1976; 58:229–240.

100. Lewis DM, Lewis JC, Loegering DA, Gleich GJ. Localization of the guinea-pig eosinophil major basic protein to the core of the granule. J Cell Biol 1978; 77:702–713.
101. Gleich GJ, Loegering DA, Maldonado JE. Identification of a major basic protein in guinea pig eosinophil granules. J Exp Med 1973; 137:1459–1471.
102. Wasmoen TL, Bell MP, Loegering DA, Gleich GJ, Prendergast FG, McKean DJ. Biochemical and amino acid sequence analysis of human eosinophil granule major basic protein. J Biol Chem 1988; 263:12559–12563.
103. Butterworth AE, Wassom DL, Gleich FJ, Loegering DA, David JR. Damage to schistosomula of *Schistosoma mansoni* induced directly by eosinophil major basic protein. J Immunol 1979; 122:221–229.
104. Davis WB, Fells GA, Sun S-H, Gadek JE, Venet A, Crystal RG. Eosinophil-mediated injury to lung parenchymal cells and interstitial matrix: a possible role for eosinophils in chronic inflammatory disorders of the lower respiratory tract. J Clin Invest 1984; 74:269–278.
105. Heutlin LM, Ackerman SJ, Gleich GJ, Thomas LL. Donor sensitivity to basophil activation by eosinophil granule major basic protein. Int Arch Allergy Appl Immunol 1985; 77:216–217.
106. Gleich GJ, Loegering D,A Kuepper F, Bajaj SP, Mann KG. Physicochemical and biological properties of the major basic protein from guinea-pig eosinophil granules. J Exp Med 1974; 140:313–331.
107. Harlin SL, Ansel DG, Lane SR, Myers J, Kephart GM, Gleich GJ. A clinical and pathologic study of chronic sinusitis. The role of the eosinophil. J Allergy Clin Immunol 1988; 81:867–875.
108. Kern P, Dietrich M. Eosinophil differentiating activity in sera of patients with AIDS under recombinant IL2 substitution. Blut 1986; 52:249–254.
109. Saito H, Hatake K, Dvorak AM. Selective induction of differentiation and proliferation of haemopoietic cells by recombinant human interleukins. Proc Natl Acad Sci USA 1988; 85:2288–2292.
110. Campbell HD, Tucker WP, Hart Y, Martinson ME, Mayo G, Clutterbuck EJ, Sanderson CJ, Young IG. Molecular cloning, nucleotide sequence and expression of the gene encoding eosinophil differentiation factor (interleukin 5). Proc Natl Acad Sci USA 1987; 84:6629–6633.
111. Metcalfe D, Begley CG, Johnson GR, Nicola NA, Vadas MA, Lopez AF, Williamson DJ, Wong GG, Clark SC, Wange EA. Biologic properties in vitro of a recombinant human granulocyte–macrophage colony-stimulating factor. Blood 1986; 67:37–45.
112. Winquist I, Olofsson T, Olsson I, Persson A-M, Hallberg T. Altered density, metabolism and surface receptors of eosinophils in eosinophilia. Immunology 1982; 47:531–539.
113. Anwar ARE, Kay AB. Enhancement of human eosinophil compelement receptors by pharmacologic mediators. J Immunol 1978; 121:1245–1250.
114. Bainton DF, Faquhar MG. Segregation and packaging of granule enzymes in eosinophil leucocytes. J Cell Biol 1970; 45:54–73.

115. Laviolette M, Picard J, Braquet P, Borgeat P. Comparison of 5- and 15-lipoxygenase activities in blood and alveolar leukocyte preparations from normal patients and patients with eosinophilia. Prostaglandins Leukotrienes Med 1986; 23:191–199.
116. Turk J, Maas RL, Brash AR, Roberts JL, Oates JA. Arachidonic acid 15-lipoxygenase products from human eosinophils. J Biol Chem 1982; 257:7068–7076.
117. Weller PF, Lee CW, Foster DW, Corey EJ, Austen KF, Lewis RA. Generation and metabolism of 5-lipoxygenase pathway leukotrienes by human eosinophils: predominant production of leukotriene C_4. Proc Natl Acad Sci USA 1983; 80:7626–7630.
118. Mygind N, Secher C, Kirkegaard J. Role of histamine and antihistamines in the nose. Eur J Respir Dis 1983; 64(suppl 128):16–20.
119. Howarth PH, Holgate ST. Comparativetrial of two nonsedative H_1-antihistamines, terfenadine and astemizole, for hay fever. Thorax 1984; 39:668–672.
120. Bedwani J, Eccles R, Jones AS. A study of the synthesis and inactivation of prostaglandin E by pig nasal mucosa. Acta Otolaryngol (Stockh) 1984; 98:308–314.
121. Bedwani J, Eccles R, Jones AS. The isolation of prostaglandin E from pig nasal mucosa. Clin Otolaryngol 1983; 8:159–163.
122. Lung MA, Phipps RJ, Want JCC, Widdicombe JG. Control of nasal vasculature and airflow resistance in the dog. J Physiol 1984; 349:535–551.
123. Walsh S, Robinson C, Howarth PH. The influence of prostaglandin D_2 (PGD_2) on nasal airways resistance in normal man. (in preparation)
124. Bisgaard H, Olsson P, Bende M. Leukotriene D_4 increases nasal blood flow in humans. Prostaglandins 19xx; 27:599–604.
125. Miadonna A, Tedeschi A, Leggiere E, Lorini M, Colco G, Sala A, Qualizza R, Froldi M, Zannussi C. Behaviour and clinical relevance of histamine and leukotrienes C_4 and B_4 in grass pollen-induced rhinitis. Am Rev Respir Dis 1987; 136:357–362.
126. Pipkorn U, Karlsson G, Bake B. Effect of platelet activating factor on human nasal mucosa. Allergy 1984; 39:141–145.
127. Proud D, Togias A, Naclerio RM, Crush SA, Norman PS, Lichtenstein LM. Kinins are generated in vitro following nasal airway challenge of allergic individuals with allergen. J Clin Invest 1983; 72:1678–1685.
128. Malm L, Petersson G. Tachykinins and nasal secretion. In: Hakanson R, Sundler F, eds. Tachykinin antagonists, Fernstrom Symposium, vol 6. Amsterdam: Elsevier, 1985:15–23.
129. Benyon RC, Robinson C, Chruch MK. Differential release of histamine and eicosanoids from human skin mast cells by IgE-dependent and non-immunological stimuli. (in press)
130. Cohen GA, MacPherson GA, Golembesky HE. Normal nasal cytology in infancy. Ann Allergy 1985; 54:112–114.

131. Jalowayski AA, Maes TE, Wasserman SI, Zeiger RS. Histochemical differentiation of human nasal mucosal mast cells from basophil leukocytes. J Allergy Clin Immunol 1983; 71:89.
132. Vaheri E. Nasal allergy with special reference to eosinophils and histopathology. Acta Allergol 1956; 10:203–214.
133. Miller RE, Paradise JL, Friday GA, Fireman P, Voith D. The nasal smear for eosinophils. Its value in children with seasonal allergic rhinitis. Am J Dis Child 1982; 136:1009–1011.
134. Murray AB, Anderson DO. The epidemiologic relationship of clinical nasal allergy to eosinophils ànd to globlet cells in the nasal smear. J Allergy 1969; 43:1–8.
135. Pipkorn U, Karlsson G, Ennerback L. The cellular response of the human allergic mucosa to natural allergen exposure. J Allergy Clin Immunol 1988; 82:1046–1054.
136. Elkhalil M, Fiore L, Bellioni P, Cantani A, Corgiolu M, Businco L. Evaluation of nasal and blood eosinophilia in children suffering from perennial allergic rhinitis treated with beclomethasone diproprionate. Allergol Immunopathol (Madr) 1983; 11:225–228.
137. Enerback L, Pipkorn U, Olafsson A. Intraepithelial migration of mucosal mast cells in hay fever: ultrastructural observations. Int Arch Allergy Appl Immunol 1986; 81:289–297.
138. Viegas M, Gomez E, Brooks J, Davies RJ. The effect of the pollen season on nasal mast cell numbers. Br Med J 1987; 294:414.
139. Bienenstock J, Befus D, Denburg J, Goto T, Lee T, Otsuka H, Shananhan F. Comparative aspects of mast cell heterogeneity in different species and sites. Int Arch Allergy Appl Immunol 1985; 77:126–129.
140. Okuda M, Ohtsuka H, Kawabori S. Studies on nasal surface basophilic cells. Ann Allergy 1985; 54:69–71.
141. Okuda M, Kawabori S, Otsuka H. Electron microscope study of basophilic cells in nasal secretions. Arch Otorhinolaryngol 1978; 221:215–220.
142. Haig DM, McKee TA, Jarrett EEE, Woodbury R, Miller HRP. Generation of mucosal mast cells is stimulated in in vitro by factors derived from T cells of helminth infected rats. Nature 1982; 300:188–190.
143. Ihle JN, Keller J, Oroszlan S, Henderson LE, Copeland TD, Fitch F, Prytsowsky MB, Goldwasser E, Schrader JW, Palaszynski E, Dy M, Lebel B. Biological properties of homogeneous interleukin 3: demonstration of WEHI-3 growth factor activity, mast cell growth factor activity, P-cell stimulating factor activity, colony-stimulating activity and histamine producing cell stimulating factor activity. J Immunol 1983; 131:282–287.
144. Otsuka H, Denburg JA, Befus AD, Hitch D, Lapp P, Rajan RS, Bienenstock J, Dolovitch J. Effect of beclomethasone diproprionate on nasal metachromatic cell sub-populations. Clin Allergy 1986; 16:589–595.

145. Gomez E, Clague JE, Gatland D, Davies RJ. Effect of topical corticosteroids on seasonally induced increases in nasal mast cells. Br Med J 1988; 296:1572–1573.
146. Volovitz B, Osur SL, Bernstein JM, Ogra PL. Leukotriene C_4 release in upper respiratory mucosa during natural exposrue to ragweed in ragweed-sensitive children. J Allergy Clin Immunol 1988; 82:414–418.
147. Blackwell GJ, Carmiccio R, Di Rossa M, Flower RJ, Parente L, Persico P. Macrocortin: a polypeptide causing the anti-phospholipase effect of glucocorticoids. Nature 1980; 287:147–149.
148. Church MK, Hiroi J. Inhibition of IgE-dependent histamine release from human dispersed lung mast cells by anti allergic drugs and salbutamol. Br J Pharmacol 1987; 90:421–429.
149. Howarth PH, Durham SR, Lee TH, Kay AB, Church MK, Holgate ST. Influence of albuterol, cromolyn sodium and ipratropium bromide on the airway and circulating mediator responses to antigen bronchial provocation in asthma. Am Rev Respir Dis 1985; 132:986–992.
150. Kay AB, Walsh GM, Mogbel R, MacDonald AJ, Nagakura T, Carroll MP, Richerson HB. Disodium cromoglycate inhibits activation of human inflammatory cells in vitro. J Allergy Clin Immunol 1987; 80:1–8.
151. Rak S, Hakansson L, Venge P. Eosinophil chemotactic activity in allergic patients during the birch pollen season: the effect of immunotheapy. Int Arch Allergy Appl Immunol 1987; 82:349–350.
152. Okuda M, Otsuka H. Basophil cells in allergic nasal secretions. Arch Otorhinolaryngol 1977; 214:85–89.
153. Creticos PS, Adkinson NF, Kagey-Sobotka A, Proud D, Meier HL, Naclerio RM. Lichtenstein LM, Norman PS. Nasal challenge with ragweed pollen in hay fever patients. J Clin Invest 1985; 76:2247–2253.
154. Malling H-J, Skov PS, Permin H, Norn S, Weeke B. Basophil histamine release and humoral changes during immunotherapy. Dissociation between basophil-bound specific IgE, serum values and cell sensitivity. Allergy 1982; 37:187–192.

2

Allergens

Martin D. Chapman, Susan M. Pollart, and Peter W. Heymann
University of Virginia Health Sciences Center, Charlottesville, Virginia

I. INTRODUCTION

Immediate hypersensitivity to inhaled allergens (e.g., pollens, dust mites, animal danders, molds, and fungi) is a common cause of seasonal or perennial rhinitis in both adults and children. Since the pioneering work of Blackley in the 19th century, pollens from grasses, weeds, and trees have been recognized as the major cause of seasonal allergic rhinitis and conjunctivitis (1). A clinical history of hay fever is usually easy to document, in part because there is a good temporal relationship between exposure to a particular pollen and exacerbation of symptoms. Although hay fever symptoms can be quite miserable and stressful, particularly in children, they can generally be controlled by drug treatment (e.g., antihistamines, local steroids, or cromolyn) and, in selected cases, by "desensitizing" injections of pollen extracts (see Chaps. 4 and 5). On the other hand, patients with perennial rhinitis generally do not associate allergen exposure as a cause of their symptoms. Many of these patients are allergic to house dust allergens [i.e., dust mites (*Dermatophagoides pteronyssinus* and *D. farinae*) and cat or dog dander]. Allergies to cockroaches, molds, and fungi should also be investigated as a possible cause of house dust-related perennial rhinitis (2). Over the past 20 years, there has been significant progress in reseach on the properties of inhalant allergens and their role in causing allergic disease. In particular, immunochemical studies have resulted in the purification of major allergens from pollens, mites, and cat dander (e.g., *Lol p* I, *Amb a* I, *Der p* I, *Fel d* I), and these purified allergens have been used in immunological, genetic, and epidemiological studies. The purpose of this chapter is to review recent evidence that exposure to inhalant allergens and the development of IgE antibody responses are important risk factors for allergic disease and to outline strategies for indoor allergen avoidance and control that can be useful for the treatment of rhinitis and asthma.

II. ROLE OF INHALANT ALLERGENS IN THE EPIDEMIOLOGY OF ALLERGIC RESPIRATORY DISEASE

Evidence that allergens play an important role in the etiology of allergic respiratory disease can be summarized as follows:

1. Patients with rhinitis or asthma show an increased prevalence of positive skin tests, serum IgE antibodies, and positive inhalation challenge tests to common allergens, when compared with nonallergic controls (3–7). This has been demonstrated in several case control and population surveys, one of the earliest of which was that of Smith and colleagues in England, who showed that 66% of children with asthma had positive skin tests to mite extracts, compared with

<10% of controls (3). Similar recent studies in Australia have shown a good correlation between positive skin tests and inhalation challenge tests in school children (8). The problem with these studies is that they do not prove a causal relationship between allergic sensitivity and disease, because one can always identify skin test-positive individuals who are asymptomatic.

2. Reductions in airway hyperreactivity have been demonstrated in asthmatics after prolonged allergen avoidance (either in "allergen-free" hospital rooms or in convalescent sanatoria at high altitudes, e.g., Davos, Switzerland; 9–11). In these studies, it took several months to sustain improvements in airway hyperreactivity, and the implication is that allergen-avoidance procedures need to be rigorous and prolonged to maintain clinical benefit.

3. The introduction of allergens into the environment is associated with an increased prevalence of asthma. The most striking example of this being in the Eastern Highlands of Papua New Guinea, where the introduction of dust mites on cotton blankets has been associated with a dramatic increase in the prevalence of asthma, from 0 to 7.3% over the past 20 years (12). Occupational exposure to allergens is also a well-documented cause of respiratory disease, a typical example being the development of rhinitis or asthma in laboratory workers exposed to rodent urinary proteins (13,14). In many occupational allergies there is a direct relationship between allergen exposure and the onset of symptoms.

4. Recent studies have shown a significantly increased prevalence of inhalant allergy in patients with acute asthma seen in hospital emergency rooms (ER), compared with patients admitted to ER with other diagnoses (15–17). These studies have been carried out in three different areas of the United States: Charlottesville, Virginia; Travis, California; and Atlanta, Georgia. In Charlottesville, most ER patients with asthma appeared in the fall (August to December) and had an increased prevalence of IgE antibodies to indoor allergens (mite, cat, and cockroach). In contrast, in Travis, in the spring (May and June) there is a well-documented "epidemic" of asthma, coincident with the rise in rye grass pollen counts, and about 94% of patients admitted to the Travis Air Force Base ER at that time show highly elevated levels of IgE antibody to rye grass pollen (Figs. 1 and 2; 15,18). Both the Charlottesville and Travis ER studies were carried out on adults; however, similar results were obtained in a pediatric ER study carried out in Grady Memorial Hospital, Atlanta. The prevalence of allergy in asthmatic children was 80%, compared with 32% in controls, and the most common sensitivities were to dust mite, cockroach, and grass pollen (17).

Together, these studies (particularly those in the ER) strongly suggest that the development of IgE antibodies to inhalant allergens is a risk factor for

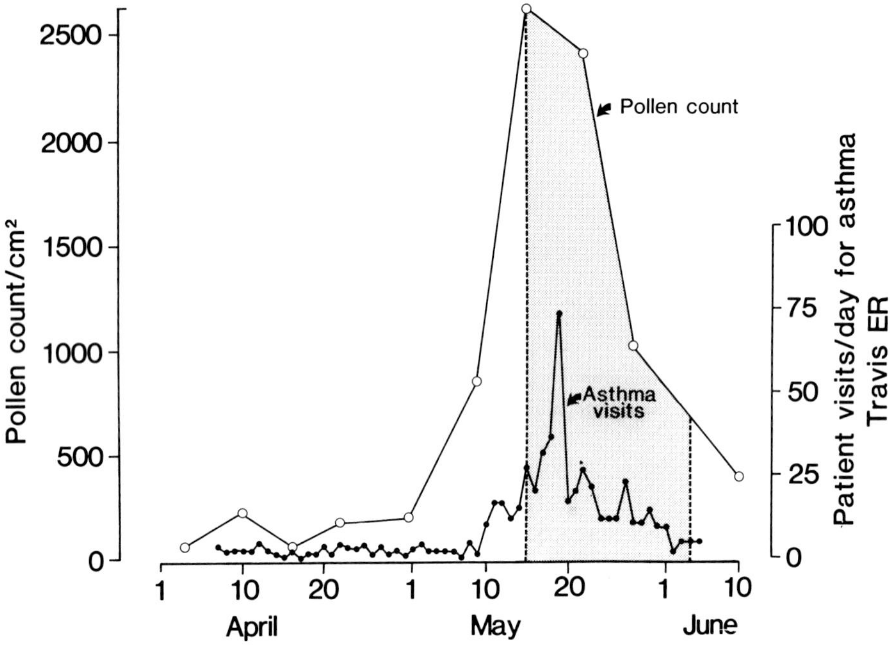

Figure 1 "Epidemic" asthma in Travis California, caused by rye grass pollen. The number of emergency room admissions with acute asthma peaks at the same time as the seasonal increase in pollen counts. The prevalence of allergy in ER patients and controls was compared in the spring of 1986. The study period is shaded. [From Pollart et al. (15)].

allergic respiratory disease and that patients with elevated IgE antibody levels are more likely to have symptoms.

There are several other reasons for believing that allergens are also involved in rhinitis (as well as asthma). Skin test-positive patients with rhinitis show the same pattern of specific IgG and IgE antibody responses to allergens as asthmatics and also show allergen-specific proliferative T-cell responses (19–23). The magnitude of these responses tends to be somewhat lower in rhinitis patients, but, in general, the immunological responses of both patient groups are similar. Moreover, there is good evidence from prospective studies that antibody responses develop early in life. Rowntree and associates showed that the development of IgG and IgE antibody responses to mite allergen,

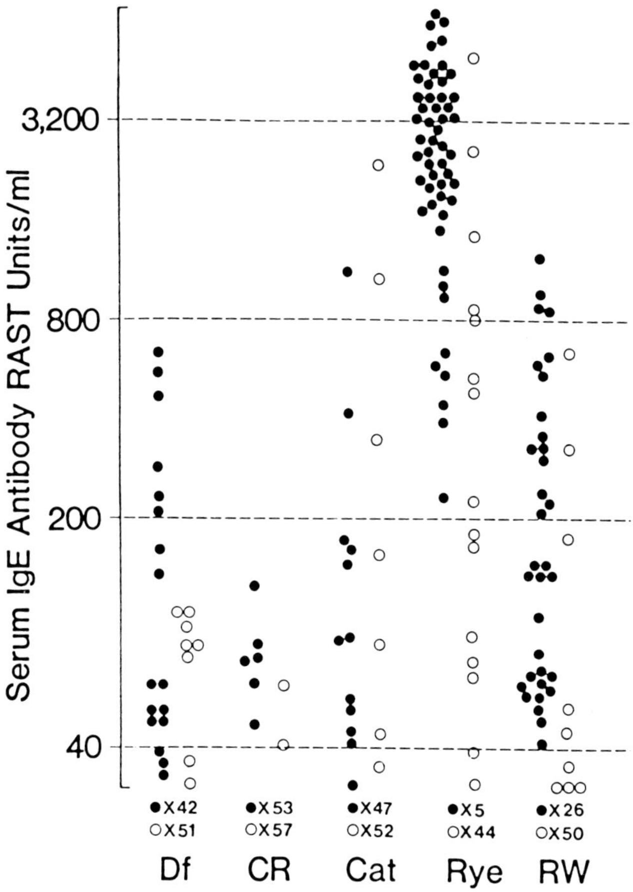

Figure 2 Serum IgE antibodies to inhalant allergens in asthmatic patients (●) and controls (○) admitted to the Travis ER. IgE antibodies to dust mite (*D. farinae*, Df), cockroach (CR), cat, rye grass pollen, and short ragweed pollen were measured by RAST. The results illustrate the high levels of IgE antibodies to rye grass pollen allergens in patients admitted with asthma. [From Pollart et al. (15)]

Der p I, and to the rye grass allergen, *Lol p* I, increased progressively from the second to the fifth year of life, in children born to at least one atopic parent (24). In addition, those children who developed IgE antibody responses also showed a higher prevalence of allergic respiratory and skin disease. It is not unusual to find children with rhinitis who have positive skin tests to inhalant allergens, detectable serum IgE antibodies, and elevated total IgE. In these children, it is reasonable to suspect that inhalant allergens are an important cause of symptoms.

III. ALLERGEN IDENTIFICATION AND QUANTIFICATION

Airborne pollen counts have been used for many years to predict the severity of symptom days for patients with seasonal hay fever. Similarly, spore counts are used in some areas (e.g., the U.S. Midwest) as indicators of exposure to *Alternaria, Cladosporium*, and other fungi. High airborne pollen and spore counts (e.g., >300 pollen grains per cubic meter) are associated with increased symptoms, and patients are advised to adjust their medications or to reduce their exposure accordingly. Unfortunately, airborne measurements are difficult to apply to house dust allergens because air circulation rates in houses are low and some allergens (e.g., mite feces) become airborne only after domestic disturbance of dust (20). Also, with the exception of mite and cat, the nature of the particles carrying dust allergens is unknown. Nonetheless, over the past 10 years, there has been considerable progress in developing tests to monitor indoor allergen exposure, to the point that exacerbations in symptons can be correlated with allergen levels in house dust samples.

Several methods have been used for measuring mite allergens in dust, including mite counts, guanine assay, and immunochemical assays [either radioallergosorbent test (RAST) inhibition or immunoassays for specific allergens such as *Der p* I)] (20). Although mite counts have been useful in epidemiological studies, they are time-consuming and unsuitable for routine use. The principle of the guanine assay is that mites are the major producer of guanine in house dust. Guanine can be measured with a simple chemical "dipstick" test, which is marketed commercially and is reported to show a good correlation with allergen assays (25). The disadvantage of this test is that guanine measurements cannot be compared with measurements of other dust allergens. Therefore, several laboratories have focused on measurements of major allergens as the most useful technique for comparing indoor allergens. Levels of the 24,000-Da group I mite allergens (*Der p* I and *Der f* I) correlate with mite counts and with RAST inhibition assays and have been used to assess mite allergen exposures in Europe and in several parts of the United States (26–31).

The technical problems in measuring specific allergens have now largely been resolved. Several major allergens have been purified and are well characterized immunochemically, and over the last 5 years, allergen-specific monoclonal antibodies (MAb) have been produced and used to develop two-site, enzyme-linked immunoassays. Most allergens are low-molecular mass (M_r) proteins or glycoproteins (5000–50,000 Da) that are readily soluble in aqueous solution. They are operationally referred to as "major" or "minor" allergens on the basis of the percentage of allergic patients in whom they stimulate an IgE antibody response (for major allergens usually >80%; minor allergens <30%). Examples of major allergens include *D. pteronyssinus* allergens, *Der p* I and *Der p* II (and the homologous allergens from *D farinae*); cat salivary allergen, *Fel d* I; and *Lol p* I and *Amb a* I from rye grass and short ragweed pollens, respectively (see Refs. 20, 32, and 33 for details of allergen immunochemistry and nomenclature).

The principle of monoclonal allergen assays is outlined in Figure 3. Plastic microtiter wells are coated with an MAb and incubated with allergen or house dust extract. Bound allergen is detected by using a second biotinylated MAb, directed against a different epitope on the allergen molecule, and the assay is developed colorimetrically. The assays are quantitated with a reference preparation of known allergen concentration to form a control curve, and the results are expressed as either nanograms or micrograms of allergen per milliliter. International Reference Preparations of several allergen extracts (e.g., *D. pteronyssinus*, short ragweed, and timothy pollen) have been prepared as part of the World Health Organization and International Union of Immunological Societies (WHO/IUIS) program in allergen standardization, and other references (e.g., cat, dog, rye grass) are current being established. National

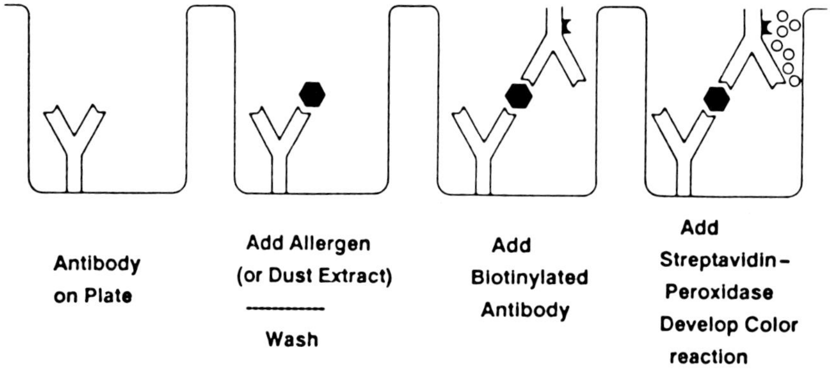

Figure 3 Principle of monoclonal ELISA assays for measuring allergen concentrations in dust samples.

agencies such as the Center for Biologics Evaluation and Research in the United States also have their own allergen references. Allergen measurements on dust samples are usually calculated as micrograms of allergen per gram of dust extracted. The advantages of these absolute values (μg/ml or μg/g) are that they allow direct comparison of the quantities of different allergens in house dust samples. Although most assays for mite and cat allergens were originally developed with polyclonal rabbit antibodies in either radioimmunoassay (RIA) or enzyme-linked immunosorbent assay (ELISA) (20,26,29), there are many advantages in using MAb. The specificity of MAb can be accurately defined, and once MAb with appropriate specificity are produced, they can be maintained indefinitely. Monoclonal assays are extremely sensitive, do not require purified allergen, and are technically straightforward—assay results on several

Table 1 Two-Site Monoclonal Immunoassays for Major Allergens[a]

Allergen	Solid-phase MAb	Labeled MAb	Reference standard	Assay
Der p I	5H8	4C1	*D. pteronyssinus* UVA 87/03 NIBSC 82/518	RIA, ELISA
Der f I	6A8	4C1	*D. farinae* UVA 87/02 OBRR E1-Df	RIA, ELISA
Der p II, *Der f* II	7A1	6D6	Affinity-purified *Der f* II	RIA
Fel d I	6F9	3E4	OBRR Cat E3	RIA, ELISA
Cockroach	10A6	Rabbit IgG ab	UVA CR extract	ELISA

[a]Assays currently being used at the University of Virginia to measure "indoor" allergens (31,34–36,73). Similar assays using either monoclonal antibodies or affinity-purified rabbit antibodies are being used by other laboratories (28–30,37,41,63,65,74). Reference standards are important in maintaining consistent allergen measurements and absolute values. NIBSC 82/518 is the WHO/IUIS International Reference Preparation of *D. pteronyssinus*, which contains 12.5 μg/ml *Der p* I (20). The OBRR mite and cat references are U.S. standards prepared by the Center for Biologics Evaluation and Research, Bethesda, Maryland. The cat reference contains 10.5 units *Fel d* I/ml. For routine use, we have prepared our own substandards from these references (UVA extracts).

Source: From Luczynska et al. (35), with permission.

hundred samples can be obtained in a few days; therefore, these assays are ideal for routine use or for epidemiological surveys. The specificity of the MAb is obviously critical in assay development. Assays for both groups of mite allergens are specific for *Dermatophagoides* spp. (Table 1; 31,34,35). Similarly, MAb assays for cat allergen, *Fel d* I, are cat-specific and do not detect allergens from other mammalian species (36,37). If only a single MAb is available, "hybrid" assays, using a combination of monoclonal and polyclonal antibodies can be used (e.g., cockroach assay, see Table 1). This type of assay is also being used to assay *Lol p* I because, although several panels of anti-*Lol p* I MAb have been produced (38–40), they do not bind well in two-site assays. This appears to be a particular problem with the antigenic structure of *Lol p* I, because there are good MAb assays for other pollen allergens (41).

Monoclonal immunoassay technology has several applications, including the standardizaiton of allergen extracts; measurement of indoor allergens in dust samples; analysis of airborne allergen distribution and particle size; and monitoring and development of allergen avoidance regimens (42). Improved standardization should result in the availability of more consistent allergen extracts for diagnosis and treatment. However, perhaps the most important feature of these assays is that they can be adapted for clinical use in doctors' offices, and, possibly by patients themselves. This offers a logical approach to the management of patients with inhalant allergy, based on accurate diagnosis and on objective assessment of indoor allergen exposure.

IV. EXPOSURE LEVELS AND ALLERGEN AVOIDANCE

A. Mite Exposure

On a worldwide basis, dust mites are the most ubiquitous indoor allergens, and most studies on household allergen exposure as a risk factor for allergic disease and on the efficacy of avoidance regimens have focused on mites. In their classic studies on mite allergy, Voorhorst and colleagues reported that mite allergic asthmatics in Holland were seen more frequently during the mites' breeding season (August through December), when mite numbers were high (up to 500 mites per gram of dust; 43,44). They were thus the first to propose a level of mite allergen exposure that was associated with exacerbation of symptoms. Subsequent studies in Europe, Japan, and North America confirmed the presence of large numbers of mites in house dust (20,27,45–48). Seasonal variation in mite allergen levels has been reported in several areas of North America: mite counts usually rise in the summer months, coincident with the rise in humidity (26,49,50). In Virginia, mite numbers rise in July and August and

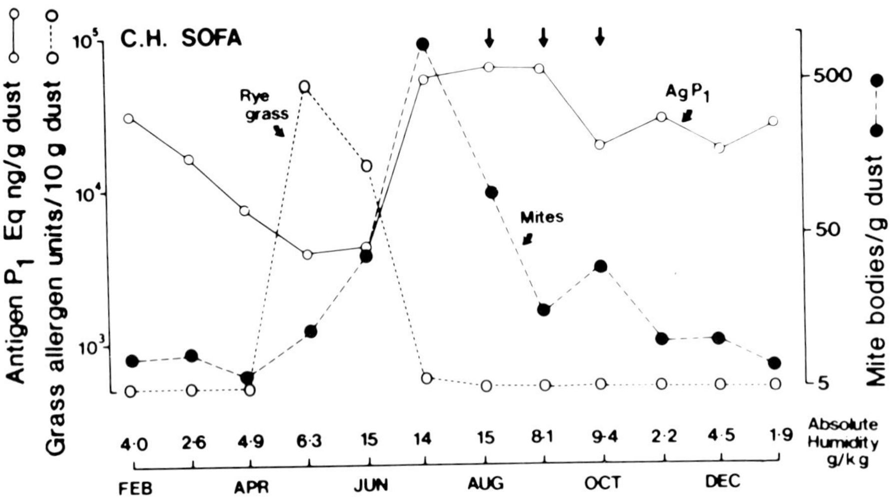

Figure 4 Seasonal variation in mite allergen levels in central Virginia and their relationship to absolute humidity. A sofa in the house of a patient with asthma (CH) was sampled monthly and the dust was assayed for mite allergen (antigen P_1Eq) (○), rye grass allergen (○---○), and mite numbers (●). The seasonal increase in mite numbers paralleled the rise in absolute humidity. Although the mite numbers fell, mite allergen levels in this sofa remained high (>5 μg/g) for most of the year. [From Platts-Mills et al. (26)].

fall rapidly in September (Fig. 4). Mite group I allergen levels also show seasonal increases and may remain high for several months after the peak in mite numbers. This probably reflects continued mite growth in sofas, mattresses, and other locally humid microenvironments (20). Mite allergen levels may vary from <1 μg/g dust to >200 μg/g dust. There is increasing evidence that levels of >10 μg/g should be regarded as clinically significant and likely to cause acute symptoms. In the seasonal variation studies (26), many patients who had exacerbations of symptoms had dust samples that exceeded 10 μg/g of mite allergen, and the levels in the houses of patients admitted to the ER with acute asthma in Atlanta ranged from 10 to 100 μg/g (51). The mean levels of *Der p* I in the houses of asthmatic patients admitted to an "allergen-free" hospital room in London, England, were 13 μg/g, and these patients showed progressive improvements in bronchial hyperreactivity during trearment, when the allergen level was maintained at or below 0.2 μg *Der p* I/g (11). Given these and other studies, a recent International Working Group, which met under the auspices of the WHO has proposed that mite allergen levels of >2 μg/g should be considered as a risk factor for sensitization (i.e., development of IgE antibody responses), and that levels of >10 μg/g (equivalent to ~500 mites per gram) should be considered as a risk factor for acute asthma (52). The important feature of these proposed risk levels is that they provide a basis for further epidemiological studies of allergen exposure in relation to both asthma and rhinitis.

B. Mite Control

Housing design has changed radically over the past 50 years. In particular, the trend to develop energy-efficient homes has resulted in increased use of central heating, airtight window and door units, and humidifiers, as well as the widespread acceptance (demand?) of fitted carpets and soft furnishings. Each of these changes has improved the conditions for mite growth by maintaining ambient temperature (about 70 °F) and indoor humidity. As their name implies, *Dermatophagoides* spp. naturally feed on human skin scales, and the highest mite numbers and allergen levels are found in mattresses, bedding, pillows, children's stuffed toys, upholstered furniture, and bedroom and living room carpeting (27,30,48,50,53). Recommended mite control measures usually involve a combination of household cleaning and attempts to reduce humidity. Several chemical methods for reducing mite growth are also currently being developed.

The most successful studies on mite avoidance in treating children have applied very strenuous efforts to cleaning of bedrooms, including removal of carpeting, covering of mattresses, and regular washing of bedding. Murray provided families with zippered vinyl covers for pillows, mattresses, and box springs and instructions for making the bedroom as easy to clean as a hospital ward. At the end of a 1-month study period, he showed a statistically significant reduction in symptoms and improved bronchial tolerance to aerosolized histamine in the group whose bedrooms had been modified (54). Excellent results were also obtained by Sarsfield and colleagues with similar mite-avoidance measures (55).

Aggressive cleaning should be the primary approach to reduce mite numbers in houses. The washing of bedding is only effective at water temperatures higher than 70 °C to kill mites. Vacuuming of carpets, although helpful in removing surface dust, should not be considered equivalent to replacing carpets with vinyl or wooden floors. Vacuuming with a poor vacuum cleaner, with inadequate suction or leaking bags, can exacerbate symptoms by increasing the concentration of airborne allergen (48). It is sensible for mite allergic patients who do their own cleaning to wear a surgical mask during and for 10–15 min after cleaning. However, masks are only partially effective because much of the air passes around the sides. There are few controlled studies on the effects of special vacuum cleaners, either on symptoms or on allergen levels. The most important aspect of cleaning regimens is that they should reduce mite counts and allergen levels. In studies for which mite control was reportedly ineffective, marked reductions in allergen levels were not achieved (56,57).

Humidity, which is difficult to control, is a requirement for mite growth. The level of absolute humidity necessary for mite growth is 8 g/kg, and Korsgaard showed that very few mites could be found in mattresses and bedroom and living room floors at an absolute humidity of less than 7 g/kg (58). He concluded that the wide differences in dust mite populations in temperate climates are related to whether or not indoor air humidity conditions permit mite survival during the dry winter months. In some new homes, the winter drying period appeared to be prevented by the use of insulation and sealants (e.g., in passive solar houses) that reduce the ventilation that normally occurs through cracks and openings in the house. Table 2 demonstrates the level of relative humidity that must be maintained at a given indoor temperature to keep the absolute humidity at 7 g/kg. Figure 4 also illustrates how changes in absolute humidity affect mite growth (typical of the southern United States). Assuming an indoor temperature of 70 °F, it is best to advise patients to try to limit relative humidity to 45% by use of air dehumidifying procedures (i.e., air conditioning) during humid summer months and not to use the type of whole-house humidifiers that are capable of increasing humidity during dry periods.

Table 2 Relationships Between Indoor Temperature, Relative Humidity, and Absolute Humidity

Indoor temperature (°F)	Absolute humidity[a] (RH = 100%)	Relative humidity[b] (AH = 7g/kg)
50	8	85%
60	11	65%
70	16	45%
80	23	30%

[a]Absolute humidity (AH) in grams of water per kilogram of dry air.
[b]Relative humidity (RH) in percentage saturation required to maintain an absolute humidity of 7 g/kg.

The use of chemical substances for house dust mite removal and prevention of reinfestation would be a useful adjunct to stringent cleaning measures and humidity control. However, most chemicals are either ineffective against mites or too toxic to recommend. Several chemicals and acaricides have been studied in the laboratory, including lindane, pirimiphos-methyl, benzyl benzoate, tannic acid, and liquid nitrogen (Table 3). Pirimiphos methyl and benzoic acid derivatives have low toxicity and good acaricidal activity and have shown promise in reducing mite allergen levels in houses (59,60). Both compounds are

Table 3 Chemicals and Acaricides Used to Control Mite Growth

Chemical	Mode of action	Comments
Lindane	Acaricide	Long-acting, too toxic for mammalian use (79)
Primiphos methyl	Insecticide	Already in use for storage mites; has been shown to reduce mite numbers in culture and to reduce mite allergen levels by up to 75% when used in home (59)
Benzoic acid ester (Acarosan)	Acaricide	Extermination rates of 95–100% in carpets and 88–100% in upholstery and mattresses; changes in allergen levels not measured (60)
Tannic acid	Denatures antigen	Washing of bedding and carpets may be effective method of reducing allergen levels (80)
Natamycin	Antifungal agent	Very low toxicity; used to prevent fungal growth on food; may reduce mite growth by effects on reproductive system; marketed in Europe (81)
Liquid nitrogen	Freezing agent	Effectively kills mites; needs special handling and application; has given promising results in a recent trial (82)

available in Europe, but not in the United States, and controlled clinical trials to investigate their effectiveness are currently underway.

C. Cat and Dog Allergens

Immunochemical studies have shown that the major cat allergen, *Fel d* I, is found in saliva and in the sebaceous glands of the skin (61,62). It presumably becomes airborne and distributed about the house during the grooming process. *Fel d* I levels in houses with cats can be very high, up to 100 FDA units/g of dust (1 unit = ~4 μg), and many commercial house dust extracts used for allergy testing contain higher *Fel d* I levels than commercial cat epithelium extracts (28,36,63,64). Crude house dust extracts are also an excellent source of *Fel d* I for allergen purification purposes (36,65). Not surprisingly, cat allergen levels show no evidence of seasonal variation; however, many houses without cats may contain readily detectable cat allergen (Fig. 5). Removal of the offending feline from the sensitized atopic individuals' environment is clearly the best means of managing cat allergy. However, cat allergen may persist in houses for several months after the departure of the cat. A recent study of 15 homes containing cats, showed that after removal of the animals it took at least 5–6 weeks and up to 20–24 weeks before *Fel d* I levels fell to those seen in control houses without cats (64). Whether vacuuming, steam cleaning, and removing carpets can make important changes in the quantity of cat allergen in a house has not been established. As with mite, some of these procedures may increase airborne cat allergen concentrations, particularly because cat allergen is associated with small airborne particles (<5 μm diameter; 66). Intense artificial dust disturbance has been shown to induce asthma in cat-sensitive patients (67). However, recent studies suggest that air filtration using high-efficiency particulate air (HEPA) filters may be effective in reducing airborne levels of cat allergen (66).

Specific major allergens have not been purified from dog dander and epithelium extracts. Dog allergens have been identified in serum, urine, and dander using serological techniques, and breed-specific as well as cross-reacting allergens have been demonstrated (68). A partially purified allergen fraction has also been used in immunoassays to assess dog allergen exposure (30). Allergen avoidance by removal of the dog from the indoor environment remains the best treatment for hypersensitivity to dog allergen.

D. Cockroach

In urban dwellings, especially in lower socioeconomic communities, cockroaches can be a major source of dust allergens and, in some inner city areas

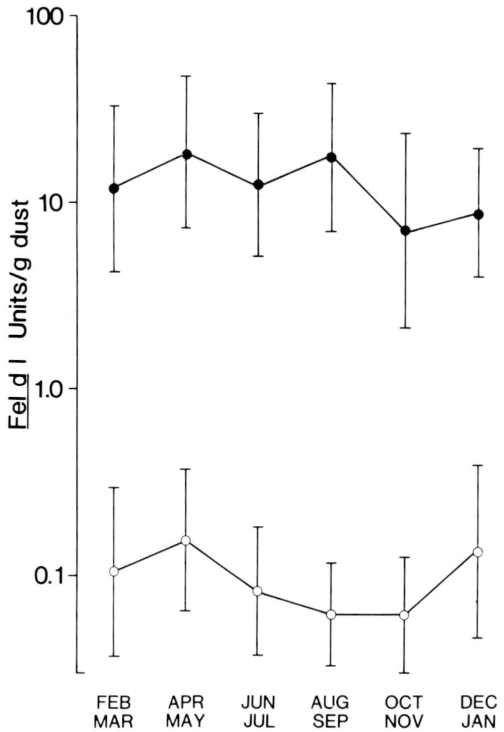

Figure 5 Year-round *Fel d* I levels in houses with (●) and without cats (○). Mean data ± 95% confidence limits of six samples from four houses with cats and five samples from houses without cats. [From Chapman et al. (36)].

(e.g., Chicago, Washington, Atlanta, New York), a high proportion (up to 70%) of dust allergic patients show positive skin tests to cockroach extracts (69–72). These patients have serum IgE antibodies to cockroach and positive immediate reactions after inhalation challenge with cockroach extract. German, American, and Oriental cockroaches are the most common causes of allergic reactions in the United States. Entomological studies suggest that cockroaches can be present in homes all year long, as long as sufficient moisture is available. Cockroaches are able to survive low ambient humidity much better than mites and can actively search for water, whereas mites cannot. Several groups have recenlty reported the use of immunochemical assays to measure German cockroach allergens (see Table 2; 73,74). Preliminary results suggest that cockroach allergens are found in highest concentration in kitchens, around the sink and in food storage cabinets and, at much lower levels, in other areas of the house (73).

Pesticides are widely available for the control of cockroaches; however reinfestation, even after professional extermination, is common and dead cockroaches or excreta of the insects may remain in the house for long periods, depending on the degree of the infestation by the cockroaches and the hygienic status of the house. Rapid movement of cockroaches from one apartment to another allows them to avoid the effects of spraying in one site. Although there are plenty of data about the effectiveness of insecticides in killing cockroaches, there are currently no reports on their effectiveness in reducing cockroach allergen levels. It is not clear in what form or under what conditions cockroach allergen becomes airborne. Thus, it is still difficult to define a simple approach to reducing cockroach exposure.

E. Pollen and Fungi as Indoor Allergens

Pollen is not usually regarded as an indoor allergen. Nevertheless, in areas in which there are large expanses of pollinating vegetation, pollen can enter houses by airborne transport (in homes ventilated by open windows and window fans) and on the clothing of the inhabitants and the coats of domestic animals. In northern California, vast areas were seeded with rye grass to prevent erosion and, in the Travis ER studies, high levels of rye grass allergen *Lol p* I were found in all parts of the homes, including bedrooms (15). Although *Lol p* I levels were as high as 150 μg/g, levels of mite and cat allergen were often much lower (<2 μg/g), and in these samples pollen was the major source of house dust allergen. It is not clear to what extent indoor pollen allergen exposure may exacerbate or prolong the symptoms of rhinitis or asthma. Measures designed to reduce airborne transport of pollen into homes may be the most reasonable way to reduce the overall pollen load (e.g., continuous use of air-conditioning during peak pollen season).

Fungi can become indoor allergens either because they grow indoors or because fungal spores enter houses from outdoor air. Fungi readily colonize interior surfaces and should be investigated as a source of perennial allergic symptoms. In addition, fungi may also play a role in acute and chronic sinusitis (75). Factors that promote indoor fungal growth are similar to those that promote mite growth: substrate moisture, locally humid air, temperature, and such. Food-storage areas, garbage containers, and soiled upholstery, all provide decaying foodstuffs that will support mold growth. The ability of fungi to break down cellulose promotes colonization of cotton, kapok, and conventional wallpaper. Synthetic foams and foam rubber tend to retain moisture and are often heavily contaminated with mold. Other surfaces that may be colonized include basement or cold outside walls, window molding, and bathroom fixtures and fittings. Poorly maintained cold mist vaporizers have been shown to emit dense fungal aerosols, and centrally installed humidifiers can occasionally harbor large fungal populations (76,77). Living plants, soil, and plant-derived material (e.g., burlap, wicker, and stored firewood) can contribute to indoor fungal levels but may require physical disturbance or active air motion for spore dispersal. Direct sampling studies suggest that a few house plants will not substantially raise indoor spore levels (78).

Given their widespread distribution, it is difficult to make cleaning recommendations that will eliminate fungi. Clearly, most effort should go toward keeping areas with obvious fungal growth clean and dry and, in general, measures used to reduce mite growth will also reduce growth of fungi. Removal of house plants and plant materials is also recommended. Many different chemicals are marketed for use in preventing fungal growth. However, although most of these chemicals are established as potent fungicides, very little data is available about their ability to reduce the load of fungal allergen in a house or to reduce symptoms. The problems with fungi are that many different species may be involved and, as yet, quantitative allergen assays are not available. Although some progress has been made in the characterization of allergens from *Alternaria, Cladosporium*, and *Aspergillus*, fungal allergens remain poorly defined. The identification and purification of allergens from the most common fungi is needed to establish the relative importance of fungi in causing chronic rhinitis and sinusitis.

V. IMPLICATIONS OF ALLERGEN EXPOSURE FOR SYMPTOMS OF RHINITIS

The treatment of children with allergic rhinitis can be improved by investigating the relationship between allergic sensitivity and allergen exposure. Currently, optimal treatment consists of allergen avoidance, proper use of medications and, in selected cases, immunotherapy. Treatment varies from patient to patient, depending on clinical history and on measurements of allergen-specific IgE antibody (e.g., by skin testing or RAST). Careful follow-up is also important for correlating changes in clinical symptoms with any of the treatment options.

There is clear experimental evidence that exposure to inhalant allergens can cause both immediate and delayed type hypersensitivity reactions in the nose. As early as 1873, Blackley challenged allergic individuals with grass pollen intranasally and produced acute symptoms of rhinitis (1). Inflammatory reactions after intranasal allergen challenge are well established (83–87), and more recent studies by Naclerio and colleagues in ragweed allergic patients, demonstrated immediate and late-phase reactions after intranasal challenge with ragweed allergen, together with release of histamine and other inflammatory mediators into nasal secretions (88,89). It is assumed that these changes also occur after natural allergen exposure. Norman and colleagues have shown an excellent correlation between daily symptom scores and quantitative ragweed pollen counts and have also demonstrated that immunotherapy can decrease these symptoms (90,91). Combined symptom and medication scores correlate significantly with seasonal ragweed pollen counts, and both ragweed and grass pollen allergic patients benefit from nasal cromolyn or local steroids when treated during the pollen season (92,93).

Studies with pollen allergens clearly show a direct relationship between nasal symptoms and allergen exposure, and this relationship is also observed in patients with domestic or laboratory animal allergy, many of whom develop immediate symptoms, for example, on entering a house with a cat or an animal vivarium. In contrast, the temporal relationship between symptoms and exposure in patients allergic to mites or cockroach is generally poor. The aerodynamic size and concentration of allergen-containing particles are probably among the most important factors that determine when symptoms will occur. Windborne pollen grains (10 to 40 μm diameter) may impact directly onto the nasal mucosa and conjunctiva at relatively high velocity. However, the air exchange rate in houses is often low (<0.5 changes per hour) and particle size, to a large extent, determines whether or not a particular allergen will remain airborne. Recent air-sampling studies suggest that the rapid onset of symptoms affecting cat allergic patients on entering a house with a cat may well be due to the significant proportion ($\sim 25\%$) of *Fel d* I carried by small particles (<5-μm diameter), which remain airborne for long periods (66,94). Rodent urinary proteins are found on small particles (mean 7-μm diameter) and also occur in very high concentrations in animal rooms (95). In contrast, mite allergens are found on fecal particles (mean 25-μm diameter) that become airborne for only short periods (20 min) after domestic activity (48,96). Thus, mite allergic patients often do not attribute their symptoms to increased dust exposure. However, mite feces contain a very high allergen concentration (~ 10 mg *Der p* I/ml) and inhalation of just a few of these particles may be sufficient to initiate and maintain inflammatory responses in allergic patients. On a practical level, studies of airborne allergens are now being used to compare the effectiveness of air-purification systems, air-conditioning units, and electrostatic filters, as methods of reducing allergen concentrations in the air.

VI. THERAPEUTIC APPROACHES

It is not uncommon in pediatric practice to make the diagnosis of allergic rhinitis based on a patients history of chronic or seasonal rhinitis alone or in conjunction with the finding of eosinophils in nasal secretions. Often, referrals for allergy evaluations are deferred because of the costs involved or unless immunotherapy appears to be indicated. In addition, recommendations on allergen avoidance are often made empirically without knowledge of a patient's specific sensitivities. In patients with persistent rhinitis, an evaluation for sensitivity to specific allergens can markedly improve their management.

Quite often, efforts to reduce allergen levels involve significant financial commitments and changes in life-style, for the patients and other family members, that may be difficult to implement unless the patient (or usually the parents) are convinced that allergens are responsible for the disease. It is much easier to convince families to make changes when it is possible to identify, or better to measure, allergens in their houses. Children may improve with use of avoidance procedures in their bedrooms alone, and this perhaps is the most pragmatic approach. Recommendations on cat or dog allegen avoidance also need to take into account the strong emotional ties between children and their pets, which may outweigh the importance of mild to moderate symptoms. Clinical experience suggests that outdoor cats may not be a serious problem. However, keeping pets in the house with children who are highly allergic to animal dander should be discouraged. Some methods available for cleaning houses may be selective for certain allergens and leave other allergen levels unaffected. The HEPA-filtered room air cleaners used together with regular vacuum cleaning of carpeting and soft furnishings may reduce airborne cat allergen levels, but not significantly alter mite allergen levels (66). Conversely, reducing humidity may effectively reduce mite and mold growth, but have little effect on cat allergen. In all cases for whom allergen avoidance is recommended, patients should be forewarned not to expect rapid clinical improvement. Optimally, recommendations to reduce indoor allergen levels should be based on assessments of the patient's sensitivities and symptoms, together with carefully planned follow-up visits to judge compliance and effectiveness.

VII. CONCLUSIONS

There is now a substantial body of evidence which suggests that the development of IgE antibodies to inhaled allergens is a risk factor for allergic respiratory disease. It is important to recognize that allergen exposure is only a risk factor in atopic individuals: nonatopic persons may be exposed to very high allergen levels, yet remain asymptomatic unless they develop IgE antibodies.

Equally, allergen exposure is only a risk factor for allergic patients if they are exposed to a relevant allergen. Thus, exposure to mite allergens was not a risk factor for ER admission at Travis in the spring and, likewise, grass pollen was not a risk factor for ER admission in Charlottesville in the fall (15–17). The evidence suggests that different allergens will be risk factors in different parts of the country, and it is important that pediatricians and allergists should be familiar with the local allergen flora and fauna in their area.

The further development of immunoassays will make it possible to analyze patients' houses for a panel of common allergens and to make more specific statements about avoidance procedures. Risk levels for exposure to mite and cat allergens can already be proposed, and many laboratories are now engaged in epidemiological studies in different parts of the world to establish the validity of the proposed levels. Clearly, the same strategies will also be applied to other allergens (e.g., fungi, dog) when suitable assays become available.These assays will also allow controlled clinical trials on the efficacy of allergen avoidance procedures that are currently being developed. Use of the combined approaches of identifying the offending allergen and carefuly monitoring avoidance procedures is a useful therapeutic strategy that should improve the management of children with rhinitis and other allergic diseases.

REFERENCES

1. Blackley CH. Experimenal researches on the cause and nature of catarrhus aestivus (hay-fever or hay-asthma). London: Baillere, Tindall and Cox, 1873; reprinted 1959 by Dawson's of Pall Mall, London.
2. Ward GW, Platts-Mills TAE. Allergic rhinitis caused by house dust and other non pollen allergens. Curr Ther Allegy Immunol Rheumatol 1988; 3:8–14.
3. Smith JM, Disney ME, Williams JP, Goels GA. Clinical significance of skin reactions to mite extracts in children with asthma. Br Med J 1969; 2:723–726.
4. Bryant DH, Burns MW. Skin test reactions to inhalant allergens in asthmatic patients. Med J Aust 1976; 1:918–920.
5. Dodge R, Cline MG, Burrows B. Comparisons of asthma, emphysema, and chronic bronchitis in a general population sample. Am Rev Respir Dis 1986; 133:981–986.
6. Mygind N, Dirkson A, Johnsen NJ, Weeke B. Perennial rhinitis: an analysis of skin testing, serum IgE and blood and smear eosinophilia in 201 patients. Clin Otolaryngol 1978; 3:189–195.
7. Burrows B, Martinez FD, Halonen M, Barbee RA, Cline MG. Association of asthma with serum IgE and skin-test reactivity to allergens. N Engl J Med 1989; 320:271–276.
8. Witt C, Stuckey MS, Woolcock AJ, Dawkins RL. Positive allergy prick tests associated with bronchial histamine responsiveness in an unselected population. J Allergy Clin Immunol 1986; 77:698–702.

9. Kerrebijn KF. Endogenous factors in childhood CNSLD. Methodological aspects in population studies. In: Orie NGM, van der Lende R, eds. Bronchitis III. Assen: The Netherlands Royal Vangorcum, 1970:38–48.
10. Charpin D, Kleisbauer JP, Lanteaume A, et al. Asthma and allergy to house dust mites in patients living in high altitude. Chest 1988; 93:758–766.
11. Platts-Mills TAE, Tovey ER, Mitchell EB, Mozarro H, Nock P, Wilkins SR. Reversal of bronchial reactivity during prolonged allergen avoidance. Lancet 1982; 2:675–678.
12. Dowse GK, Turner KJ, Stewart GA, Alpers MP, Woolcock AJ. The association between *Dermatophagoides* mites and the increasing prevalence of asthma in village communities within the Papua New Guinea Highlands. J Allergy Clin Immunol 1985; 75:75–80.
13. Cockroft A, Edwards J, McCarthy P, Andersson N. Allergy in laboratory animal workers. Lancet 1981; 1:827–829.
14. Platts-Mills TAE, Longbottom J, Edwards J, Cockroft A, Wilkins S. Occupational asthma and rhinitis related to laboratory rats: serum IgG and IgE antibodies to the rat urinary allergen. J Allergy Clin Immunol 1987; 79:505–515.
15. Pollart SM, Reid MJ, Fling JA, Chapman MD, Platts-Mills TAE. Epidemiology of emergency room asthma in northern California: association with IgE antibody to rye grass pollen. J Allergy Clin Immunol 1988; 82:224–230.
16. Pollart SM, Chapman MD, Fiocco GP, Rose G, Platts-Mills TAE. Epidemiology of acute asthma: IgE antibodies to common inhalant allergens as a risk factor for emergency room visits. J Allergy Clin Immunol 1989; 83:875–882.
17. Chapman MD, Pollart SM, Luczynska CM, Platts-Mills TAE. Hidden allergic factors in the etiology of asthma. Chest 1988; 94:185–190.
18. Reid MJ, Moss RB, Hsu YP, Kwasnicki JM, Commerford TM, Nelson BL. Seasonal asthma in northern California: allergic causes and efficacy of immunotherapy. J Allergy Clin Immunol 1986; 78:590–600.
19. Chapman MD, Rowntree S, Mitchell EB, DiPrisco de Fuenmajor MC, Platts-Mills TAE. Quantitative assessments of IgG and IgE antibodies to inhalant allergens in patients with atopic dermatitis. J Allergy Clin Immunol 1983; 72:27–33.
20. Platts-Mills TAE, Chapman MD. Dust mites: immunology, allergic disease and environmental control. J Allergy Clin Immunol 1987; 80:755–777.
21. Marsh DG, Hsu SH, Roebber M. HLA-DW2: a genetic marker for human immune response to short ragweed pollen allergen Ra5. I. Response resulting primarily from natural allergen exposure. J Exp Med 1982; 155:1439–1450.
22. Brostoff JB, Greaves MF, Roitt IM. IgE in lymphoid cells from pollen stimulated cultures. Lancet 1969; 1:803–805.
23. Rawle FC, Mitchell EB, Platts-Mills TAE. T cell responses to the major allergen from the house dust mite, *Dermatophagoides pteronyssinus*, antigen P[1]: comparison of patients with asthma, atopic dermatitis and perennial rhinitis. J Immunol 1984; 133:195–201.
24. Rowntree S, Cogswell JJ, Platts-Mills TAE, Mitchell EB. Development of IgG and IgE antibodies to food and inhalant allergens in children at risk of allergic disease. Arch Dis Child 1985; 60:727–735.

25. Pauli G, Tenabene A, Bessot JC, Bischoff E. Guanine dosage in house dust samples and quantification of mite allergens. In: Advances in aerobiology, Basel: Berkhauser Verlag, 1987:203–209, 189–196.
26. Platts-Mills TAE, Hayden ML, Chapman MD, Wilkins SR. Seasonal variation in dust mite and grass pollen allergens in dust from the houses of patients with asthma. J Allergy Clin Immunol 1987; 79:781–791.
27. Smith TF, Kelly LB, Heymann PW, Wilkins SR, Platts-Mills TAE. Natural exposure and serum antibodies to house dust mite of allergic children in Atlanta. J Allergy Clin Immunol 1985; 76:782–788.
28. Wood RA, Eggleston PA, Lind P, Ingemann L, Schwartz B, Graveson S, Terry D, Wheeler B, Adkinson NF. Antigenic analysis of household dust samples. Am Rev Respir Dis 1988; 137:358–363.
29. Lind P, Norman PS, Newton M, Lowenstein H, Schwartz B. The prevalence of indoor allergens in the Baltimore area: house dust mite and animal dander antigens measured by immunochemical techniques. J Allergy Clin Immunol 1987; 80:541–546.
30. Lind P. Enzyme linked immunosorbent assay for determination of major excrement allergens of house dust mite species *D. pteronyssinus, D. farinae* and *D. microceras*. Allergy 1986; 41:442–450.
31. Chapman MD, Heymann PW, Wilkins SR, Brown MB, Platts-Mills TAE. Monoclonal immunoassays for measure major dust mite (*Dermatophagoides*) allergens, *Der p* I and *Der f* I, and quantitative analysis of the allergen content of mite and house dust extracts. J Allergy Clin Immunol 1987; 80:184–194.
32. Marsh DG, Goodfriend L, King TP, Lowenstein H, Platts-Mills TAE. Allergen nomenclature. J Allergy Clin Immunol 1987; 80:639–645.
33. Chapman MD. Purification of allergens. Curr Opin Immunol 1989; 1:647–653.
34. Heymann PW, Chapman MD, Aalberse RC, Fox J, Platts-Mills TAE. Antigenic and structural analysis of group II allergens (*Der f* II and *Der p* II) from house dust mites (*Dermatophagoides* spp.). J Allergy Clin Immunol 1989; 83:1055–1067.
35. Luczynska CM, Arruda LK, Platts-Mills TAE, Miller JD, Lopez M, Chapman MD. A two-site monoclonal antibody ELISA assay for the quantification of the major *Dermatophagoides* spp. allergens, *Der p* I and *Der f* I. J Immunol Methods 1989; 118:227–235.
36. Chapman MD, Aalberse RC, Brown MB, Platts-Mills TAE. Monoclonal antibodies to the major feline allergen *Fel d* I. II. Single step affinity purification of *Fel d* I, N-terminal sequence analysis and development of a sensitive two site immunoassay to assess *Fel d* I exposure. J Immunol 1988; 140:812–818.
37. Lombardero M, Carreira J, Duffort O. Monoclonal antibody based radioimmunoassay for the quantitation of the main cat allergen (*Fel d* I or cat-1). J Immunol Methods 1988; 108:71–76.
38. Bose R, Rector ES, Fischer J, Taronno R, Delespesse G. Production and characterization of mouse monoclonal antibodies to allergenic epitopes on *Lol p* I (rye I). Immunology 1986; 59:309–315.

39. Mourad W, Mecheri S, Peltre G, David B, Herbert J. Study of the epitope structure of purified *Dac g* I and *Lol p* I, the major allergens on *Dactylis glomerata* and *Lolium perenne* pollens, using monoclonal antibodies. J Immunol 1988; 141:3486–3491.
40. Esch RE, and Klapper DG. Identification and localization of allergenic determinants on grass group I antigens using monoclonal antibodies. J Immunol 1989; 142:179–184.
41. Corbi AL, Ayuso R, Lombardero M, Carreira J, Duffort O. A competitive solid phase radioimmunoassay for quantitation of the major allergen of *Parietaria* pollen. J Immunol Methods 1985; 83:83–88.
42. Chapman MD. Allergen specific monoclonal antibodies: new tools for the management of allergic disease. Allergy 1988; 43(5):7–14.
43. Voorhorst R, Spieksma FTM, Speksma-Boezeman MIA. Is a mite (*Dermatophagoides* sp) the producer of the house dust allergen. Allergie Asthma 1964; 10:329–334.
44. Voorhorst R, Spieksma FTH, Varekamp H, Leupen MJ, Lyklema AW. The house dust mite (*Dermatophagoides pteronyssinus*) and the allergens it produces: identity with the house dust allergen. J Allergy 1967; 39:325–334.
45. Miyamoto T, Oshima S, Ishizaki T, Sano S. Allergenic identity between the common floor mite (*Dermatophagides farinae* Hughes, 1961) and house dust as a causative agent in bronchial asthma. J Allergy 1968; 42:14–28.
46. Van Bronswijk JEMH, Sinha RN. Pyroglyphid mites (acari) and house dust allergy: a review. J Allergy 1971; 47:31–52.
47. Bullock JD, Frick OL. Mite sensitivity in house dust allergic children: evaluation by clinical and laboratory methods. Am J Dis Child 1972; 123:222–226.
48. Tovey ER, Chapman MD, Wells CW, Platts-Mills TAE. The distribution of dust mite allergen in the houses of patients with asthma. Am Rev Respir Dis 1981; 124:630–635.
49. Murray AB, Ferguson AC, Morrison B. The seasonal variation of allergic respiratory symptoms induced by house dust mites. Ann Allergy 1980; 45:347–352.
50. Arlian LG, Bernstein IL, Gallagher JS. The prevalence of house dust mites, *Dermatophagoides* sp, and associated environmental conditions in homes in Ohio. J Allergy Clin Immunol 1982; 69:527–535.
51. Pollart SM, Chapman MD, Platts-Mills TAE. Allergen levels inside homes: risk factors for acute asthma attacks. J Allergy Clin Immunol 1988; 81:242.
52. Dust mite allergens and asthma—a worldwide problem. Report of an International Workshop in Bad Kreuznach, FRG, Sept 1987. J Allergy Clin Immunol 1989; 83:416–427.
53. Carpenter MD, Win GH, Furumizo RT, Massey DG, Ortiz AA. Air conditioning and the house dust mite. J Allergy Clin Immunol 1985; 75:121.
54. Murray AB, Ferguson AC. Dust-free bedrooms in the treatment of asthmatic children with house dust mite allergy: a controlled trial. Pediatrics 1983; 71:418–425.

55. Sarsfield JK, Gowland G, Toy R, Norman AL. Mite sensitive asthma of childhood: trial of avoidance measures. Arch Dis Child 1974; 49:711–716.
56. Korsgaard J. Preventative measures in house dust allergy. Am Rev Respir Dis 1982; 125:80–84.
57. Burr ML, Dean BV, Merrett TG, Neale E, St Leger AS, Verrier-Jones ER. Effects of anti-mite measures on children with mite-sensitive asthma: a controlled trial. Thorax 1980; 35:506–512.
58. Korsgaard J. House dust mites and absolute indoor humditiy. Allergy 1983; 38:85–92.
59. Mitchell EB, Wilkins S, McCallum Deighton J, Platts-Mills TAE. Reduction of house dust mite allergen levels in the home: use of the acaricide, pirimiphos methyl. Clin Allergy 1985; 15:235–240.
60. Bischoff E, Fischer A. A new method of counting mites to establish the efficacy of water based acaricides, and their application. J Allergy Clin Immunol 1987; 79:194.
61. Brown PR, Leiterman K, Ohman JL. Distribution of cat allergen 1 in cat tissues and fluids. Int Arch Allergy Appl Immunol 1984; 74:67–70.
62. Bartholome K, Kissler W, Baer H, Kopietz-Schulte E, Wahn U. Where does cat allergen 1 come from? J Allergy Clin Immunol 1985; 76:503–506.
63. Ohman JL, Lorusso JR, Lewis SR. Cat allergen content of commercial house dust extracts: comparison of dust extracts from a cat containing environment. J Allergy Clin Immunol 1987; 79:955–959.
64. Wood RA, Chapman MD, Adkinson NF, Eggleston PA. The effect of cat removal on *Fel d* I content in household dust samples. J Allergy Clin Immunol 1989; 83:730–734.
65. DeGroot H, Van Swieten P, Van Leeuwen J, Lind P, Aalberse RC. Monoclonal antibodies to the major feline allergen, *Fel d* I. I. Serologic and biologic activity of affinity purified *Fel d* I and of *Fel d* I depleted extract. J Allergy Clin Immunol 1988; 82:778–786.
66. Luczynska CM, Li Y, Chapman MD, Platts-Mills TAE. Factors controlling airborne concentrations and particle size distribution of allergen derived from domestic cats (*Felis domesticus*): measurement using cascade impactor, liquid impinger and a two site monoclonal antibody assay for *Fel d* I. Am Rev Respir Dis 1989; (in press).
67. Van Metre TE, Marsh DG, Adkinson NF, Fish JE, Kagey-Sobotka A, Norman PS, Radden EB, Rosenberg GL. Dose of cat (*Felis domesticus*) allergen I (*Fel d* I) that induces asthma. J Allergy Clin Immunol 1986; 78:62–72.
68. McLean AC, Glovsky MM, Hoffman DR, Glekiger LM. Identification of allergens in dog dander extract. I. Clinical and immunological aspects of allergenicity activity. Ann Allergy 1980; 45:199–200.
69. Bernton HS, Brown H. Insect allergy—preliminary studies of the cockroach. J Allergy 1964; 35:506.

70. Twarog FJ, Picone FJ, Strunk RS, So J, Colten HR. Immediate hypersensitivity to cockroach: isolation and purification of the major antigens. J Allergy Clin Immunol 1977; 59:154–160.
71. Kang B. Study on cockroach antigen as a probable causative agent in bronchial asthma. J Allergy Clin Immunol 1976; 58:357–365.
72. Hulett AC, Dockhorn RJ. House dust mite (*D. farinae*) and cockroach allergy in a Midwestern population. Ann Allergy 1979; 42:160–165.
73. Pollart SM, Platts-Mills TAE, Chapman MD. Identification, quantification and purification of cockroach allergens using monoclonal antibodies. J Allergy Clin Immunol 1989; 83:293.
74. Schou C, Fernandez-Caldas E, Lockey RF, Lowenstein H. Environmental assay for cockroach allergen. J Allergy Clin Immunol 1989; 83:258.
75. Gumowski P, Lech B, Chaves I, Girard JP. Chronic asthma and rhinitis due to *Candida albicans, Epidermaphyton* and *Trichophyton*. Ann Allergy 1987; 59:48–51.
76. Burge HA, Solomon WR, Borsi JR. Microbial prevalence in domestic humidifiers. Appl Environ Microbiol 1980; 39:340.
77. Solomon WR. Fungal aerosols arising from cold mist vaporizers. J Allergy Clin Immunol 1975; 54:222.
78. Jelks ML, Solomon WR. Airborne allergens. In: Kaplan AP, ed. Allergy. New York: Churchill-Livingston, 1985:225–320.
79. Heller-Haupt A, Busvine JR. Tests of acaricides against house dust mites. J Med Entomol 1974; 2:551–558.
80. Green WF. Abolition of allergens by tannic acid. Lancet 1984; 1:3895.
81. Van Bronswijk JEMH, Sinha RN. Role of fungi in the survival of *Dermatophagoides* in house dust environment. Environ Entomol 1973; 2:142–145.
82. Dorward AJ, Colloff MJ, MacKay NS, McSharry C, Thomson NC. Effect of house dust mite avoidance measures on adult atopic asthma. Thorax 1988; 43:98–105.
83. Taylor G, Shrivalkar PR. Changes in nasal airways resistance on antigenic challenge in allergic rhinitis. Clin Allergy 1971; 1:63–69.
84. Connell J. Quantitative intranasal pollen challenge. J Allergy 1968; 41:123–139.
85. Dolovich J, Bach N, Arbesman C. Kinin like activity in nasal secretions of allergic patients. Int Arch Allergy Appl Immunol 1970; 38:337–344.
86. Okazaki T, Reisman R, Arbesman C. Prostaglandin E in the secretions of allergic rhinitis. Prostaglandins 1977; 13:681–690.
87. Eggleston P, Hendley J, Gwaltney J, Eggleston A, Leavell B. Histamine in nasal secretions. Int Arch Allergy Appl Immunol 1978; 57:193–200.
88. Naclerio RM, Proud D, Togias AG, Adkinson NF, Meyers DA, Kagey-Sobotka A, Plaut M, Norman PS, Lichtenstein LM. Inflammatory mediators in late antigen induced rhinitis. N Engl J Med 1985; 313:65–69.
89. Naclerio RM. The pathophysiology of allergic rhinitis: impact of therapeutic intervention. J Allergy Clin Immunol 1988; 82:927–934.

90. Norman PS, Winkenwerder MD, Lichtenstein LM. Trials of alum precipitated pollen extracts in the treatment of hayfever. J Allergy Clin Immunol 1972; 50:31–44.
91. Van Metre TE, Adkinson NF, Amodio FJ, Lichtenstein LM, Mardiney MR, Norman PS, Rosenberg GL, Sobotka AK, Valentine MD. A comparative study of the effectiveness of the Rinkel method and the current standard method for immunotherapy for ragweed pollen hayfever. J Allergy Clin Immunol 1980; 66:500–513.
92. Handelman NI, Friday GA, Schwartz HJ, Kuhn FS, Lindsay DE, Koons PG, Moyer RP, Smith CS, Kemper CF, Nagel JR, Rosch J, Murphy S, Miller DL. Cromolyn sodium nasal solution in the prophylactic treatment of pollen induced seasonal allergic rhinitis. J Allergy Clin Immunol 1977; 59:237–242.
93. Norman PS. Allergic rhinitis. J Allergy Clin Immunol 1985; 75:531–550.
94. Swanson MA, Agarwal MK, Reed CE. An immunochemical approach to indoor aeroallergen quantitation with a new volumetric air sampler: studies with mite, roach, cat, mouse and guinea pig antigens. J Allergy Clin Immunol 1985; 76:724–731.
95. Platts-Mills TAE, Heymann PW, Longbottom J, Wilkins SR. Airborne particles carrying dust mites and rat allergens. J Allergy Clin Immunol 1986; 77:850–857.
96. Tovey ER, Chapman MD, Platts-Mills TAE. Mite faeces are a major source of house dust allergens. Nature 1984; 289:592–593.

3

Air Pollution and the Upper Respiratory Tract

Eli O. Meltzer
University of California—San Diego and Allergy and Asthma Medical Group and Research Center, San Diego, California

I. INTRODUCTION

Upper airway symptoms are produced by effector nerves, blood vessels, and glands. Triggering factors for the symptoms include irritant, physical, and chemical stimuli, and inflammation caused by infections and allergens. Any state of autonomic imbalance or hyperreactivity will further potentiate the clinical disease (Fig. 1). This chapter will focus on the irritant stimuli. We will review sources, their health effects, and the measures to help control them in our environment.

II. OUTDOOR AIR POLLUTION

Respiratory disease, exacerbated by air pollution, is a problem of growing recognition. *Air pollution* is defined as the atmospheric accumulation of

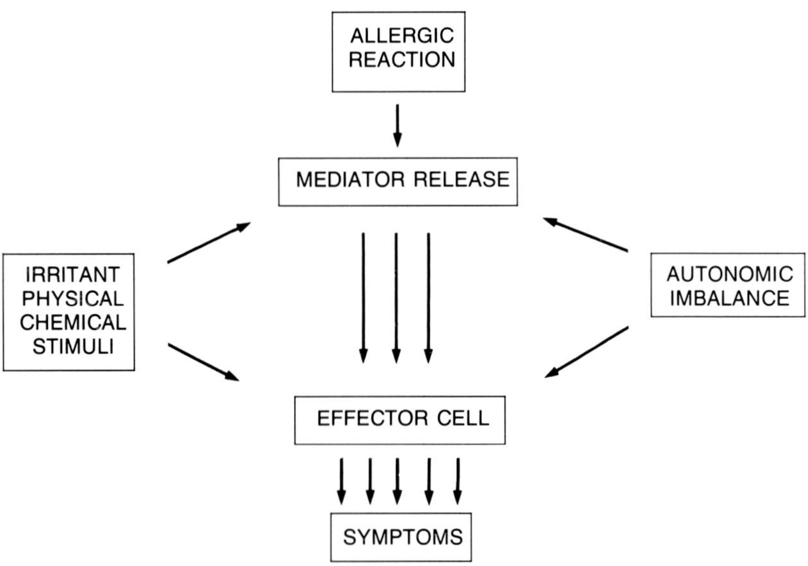

Figure 1 Pathophysiology of rhinitis.

substances to a degree that becomes injurious to humans, animals, or plants (Table 1) (1). There are two main types of outdoor smog pollution (*smog* is a combination of the words smoke and fog). Industrial smog results from the combustion of sulfur-containing fossil fuel (e.g., coal and oil). Photochemical smog is due to the chemical reaction of sunlight with hydrocarbons and nitrogen oxides from automobile exhaust emissions. These two types can coexist in a given area at the same time.

The levels of air pollutants are affected by many weather conditions; low wind velocity especially hinders their horizontal dispersion and high-pressure and temperature inversions limit their vertical dispersion. Local geographic features that confine pollutants that are emitted into the air also contribute to air stagnation.

Although the overall concentrations of outdoor air pollutants have decreased since the Clean Air Act was passed in 1970, certain communities have increased their pollution as a result of urbanization. Recent air quality data indicate that more than 30% of the United States population live in an area where they are potentially exposed to peak ozone concentrations that exceed standards (2). Figure 2 maps the United States areas violating ozone and carbon monoxide air quality standards (3). The National Air Quality Standards for pollutants and the adverse health effects attributed to their increased concentration are listed in Table 2 (4).

For nonsusceptible children without allergy or increased airway hyperreactivity, the current standards may be adequate. Ordinary exogenous stimuli effect only slight changes in nasal blood vessels and the secretory activity of the 250 large serous glands in the anterior part of the nose and the 120,000 small seromucous glands (5). In the normal nose, these changes are not usually perceived (Fig. 3; 6).

In contrast with the minimal symptoms noted with modest exposures, almost all noses will react with significant symptoms to a challenge of large amounts of dust, high levels of water-soluble gas, such as sulfur dioxide (7), or an extreme temperature change. The symptoms are nasal irritation, sneezing, moderate discharge, and some congestion (Fig. 4; 6). The magnitude of the symptoms will depend, in part, on the anatomy of the nose. A child who has a narrow nasal airway will block more readily than will a normal adult.

The magnitude of the nasal symptoms depends not only on the type and quality of exogenous stimulation and the anatomy of the nose. The severity of disease is also compounded by the degree of the child's nasal airway reactivity. Hyperreactivity can be due to (1) increased epithelial permeability, as occurs with airway inflammation; (2) increased number or increased sensitivity of the mediator cells (e.g. mast cells and basophils); (3) increased sensitivity

Table 1 Summary of Air Pollution Sources

Pollutants	Source
Group I: sources predominantly outdoor	
Sulfur oxides (gases, particles)	Fuel combustion, nonferrous smelters
Ozone	Photochemical reactions
Pollens	Trees, grass, weeds, plants
Lead, manganese	Automobiles
Calcium, chlorine, silicon, cadmium	Suspension of soils or industrial emissions
Organic substances	Petrochemical solvents, natural sources, vaporization of unburned fuels
Group II: sources both indoor and outdoor	
Nitric oxide, nitrogen dioxide	Fuel burning
Carbon monoxide	Fuel burning
Carbon dioxide	Metabolic activity, combustion
Particles	Resuspension, condensation of vapors and combustion products
Water vapor	Biologic activity, combustion, evaporation
Organic substances	Volatilization, combustion, paint, metabolic action, pesticides, insecticides, fungicides
Spores	Fungi, molds
Group III: sources predominantly indoor	
Radon	Building construction materials (concrete, stone) water, soil
Formaldehyde	Particleboard, insulation, furnishings, tobacco smoke, gas stoves
Asbestos, mineral and synthetic fibers	Fire-retardant, acoustic, thermal or electric insulation
Organic substances	Adhesives, solvents, cooking, cosmetics
Ammonia	Metabolic activity, cleaning products
Polycyclic hydrocarbons, arsenic, nicotine acrolein, etc.	Tobacco smoke
Mercury	Fungicides in paints, spills in dental care facilities or laboratories, thermometer breakage
Aerosols	Consumer products
Viable organisms	Infections
Allergens	House dust, animal dander

Source: From Yocom JE (1), cited in Koenig JQ. J Allergy Clin Immunol 1988; 81:1055, with permission.

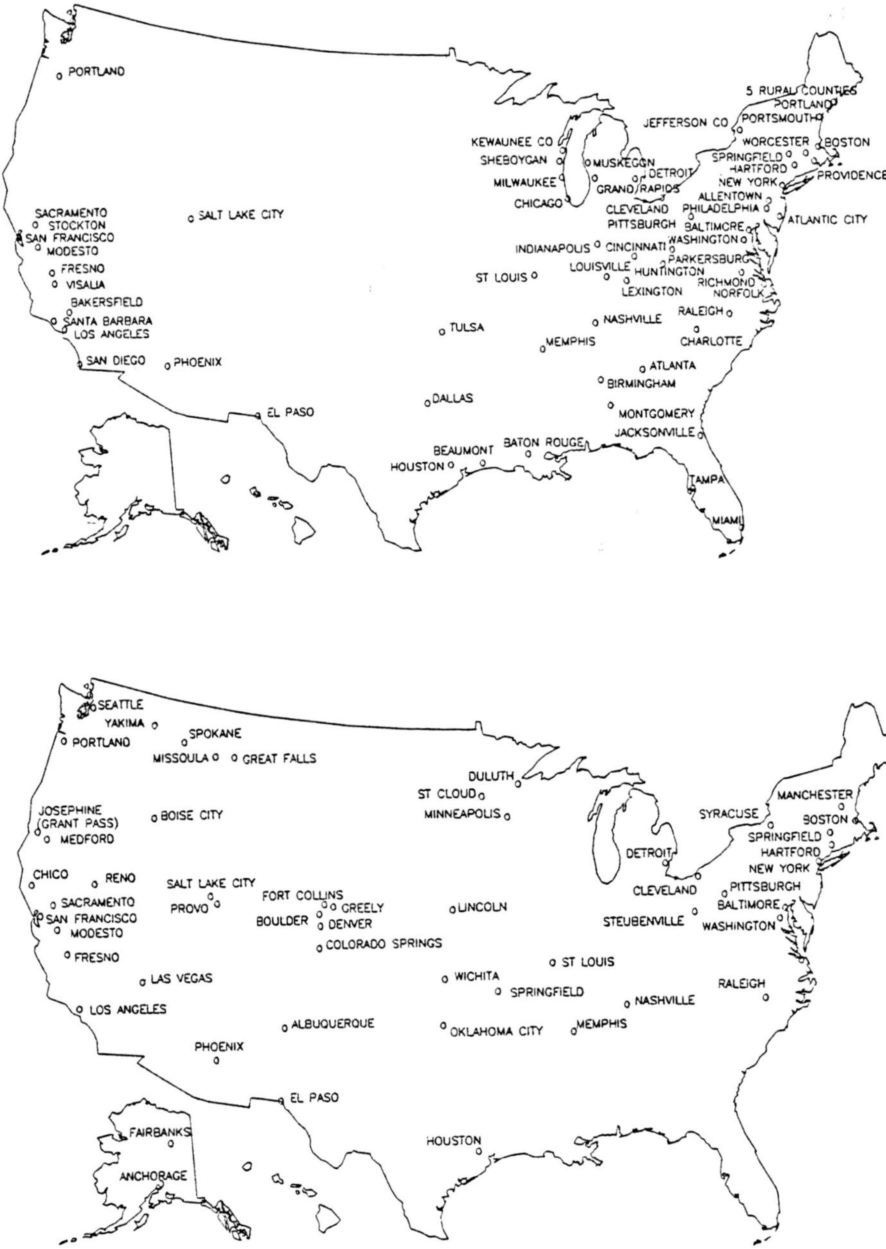

Figure 2 U. S. areas violating air quality standards. [From Marwick (3), with permission]

Table 2 National Primary Air Quality Standards and Principal Health Effects Attributed to Increased Concentrations of Pollutants

Pollutant	Standard	Standard averaging time	Health effects of concentration greater than standard
Sulfur dioxide	0.03 ppm	Annual arithmetic mean[a]	Exacerbation of chronic airways disease
			Decreased nasal mucus flow
	0.14 ppm	Maximal 24-hr average[b]	Increased nasal airway resistence
Total suspended particulates	75 g/m^3	Annual geometric mean [a]	Altered lung function in children
	260 g/m^3	Maximal 24-hr average[b]	
Photochemical oxidants (ozone)	0.08 ppm	Maximal 1-hr average	Eye irritation, respiratory impairment
Nitrogen dioxide (NO_2)	0.05 ppm	Annual arithmetic mean	Risk of acute and chronic lung disease

[a] Peak leveals for each day are averaged for the whole year, and the average cannot exceed this value.
[b] Peak levels for each hour of a given day averaged, and the average cannot exceed this value.

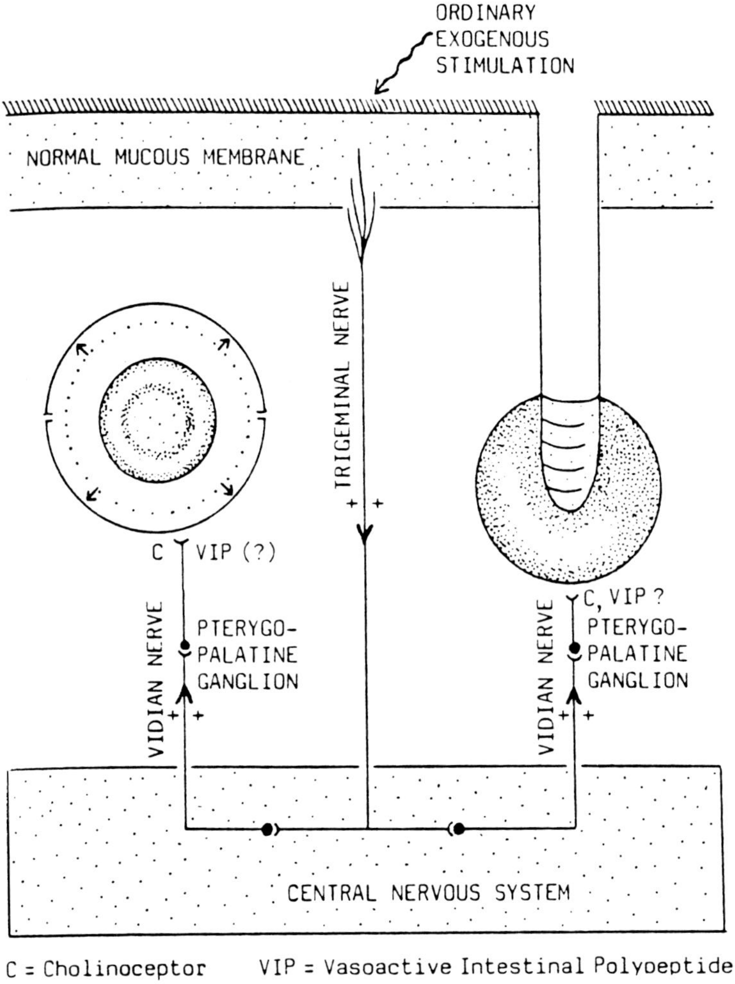

Figure 3 Normal parasympathetic reflexes. The sensory nerves in the nose are slightly stimulated by ordinary inhaled air due to this unphysiological condition (dry, polluted, cold). This stimulation will result in reflex activity producing mild hypersecretion and vascular changes not noted by the normal subject. [From Mygind (6), with permission.]

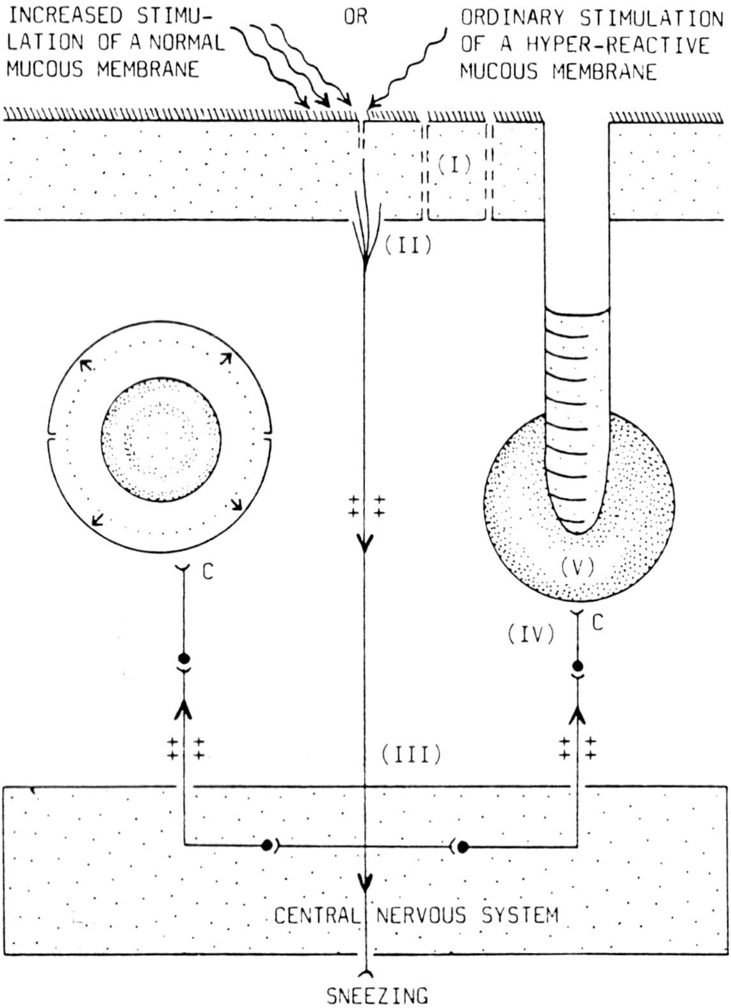

Figure 4 Increased reflex activity. High concentrations of irritant gases or dust and extreme temperature changes result in sneezing, moderate discharge, and slight vasodilation in the normal nose. The same symptoms can be evoked in the hyperreactive mucous membrane by ordinary exogenous stimuli. [From Mygind (6), with permission.]

of sensory nerves; (4) changed modulation of afferent impulses in the central nervous system; and (5) increased number or sensitivity of receptors on effector cells in blood vessels and glands (6). One example is a nonallergic form of rhinitis that is induced by cold dry air. An elevation in the osmolality of the nasal secretions in these individuals activates the mast cells and releases mediators (8).

Not only do outdoor pollutants affect the upper airway, it has also been demonstrated that pollutants, such as sulfur dioxide, can cause substantial bronchoconstriction in asthmatic subjects. Moreover, in animal experiments, sulfur dioxide has been shown to enhance IgE antibody formation (9). A normally functioning nasal airway may mitigate the impact outdoor pollution exposures have on the health of the entire airway (10).

III. INDOOR AIR POLLUTION

A. Tight Building Syndrome

Studies of time–activity patterns demonstrate that adult residents of more developed countries spend, on average, less than 3% (1/2 hr) of their day outside (11). Even though most children have greater outdoor time, indoor air pollutants are the predominant pollutant exposure. The principal sources of irritant pollution are due to combustion from tobacco smoking, gas cooking, unvented kerosene heaters, and wood-burning stoves. The problem of indoor pollution may be even more serious than in the past because energy-conserving measures in new construction have made structures more resistant to indoor–outdoor air exchange. Mobile homes, prefabricated housing units, and energy-efficient homes are especially prone to these indoor air problems. Whereas the average house has a 100% turnover of indoor air in 1 hr, the newer, "tighter" insulated structures have only a 50% turnover of indoor air in 1 hr. This can result in inadequate and poorly distributed fresh air and the accumulation of outdoor contaminants, bacteria, fungi, and gaseous substances. This may lead to what has been called the "tight or sick building syndrome" in which occupants develop such symptoms as lethargy, headache, nasal blockage, and irritation of mucous membranes.

Outbreaks of illness in public buildings related to some of the foregoing ecological factors have occurred for many years and are classified in Table 3 (12).

Table 3 Classification[a] of the Etiology of Building-Related Illnesses in 356 Health Hazard Evaluations Conducted by the National Institute for Occupational Safety and Health Through December 1985

Etiology	(n)	(%)
Inside contaminants	67	19
Outside contaminants	38	11
Contaminants from building materials	14	4
Biological contaminants	19	5
Inadequate ventilation	179	50
Unknown	39	11

[a] Data provided by Kenneth Wallingford, personal communications.
Source: From Samet et al. (12), with permission.

Various moderate outdoor and indoor environmental pollutants may act together to increase respiratory disease, especially in children with a family history of allergy. Swedish workers have reported that children who live in rural areas have a cumulative prevalence of bronchial hyperreactivity of 9.7% and of allergic asthma of 5.2%. Children who live near an outdoor-polluting paper pulp plant more often had symptoms suggesting bronchial hyperreactivity (13%) and allergic asthma (7.1%). In children living in modern, well-insulated houses with damage caused by dampness, bronchial hyperreactivity was found in 19% and allergic asthma in 8.7% of the children. If, in one of these well-insulated, but damp houses, the parents were tobacco smokers, adding further environmental injury, the prevalence of bronchial hyperreactivity climbed to 23.5% and allergic asthma to 11.6%. This group also had the highest prevalence of allergic rhinitis (13).

B. Tobacco Smoke

Tobacco smoke is the major indoor air pollutant. Although fewer than 30% of American adults smoke, more than 40% of all children are affected by passive smoke (14). Tobacco combustion contributes to concentrations of respirable particles, polycyclic hydrocarbon, carbon monoxide, nicotine, nitrogen dioxides, and acrolein. The level of airborne particles in homes with no smokers is slightly above the level of the surrounding outdoor concentration. One smoker in the house raises the particulate matter level from 20 to 30-$\mu g/m^3$ above the outdoor level. Two or more smokers in the home cause particle concentrations that are in violation of outdoor federal standards. The small particle size of environmental tobacco smoke will follow airstreams, and its distribution will occur rapidly throughout a room. Therefore, the simple separation of smokers from nonsmokers within the same airspace may reduce, but will not eliminate, exposure to environmental tobacco smoke.

Currently, the most sensitive and specific markers for tobacco smoke exposure are nicotine and its metabolite, cotinine. The cotinine levels provide information about more chronic exposure in both active and involuntary smokers. Luck and Nau have shown that the nicotine and cotinine levels measured in infants breast-fed by mothers who smoke reflect both the doses received from the breast milk and from involuntary smoking (15). In another study of infants, the serum cotinine levels increased with the number of cigarettes smoked by the mother (16). In a study of schoolchildren in England, salivary cotinine levels rose with the number of parents who smoke in the home, from a median of 0.20 ng/ml, without household exposure, to greater than ten times the median of 2.70 ng/ml, if both parents smoked (17).

About 75% of the smoke from a cigarette wafts into the air without being inhaled by the smokers. This "side stream" smoke burns hotter and is considerably more toxic than the smoke inhaled by the cigarette user; for example, the concentration of ammonia is 50 times greater, and there are more respirable particles in the smoke. The acute effects of exposure to environmental tobacco smoke are due to its many irritant substances. These cause headache, eye irritation, nasal discomfort, sneezing, sore throat, and cough (18). This exposure experimentally results in pathological changes in mucociliary transport and cellular composition of the respiratory tract.

Chronic tobacco smoke exposure exerts numerous deleterious effects on the airway's defense mechanisms. These include decilitation, ranging from patchy areas to complete loss, especially in the upper airway (19), toxic effects on ciliary function, with decrease in mucociliary clearance of inhaled materials; epithelial changes of squamous metaplasia; basal cell hyperplasia and goblet cell hypertrophy; and depression of macrophage phagocytic and bactericidal activity (19,20).

The loss of effectively beating cilia and goblet cell hyperplasia seen with passive smoking parallel the pathological findings in animals with persistent middle ear effusion and sinusitis (21,22). Appropriate mucociliary clearance in the middle ear and sinuses is vital for the normal resistance to infection and function of these anatomical regions (23). The rheological or viscoelastic properties of mucus are altered by the cell changes caused by a toxin such as tobacco smoke. This abnormal mucus potentiates the likelihood of both acute otitis media and acute sinusitis. The increased levels of carbon monoxide and carbon dioxide in environmental tobacco smoke also affect the cellular differentiation toward a cell population favoring more mucus-producing cells in the respiratory mucosa (24).

It is clear that chronic environmental tobacco smoke exposure has an untoward effect on the upper respiratory passages of children. This can be indirectly shown in the increased rate of nasal complaints, cough, acute otitis media, and persistent middle ear effusions in children exposed to smoke, when compared with a control population (25–27). It has also been indicated as a risk factor for adenotonsillar disorders requiring surgery (28).

The mechanisms that lead to these problems is probably a combination of factors that include the altered mucociliary transport and diminished phagocytic response caused by the smoke exposure, concomitant with upper respiratory tract infections. Tobacco smokers are known to develop more viral infections than nonsmokers. An inflammatory process, such as an allergic reaction or another cause of airway hyperreactivity, would result in further dysfunction (Table 4;29).

Because the human genotype and, hence, the genetically determined predisposition for allergic disease, has not changed, environmental influences must account for the increased prevalence of atopic diseases in industrialized countries. Andrae and co-workers from Sweden have reported a higher prevalence of pollen allergy in children living near an air-polluting paper pulp plant than in children living in a nonindustrialized area about 25 miles away (13). This finding corroborates a growing body of evidence about the role of environmental pollutants in facilitating sensitization to allergens. Tobacco smoke in adults is associated with increased IgE levels and increases the risk of occupational asthma. Exposure to their parents tobacco smoke causes allergic children to become symptomatic earlier and more frequently (30).

C. Nitrogen Dioxide, Carbon Monoxide, Woodsmoke

In about 50% of homes in the United States, natural gas or liquid propane are used for cooking. The combustion of fuels can be a source of CO, CO_2, SO_2, hydrocarbons, and nitrogen oxides. Numerous studies have reported that when these cooking appliances are unvented, elevated indoor levels of CO, CO_2, NO, and NO_2 are found (31). Homes with gas stoves can have NO_2 levels five times higher than the outside air or homes without gas stoves, and levels in the kitchen with unvented gas stoves can reach 100 times the outside air for brief periods.

Elevated concentrations of nitrogen dioxide and carbon monoxide have also been reported in homes and schools with unvented gas or kerosene heaters.

Table 4 Combined Effects for Risk Factors for Persistent Middle Ear Effusion

Factors	PMEE patients (n = 76) (%)	Surgical controls (n = 76) (%)	Relative risk[a,b]	95% confidence interval[c]
None	21.0	40.8	1.0	
One factor	36.8	43.4	1.6	0. 7–3.6
Congestion (>1 day/mo)	18.4	9.2	3.9	1.3–11.3
Smoking (> 0.5 PPD)	17.1	28.9	1.1	0.5–2.9
Atopy (> 1 day/mo)	1.3	5.3	0.5	0.05–4.6
Two factors	25.0	10.5	4.6	1.7–12.5
Smoking + congestion	14.5	6.6	4.3	1.3–13.9
Smoking + atopy	1.3	0.9		
Congestion + atopy	9.2	3.9	4.5	1.1–18.7
Three factors	17.2	5.3	6.3	1.9–21.1

PMEE, persistent middle ear effusion, PPD, packs per day.
[a] Standardized for age and sex by method of Mantel and Haenszel.
[b] Test for linear trend comparing none, one, two and three factors ($p < 0.001$).
[c] Approximate limits, calculated by the method of Miettinen.
Source: From Kraemer et al. (29), cited in Richardson MA. J Allergy Clin Immunol 1988; 81:1032, with permission.

A study of gas stove use in an area of urban poverty in New York, documented that 50% of families used their gas stove as a source of heat (32). Exposures to NO_2 have been associated with bronchoconstriction and increased infection rates (33), although this relationship is not consistent. The effects of the lower levels of carbon monoxide exposure generally encountered in indoor environments are controversial at present.

There has been a national trend away from cleaner space-heating fuels such as gas and electricity and a resurgence of wood- and coal-burning stoves, along with kerosene heaters. The number of wood-burning stoves is in excess of 12 million, and there are over 13 million kerosene heating units in use during the winter months. When they are not cleaned or drafted properly, they emit toxic and carcinogenic particles and gases. Indoor heating with wood-burning stoves has been associated with increased frequency and severity of respiratory irritation, cough, and wheezing, compared with homes heated by other means. In Honicky's study, 84% of children in a wood-burning stove group reported the occurrence of at least one severe symptom, compared with only 3% of the control group (34). Wood stoves may contribute to outdoor air pollution as well. On cold winter mornings, chimney smoke may become trapped around the house by a "radiant inversion." This pocket of toxic gases and particulates may cause exacerbations of airway symptoms in sensitive individuals. Major pollutant emissions of wood combustion from these stores include carbon monoxide, nitrogen dioxide, sulfur dioxide, and respirable particulates.

D. Formaldehyde and Other Volatile Organic Compounds

Formaldehyde exposure has also been viewed as problematic. It is a far more ubiquitous product than might be thought. It is contained in foams and resins used in the manufacture of plastics, plywood, particle board, wrinkle-proof clothing, and insulation. Formalin is used as a tissue preservative, as a disinfectant, and is found in shampoo and in 800 other cosmetics. Outgasing of formaldehyde from these products can occur over a considerable period of years and the levels are directly proportional to the relative humidity.

Exposure from cosmetics or fabrics is usually less than 0.03 parts per million (ppm). However, homes with urea formaldehyde foam insulation frequently have levels of from 0.05 ppm to 2.0 ppm, which can cause headaches, irritability, dermatitis, irritation of the eyes and upper airways and, in some patients, brochospasm (Table 5; 35). The wide range of concentrations at which individual symptoms occur suggests a large variation in individual sensitivity to formaldehyde irritation, but it should be considered in residents of mobile homes, new homes, and homes with potentially strong sources, such as new

Table 5 Acute Human Health Effects of Formaldehyde at Various Concentrations

Reported effects	Formaldehyde concentration (ppm)
None reported	0.0–0.5
Neurophysiological effects[a]	0.05–1.5
Odor threshold	0.05–1.0
Eye irritation[b]	0.01–2.0
Upper airway irritation	0.10–25
Lower airway and pulmonary effects	5–30
Pulmonary edema, inflammation, pneumonia	50–100
Death	> 100

[a] As measured by determination of optical chronaxy, electroencephalography, and sensitivity of dark-adapted eyes to light.
[b] The low concentration (0.01 ppm) was observed in the presence of other pollutants that may have been acting synergistically.
Source: From National Research Council, Committee on Aldehydes (35), cited in Samet et al. (12), with permission.

carpeting. The health effects of chronic formaldehyde exposure still remain inconclusive and, until further studies clarify this issue, limiting exposure would seem prudent.

Hundreds of volatile organic compounds exist in both residences and public buildings with such sources as paints, adhesives, cleansers, cosmetics, furnishings, cigarettes, gasoline, and printed materials. In all exposure assessment studies performed, to date, concentrations of individual compounds have been below the permissible levels established for industrial environments (12). However, concern has been raised about their potential, even at low concentrations, to cause both acute and chronic effects. Some of the most commonly measured volatile organic compounds are established or suspected mutagens, and many are mucous membrane irritants. Additionally, some have been implicated as a cause of building-related illness. Furthermore, synergistic interactions among compounds may result in greater health impact than would be anticipated from simple additivity of effects. Future studies are needed to more fully describe sources, concentrations, and distributions of these chemicals to provide estimates of risk and the formulation of environmental policies.

IV. CONTROL OF AIR POLLUTION

Children are regularly exposed to environmental irritants and multiple exposures can cause both acute and long-term health effects. The presence of official standards of "acceptable" levels does not guarantee safety. It is important for health professionals to participate in developing local and national environmental policies.

A. Resource Agencies and Organizations

1. Federal Agencies

Many of these agencies have regional and local offices.

Environmental Protection Agency (EPA)
Public Information Center, PM211B
401 M St., S. W.
Washington, DC 20460
(202) 382-2090
Sponsors research, sets standards, enforces regulations and monitors compliance with respect to pesticides, toxic wastes, commercial chemicals, air water pollution and noise

Food and Drug Administration (FDA)
5600 Fishers Lane
Rockville, MD 20857
(301) 443-2410
Regulates drugs, foods and pesticide residues on food, cosmetics, and personal hygiene products

Consumer Product Safety Commission (CPSC)
Office of Information
5401 Westbard Ave.
Bethesda, MD 20207
(800) 638-CPCS
Regulates some consumer products that are not covered by the FDA or the EPA, including heating and cooking devices that may produce indoor air pollution

Center for Disease Control (CDC)
Atlanta, GA 30333
(404) 639-3311
Develops programs dealing with environmental health problems, including measures for responding to environmental, chemical, and radiation emergencies

Agency for Toxic Substances and Disease Registry (ATSDR)
Atlanta, GA
(404) 454-4590
Collects information on toxic hazards, consults with health care providers caring for exposed individuals, helps identify hazardous substances for regulation by the EPA; 24-hr emergency number: (404) 329-2888

National Health Information Clearinghouse (NHIC)
P.O. Box 1133, ODPHP
Washington, DC 20013-1133
(800) 336-4797
Helps the general public and health professionals locate health information resources; does not provide medical advice, diagnosis, or physician referral

2. *Citizen Activist Organizations*

Golden Empire Health Planning Center
2100 21st Street
Sacramento, CA 95818
Works to prevent public exposure to toxic materials, expand community input in making decisions on hazardous material handling, and educate school children on environmental issues

Sierra Club
730 Polk St.
San Francisco, CA 94109
Promotes the preservation of natural resources, including clean air and water

US Public Interest Research Group
215 Pennsylvania Ave., S. E.
Washington, DC 20003
Conducts research, issues reports, drafts legislation, and lobbies for environmental regulation; assists and coordinates efforts of state-level public interest research groups

B. Recommendations to Decrease Exposure

Sources of pollution may be removed, relocated or mitigated (see Table 6; 12). Ventilation may be increased to reduce pollutant concentrations throughout a structure or in specific areas. Pollutant concentration may also be reduced by air-cleaning devices, which operate by filtration, adsorption, absorption, or

Table 6 Control Measures for Pollutants

Pollutant	Control measures	
	Equipment and Materials	Ventilation and design
Respirable particles	High-efficiency filters Tight-sealing doors and grates Properly drafting chimney Electrostatic precipitators	Zone and ventilate for smoking Supply outside combustion air to heater and fireplace Relocate air intakes Maintain filter system
NO_1,NO_2	Remove gasoline engine Pilotless ignition	Effective hood vent over source Isolate garage from indoor space
CO	Pilotless ignition Restrict heater use to uninhabited space Use catalytic converter Replace indoor gasoline engines with electric	Supply outside combustion air Vent emission outside Kitchen/hood vent Relocate vents Provide smoking zones Isolate garage from indoor space
CO_2	Check static pressure in return air ducts to make sure return is not overriding fresh air intake	Isolate garage from indoor space

Formaldehyde	Substitute products such as phenolic resin plywood Seal sources Removal of materials	Increase air exchange to house or office
Radon and radon daughters	Vapor barrier around foundation Damp-proof basement and crawl space Seal cracks and holes in floor traps and drains Install charcoal water-scrubber for well water Completely seal foundation	Vent crawl space Vent sumphole to exterior Subslab depressurization Vent bathroom and laundry to exterior
Volatile organic compounds	Substitute products Isolate storage area Apply only according to specifications Do not locate transformers indoors	Use only with adequate ventilation Ventilate laundry, shop Provide separate ventilation to storage area
Asbestos	Removal Injection sealant Wrap pipes with plastic and duct tape	Ventilation does not provide adequate protection

Source: From Samet et al. (12), with permission.

electrostatic precipitation. Specific recommendations to decrease exposure to tobacco smoke, nitrogen dioxide, carbon monoxide, woodsmoke, formaldehyde, and other volatile organic compounds follow.

1. Environmental Tobacco Smoke

A. Gather data
   1. Include all sources: parents, baby sitters, day-care workers.

B. Educate
   1. Encourage parents to stop smoking, inform parents about local smoke cessation programs. Physicians have the potential to reach a large segment of the United States population, since it is estimated that about 70% of residents in this country see a physician yearly (36). The public health impact of reducing smoking among the 38 millions adults in the United States who smoke and see a physician yearly would be enormous, even if only 5–10% of these persons quit on a long-term basis because of physician intervention. There are techniques that any physician can use during a busy work day to help patients and parents quit smoking (37).
   2. Identify the smoking habit
      a. Ask about the duration of smoking, the amount smoked and the brand smoked.
      b. Make the diagnosis of tobacco dependence.
   3. Give cessation advice
      a. Inform the smoker that smoking is harmful to their health and their child's health and that they should quit now. This counseling, together with at least a 6-month follow-up has resulted in quit rates between 3 and 20%.
      b. Describe the main risks of smoking, use of the child's clinical condition will increase the effectiveness of the message.
      c. Suggest undesirable social aspects and remind parent of being a role-model.
      d. Talk about the cost. Smoking one pack a day costs about 500.00 dollars a year.
      e. Set a goal
   4. Suggest a self-help program
      a. "Freedom from Smoking in 20 Days" and "A Lifetime of Freedom from Smoking," American Lung Association, 1740 Broadway, New York, NY 10019
      b. "I Quit Kit," American Cancer Society, 4 West 35th St, New York, NY 10001

5. Prevent relapse
   a. Enlist family support.
   b. Counsel to identify and avoid situations that are relapse scenarios, for example, with a social drink, with relaxation after a meal, during anxiety-provoking situations, with depression and loneliness.
   c. Boost patient confidence in the ability to quit.
   d. Review the three most common obstacles to quitting: nicotine addiction (nervousness is a sign, explain that the symptom will abate over time), weight gain (only one-third of those who gain weight keep that weight longer than a year), failure in prior attempts to quit (the odds of success increase with each attempt).
   e. Actively follow.
   f. Consider specialized smoking cessation program (with or without nicotine gum).

C. Limit exposure
1. In car, in rooms in which child spends appreciable amounts of time.
2. Improve local ventilation, increase air-exchange rates.
3. Use purifiers or filters.
4. Reduce public use.
5. Increase excise tax: The state of California passed The Tobacco Tax Initiative in November 1988. This initiative can possibly raise 650 million dollars per year by adding a tax of 25 cents to every package of cigarettes sold. The money will be distributed as follows: 45% for health services, 20% for health education in the schools (90% of all individuals start smoking by the age of 19), 5% to an environmental account to help replace areas damaged by cigarette-caused fires, and 25% into a nonallocated account for use when needed.

2. *Nitrogen Dioxide, Carbon Monoxide, Woodsmoke*

A. Gather data
1. Include all sources: family home, day care, and school buildings.
2. Determine whether stove is used for cooking only or also for heating.
3. Determine number of hours of use.

B. Educate
1. Discourage family for using gas or wood-burning stove as source of heat.

C. Limit exposure: In November 1988, the United States joined with 24 other industrialized nations in signing an international protocol to freeze emissions of nitrogen oxides. Under the agreement signed in Bulgaria, participating nations will limit nitrogen oxide to levels no higher than those prevailing in 1987. This signing marked the first time the United States had entered into a binding international agreement to limit nitrogen oxide pollution.
   1. If the family can afford it, advise replacement of gas or wood-burning stove with an electric one.
   2. If family cannot replace, advise parents to increase air-exchange rates by using a venting hood, fans, and opening windows.
   3. Stoves should be properly installed and preferably equipped with a catalytic converter that reduces emissions. Chimneys should be regularly cleaned.
   4. Children should be kept out of the area when the gas or wood-burning stove is in use.
   5. If a child has respiratory symptoms that may be caused by wood smoke and the family has an alternative way of heating the house, a "wood elimination trial" is indicated.

3. *Formaldehyde and Other Volatile Organic Compounds*

A. Gather data
   1. Determine whether the family lives in a mobile home, whether urea formaldehyde foam was used for insulation, whether cabinet work is made of particle board, whether carpeting was recently installed, how often the child is exposed to cleaners, polishes, air freshners, and mothballs.
   2. If symptoms of irritation exist and a source of formaldehyde is present, obtain formaldehyde levels from the local health department or a private laboratory that the department recommends.

B. Limit exposure
   1. Discourage excessive use of aforementioned products.
   2. If formaldehyde levels are higher than 0.05 ppm, suggest removal of the source from the household.
   3. If removal is not possible, suggest reducing exposure by improving ventilation or painting with vapor-barrier paint, or both.

REFERENCES

1. Yocom JE. J Air Pollut Control Assoc 1982; 32:500.
2. Environmental Health Newsletter, July 1, 1987.
3. Marwick C. As nation's long, hot summer drags on, so does war against forms of air pollution. JAMA 1988; 260:603.
4. Weiss ST. Indoor and outdoor air pollution and airway disease. Mediguide Pulmonary Med 1986; 3:1.
5. Tos M. Mucous elements in the nose. Rhinology 1976; 14:155.
6. Mygind N. Mediators of nasal allergy. J. Allergy Clin Immunol 1982; 70:149.
7. Koenig JQ, Pierson WE. Nasal responses to air pollutants. Clin Rev. Allergy 1984; 2:255.
8. Togias A, Naclerio RM, Proud D, Pipkorn U, Bascom R, Illiopoulos O, Kagey-Sobotka A, Norman PS, Lichtenstein LM. Studies on the allergic and nonallergic nasal inflammations. J Allergy Clin Immunol 1988; 81:782.
9. Osebold JW, Gerschwin LJ, Zee YC. Studies on the enhancement of allergic lung sensitization by inhalation of ozone and sulfuric acid aerosol. J Environ Pathol Toxicol 1980; 3:221.
10. Koenig JQ, Morgan JS, Horike M, Pierson WE. The effects of sulfur dioxides on nasal and lung function in adolescents with extrinsic asthma. J Allergy Clin Immunol 1985; 76:813.
11. Szalai A, ed. The use of time: daily activities of urban and suburban populations in twelve countries. The Hague; Mouton, 1972.
12. Samet JM, Marbury MC, Spengler JD. Health effects and sources of indoor air pollution. Part II. Am Rev Respir Dis 1988; 137:221.
13. Andrae S, Axelson O, Bjorksten B, Fredriksson M, Kjellman N-IM. Symptoms of bronchial hyperreactivity and asthma in relation to environment factors. Arch Dis Child 1988; 63:473.
14. Office on Smoking and Health. The health consequences of involuntary smoking: a report of the Surgeon General. Rockville, MD; US Public Health Service, 1986.
15. Luck, W, Nau H. Nicotine and cotinine concentrations in serum and urine of infants exposed via passive smoking or milk from smoking mothers. J Pediatr 1985; 107:816.
16. Pattishall EN, Strope, GL, Etzel RA, Helms, RW, Haley, NJ, Denny FW. Serum cotinine as a measure of tobacco smoke exposure in children. Am J Dis Child 1985; 139:1011.
17. Jarvis MJ, Russell MA, Feyerbend C, et al. Passive exposure to tabacco smoke: saliva cotinine concentrations in a representative population sample on non-smoking school children. Br Med J 1985; 291:927.
18. US Department of Health, Education and Welfare. Smoking and health, a report of the Surgeon General. Publ, (PHS) 79-50066, 1979.
19. Coggins CRE, Fouillet XLM, Lam R, Morgan KT. Cigarette smoke induced pathology of the rat respiratory tract: a comparison of the effects of the particulates

and vapour phases. Toxicology 1980; 16:83.
20. Park SS, Kikkawa Y, Goldring IP, et al. An animal model of cigarette smoking in beagle dogs: correlative evaluation of effects on pulmonary function, defence, and morphology. Am Rev Respir Dis 1977; 115:971.
21. Sade J. Inflammatory and non-inflammatory factors related to secretory otitis media. Int J Pediatr Otolaryngol 1979; 1:41.
22. Reimer A, Von Mecklenburg C, Toremalm NG. The mucociliary activity of the upper respiratory tract. III. A functional and morphological study on human and animal material with special reference to maxillary sinus disease. Acta Otolaryngol Supp. 1978; 355:1.
23. Sade J. Cilary activity and middle ear clearance. Arch Otolaryngol 1967; 86:128.
24. Stecenko A, McNicol K, Sauder R. Effect of passive smoking on the lung of young lambs. Pediatr Res 1986; 20:853.
25. Weiss ST, Tager IB, Schenker M, Speizer FE. The health effects of involuntary smoking. Am Rev Respir Dis 1983; 128:933.
26. Pukander J, Luotonen J, Timonen M, Karmer P. Risk factors affecting the occurrence of acute otitis media among 2–3 year old urban children. Acta Otolaryngol 1985; 100:260.
27. Teele DW, Rosner BA, Klein JO. Epidemiology of otitis media in children. Ann Otorhinolaryngol 1980; 89(suppl 68):5.
28. Said G, Zalokar J, Lellouch J, Patois E. Parental smoking related to adenoidectomy and tonsillectomy in children. J Epidemiol Commun Health 1978; 32:97.
29. Kraemer MJ, Richardson MA, Weiss NS, et al. Risk factors for persistent middle-ear effusions: otitis media, catarrh, cigarette smoke exposure, and atopy. JAMA 1983; 249:1022.
30. Bjorksten B, Kjellman N-IM. Perinatal fators influencing the development of allergy. Clin Rev Allergy 1987; 5:339.
31. Committee on Indoor Pollutants, National Research Council. Indoor pollutants. Washington, DC: National Academy Press, 1981.
32. Sterling TD, Kobayashi D. Use of gas ranges for cooking and heating in urban dwellings. J Air Pollut Control Assoc 1981; 31:162.
33. Jakab GJ. Nitrogen dioxide-induced susceptibility to acute respiratory illness: a perspective. Bull NY Acad Med 1980; 56:847.
34. Honicky RE, Osborne JS III, Akpom CA. Symptoms of respiratory illness in young children and the use of wood burning stoves for indoor heating. Pediatrics 1985; 75:587.
35. National Research Council, Committee on Aldehydes. Formaldehyde and other aldehydes. Washington, DC: National Academy Press, 1981.
36. The health consequences of smoking: chronic obstructive lung disease - a report of the Surgeon General. DHHS publication No (PHS) 84-50205. Office on Smoking and Health, 1984:455.
37. Prochazka AV, Boyko EJ. How physicians can help their patients quit smoking: a practical guide. West J Med 1988; 149:188.

4

Basic Principles of Therapeutics: Allergic Rhinitis and Sinusitis

Charles K. Naspitz
Escola Paulista de Medicina, São Paulo, Brazil

David G. Tinkelman
Medical College of Georgia, Augusta, Georgia, and Atlanta Allergy Clinic, Atlanta, Georgia

I. INTRANASAL MEDICATIONS

A. Physiological Saline

The application of a physiological saline solution (sodium chloride diluted in water, 9%) to the inflamed nasal mucosa can debride tenacious mucus, soothe irritated tissue, moisturize dry membranes and, thereby, reduce nose bleeding, improve mucociliary flow, and aid olfaction. The regular use of intranasal saline is of benefit to patients with chronic rhinitis and sinusitis. Saline solution can be prepared at home by adding 1 tsp of salt to 1 L of warm water. There are also commercial buffered saline preparations, and one of the most effective ways of delivering saline to the nose is through an adaptor to a Water Pik (1,2).

The correct administration of intranasal medication is very important, and the patients should be properly instructed (3).

B. Vasoconstrictor Sympathomimetics

Topical administration of vasoconstrictor sympathomimetic agents has the advantage of a more rapid onset of action. They can be divided in catecolamines (epinephrine, phenylephrine), which act preferentially on α_1-adrenoceptors, and imidazole derivatives (naphazoline, oxymetazoline, xylometazoline, tetrahydrozoline), which act more selectively on α_2-adrenoceptors (Table 1).

It is probable that both α_1- and α_2-adrenoceptors exist on the nasal vessels responsible for mucosal swelling, because clinical trials have confirmed that both types of drugs are very effective as nasal decongestants (4). Nasal aeration and ventilation are improved temporarily after intranasal application of these drugs, and local vasoconstriction occurs within 2–5 min. This action on the vessels induces a reduction in blood flow and edema of the nasal mucosa. The

Table 1 Nasal Decongestants That May Be Applied Topically or Used Orally

Drug	Oral	Topical
Epinephrine hydrochloride		X
Naphazoline hydrochloride		X
Oxymetazoline hydrochloride		X
Phenylephrine hydrochloride	X	X
Propylhexedrine hydrochloride		X
Tetrahydrozoline hydrochloride		X
Xylometazoline hydrochloride		X
Phenylpropanolamine hydrochloride	X	
Propadrine hydrochloride	X	
Pseudoephedrine hydrochloride	X	
Pseudoephedrine sulfate	X	X
Ephedrine sulfate	X	

topical decongestants can be short-acting, 1–2 hr (phenylephrine, naphazoline), or long-acting, 6–8 hr (oxymetazoline, xylometazoline) (1).

Topical therapy avoids undesired systemic effects elsewhere in the body, but should not be used for more than 3–5 days; prolonged therapy will result in more severe nasal obstruction owing to a rebound phenomenon in which nasal vascular congestion not only recurs but increases in severity as the effect of each application wears off, thereby inducing repeated usage at shorter intervals. This rhinitis medicamentosa is characterized by chronic swelling of the nasal mucosa, being additive to the swelling of the allergic rhinitis (5). Therefore, these vasoconstrictor topical medications are contraindicated for the long-term treatment of allergic rhinitis. Furthermore, rebound congestion is particularly hazardous and may produce obstructive apnea in infants, who are obligate nasal breathers. Fortunately, the iatrogenic rhinitis medicamentosa is usually reversible after the medication has been withdrawn for a few days.

The topical application of nasal decongestants may cause sneezing and nasal stinging, burning, and mucosal dryness or ulceration, interfering with ciliary action. These adverse effects can be attributed to the pH of the substance or to the presence of an antioxidant or preservative.

In infants and children, particularly, topical decongestants may produce systemic reactions. The topical forms include drops and sprays. Proper use of nasal sprays may be the best way to avoid systemic absorption, which may be significant and occurs at the nasal mucosa or in the gastrointestinal tract. The systemic effects include transient hypertension, nausea, dizziness, nervousness, and palpitations. Severe reactions have been described in children following systemic absorption after overdosage of naphazoline: sweating, drowsiness, deep sleep, and coma (6).

Solutions of topical nasal decongestants quickly become contaminated after use. To minimize the risk of spreading infections, the dropper or spray tip should be rinsed with hot water after use. More than one person should not use the same dropper or spray dispenser.

C. Cromolyn Sodium

Cromolyn was initially synthesized in 1965 from khellin, a naturally occurring plant hormone. It is a *bis*-chromone, the disodium salt of 1,3-*bis*-(2,carboxychromon-5-yloxy)-2-hydroxypropane.

Cromolyn sodium (CS) is a potent and effective inhibitor of mast cell degranulation in the rat. In human mast cells—passively sensitized human lung fragments challenged with antigen—the inhibitory activity of CS is partial and variable. A possible mechanism of action by which CS may regulate the release of mediators stored in mast cell granules is the inhibition of cyclic AMP phosphodiesterase. Compound 48/80, ionophore A23817, and antirat IgE can induce a similar pattern of protein phosphorylation of rat peritoneal mast cells. The phosphorylation of three initial proteins is followed by phosphorylation of a fourth protein, with a molecular mass of 78,000, which might be associated with the termination of secretion and restabilization of the cell. Phosphorylation of this 78,000 Da protein is induced by CS, which inhibits histamine release. Thus, CS appears to activate an endogenous control mechanism for switching off mediator release, by a mechanism mediated by cyclic GMP, probably by a stimulation of guanylate cyclase. A CS-binding protein was isolated from rat basophils, and the findings, thus far, suggests that this protein may be either part of, or closely related to, the calcium gate and has a role in the transmembrane calcium influx that induces degranulation (7). There is still controversy, however, on whether or not the effects of CS are due to its inhibition of mast cell mediator release. Although CS could stabilize mast cells, there are many basophils (more than one type) in the nasal mucosa, and CS is less effective at preventing basophil degranulation.

Topical CS is of clinical benefit in the treatment of allergic rhinitis and is effective for prevention of the immediate and late nasal responses associated with allergen challenge in patients with allergic rhinitis. The drug is most effective when used before the onset of symptoms; its effects are of short duration; therefore, it must be administered frequently, throughout the period of allergen exposure in the treatment of seasonal rhinitis and continuously in perennial allergic rhinitis.

Cromolyn is effective only for prophylactic treatment, and its efficacy is greatest in those patients with positive skin tests to allergens, high titers of specific IgE, and eosinophils in nasal secretions. Clinical data showed that CS is more helpful for nasal itching, sneezing, and rhinorrhea than for nasal obstruction (2). When the nasal passages are very blocked, the prior use of a decongestant for a short period may be needed until a reasonable clinical response is achieved (8). The combination of 2% cromolyn and a low concentration (0.025%) of xylometazoline used as a starter treatment for 1 or 2 weeks before the use of CS alone, appears to provide a practical answer (9).

In general, intranasal CS has been remarkably free of side effects, and it is well tolerated by virtually all patients (10). Side effects occur in fewer than 10% of patients, are generally quite transient, and are limited to mild nasal irritation, sore throat, headache, and an unpleasant taste. Tachyphylaxis to the effects of intranasal CS has not been reported.

The recommended dose of the 4% solution is one spray in each nostril four times a day. Each spray of the metered–dose device will deliver a 5.2-mg dose of CS. Approximately 7% of the intranasally dose is absorbed; this is excreted in bile and urine, with the remainder either swallowed or exhaled (8). The dosage of intranasal CS can be reduced to two or three times daily when symptomatic relief becomes apparent.

D. Nedocromil Sodium

Nedocromil sodium (NS) is the disodium salt of pyranoquinoline dicarboyxlic acid. It acts like CS, and studies on release inhibition of chemical mediators from respiratory cells after stimulation with antigen, showed that CS has less than 0.02 the potency of NS (2). The efficacy of NS for the treatment of asthma has been confirmed (early and late responses), and the metered-dose inhalation for asthma treatment is 4.0 mg, given two or four times daily.

There are few studies in allergic rhinitis. In human studies a 1 or 2% solution of the drug has been used, delivering 0.13 ml/nostril. In the treatment of ragweed seasonal allergic rhinitis, a 1% nasal solution of NS, administered qid for an 8-week period, was clearly effective in reducing major symptoms during peak pollen exposure (11).

The role of NS in the topical treatment of allergic rhinitis remains to be established.

E. Azatadine

Azatadine is a tricyclic antihistamine of the piperidine class. The effect of topical administration of azatadine (0.125 ml of a 0.4% solution administered to each nostril) was tested on the experimental nasal response to nasal provocation with antigen, with histamine, and with cold dry air, in patients with allergic rhinitis. Azatadine inhibited the release of chemical mediators and effectively reduced symptoms and increased vascular permeability after histamine and antigen challenges. Although all the symptoms were reduced, the reduction in nasal congestion was less. Topical azatadine did not inhibit the release of mediators after cold dry air stimulus suggesting that mediators other than histamine play a role in this form of rhinitis (12). This preparation of the drug is still experimental.

F. Levocabastine

Levocabastine is a new specific H_1-receptor antagonist, without anticholinergic or antiserotonin effects. The effect of the drug administered locally in the nose was compared with placebo in a quantified nasal provocation test with allergens in rhinitis patients allergic to grass pollen. Two puffs of levocabastine (100 μl/puff) were administered in each nostril by means of a metered spray. In the nasal provocation test, levocabastine was able to increase the "reaction threshold" (dose of allergen necessary to trigger allergic symptoms) in 9 of 12 patients; the drug inhibited rhinorrhea and sneezing, but not nasal obstruction (13). Recently, levocabastine was used as a nasal spray in nasal provocation tests with allergens in 44 patients. One single topical administration of levocabastine (0.5 mg/ml) significantly inhibited the nasal reaction to allergen challenges and seems to have a long-lasting topical effect in allergic patients. The local administration of levocabastine might be useful in allergic rhinitis, but further clinical studies should be performed.

G. Inhaled Corticosteroids

The treatment of allergic and nonallergic rhinitis had a dramatic change with the introduction of topical corticosteroids. It has long been recognized that systemic steroids were efficacious in the treatment of rhinitis. However, their potential for significant side effects prevented their widespread use for this problem. Topical administration, with limited absorption and side effect potential, reduced this risk. Numerous studies have been performed documenting the safety and efficacy of a variety of these preparations in allergic rhinitis (14,15).

The first topical preparation introduced onto the market was dexamethasone. Although effective as a site-specific agent, systemic absorption of sufficient quantity to demonstrate suppression of the hypothalamus–pituitary–adrenal axis prevented its widespread use (16). Further development of these agents has led to the introduction of several other topically active site-specific steroid preparations. These include presently available beclomethasone and flunisolone. Others are currently being tested in both the United States and Europe and should be available for use in the near future.

Beclomethasone has been studied and found to be effective in children 5 years of age and older (17). The recommended starting dose for beclomethasone is one spray in each nostril three times a day (18). It needs to be recognized that nasal steroids do not produce any immediate relief of symptoms, as do topical vasoconstrictor agents. Thus, the spray needs to be administered for several days to 2 weeks before deciding whether or not the preparation has given significant relief of symptoms. Beclomethasone is available in two different formulations: the pressurized aerosol and an aqueous nasal spray. Studies in children have demonstrated no difference in efficacy between the preparations. Complaints of local adverse experience were more frequently seen with the aerosol. These were felt to be due to the force of the aerosol, rather than the active medication. There was a preference for the aqueous spray (17,19). To avoid the local irritation and drying effect of freon-propelled aerosols, a solution of flunisolide was developed. This newer type of topical corticosteroid has also been effective in the treatment of allergic rhinitis (20). One common complaint with the flunisolide preparation is stinging, of short duration, immediately upon use. This is due to the dissolving agent, polyethylene glycol (21). A newer preparation without this stinging property is currently being studied.

Another topical corticosteroid preparation available in Europe and South America is budesonide. Although studies with this agent in children are lacking, there is good evidence in adult populations to suggest that it is equivalent in efficacy to beclomethasone and flunisolide (22–24). Budesonide is applied in a freon-propelled inhaler and, thus, has the irritating effect of a high-speed spray delivery system.

With newer and more topically effective agents becoming available, this form of therapy will probably become first-line therapy in most children with chronic allergic and nonallergic rhinitis who require long-term daily medication.

H. Anticholinergic Agents

Anticholinergic agents have been demonstrated to have some effect on serous and seromucous secretions. This has not been associated with a similar reduction in the typical histamine release symptoms of sneezing and nasal congestion. The lining of the nasal mucosa has significant parasympathetic innervation, and this has been proposed as a mechanism for the rhinorrhea associated with allergic rhinitis (25). Several studies in adults have demonstrated effectiveness of an inhaled anticholinergic agent, ipratropium bromide, in reducing this rhinorrhea (26–28). There have been the expected anticholinergic side effects, such as drying of the nasal mucosa, crusting in the nose, and epistaxis. These studies have been performed in adults, and few data are available for children. This product is currently available in a metered-dose inhaler for use in the lung, but as yet, it has not been approved for the indication of treating rhinitis.

II. ORAL MEDICATION

A. Sympathomimetics (Decongestants)

Oral sympathomimetic amines (phenylephrine, phenylpropanolamine, pseudoephedrine, and ephedrine) have been shown to reduce nasal congestion effectively, causing vasoconstriction by a direct effect on α-adrenergic receptors. The constriction of arterioles within the nasal mucosa reduces blood flow in the engorged, edematous tissues, reducing edema and nasal congestion, thereby opening the obstructed nasal passages.

Pseudoephedrine and phenylpropanolamine are the two α-adrenergic agents most frequently employed (4). These drugs are used to relieve nasal congestion associated with acute or chronic rhinitis, including allergic rhinitis. The nasal decongestion after oral administration of the α-adrenergic agonists occurs within 30 min and persists up to 6 hr (2). These oral medications produce little if any rebound congestion.

Phenylpropanolamine has pharmacologic properties analagous to those of ephedrine, being equal in potency, but causing less central nervous system stimulation. The oral dosage for children 8–12 years is 20–25 mg three times daily.

Pseudoephedrine is a physiologically active stereoisomer of ephedrine, with similar properties and use. The oral dosage for children is 4 mg/kg daily, in four divided doses.

Systemic effects, such as restlessness, insomnia, tremor, tachycardia, palpitations, and increase in blood pressure, may occur and be troublesome.

B. Oral Antihistamines

Antihistamines are chemical agents that exert their effect primarily by preventing or blocking the action of histamine at receptor sites (29). Antihistamines, primarily the H_1-antagonist type are beneficial in the management of seasonal and perennial allergic rhinitis, relieving the rhinorrhea, sneezing, and itching, but nasal congestion is often unchanged (30). Symptomatic relief experienced by patients with allergic rhinitis sometimes can be attributed to the drying effect on nasal mucosa caused by the anticholinergic action of some antihistamines. There is no evidence that combinations containing two or more antihistamines (in therapeutic or subtherapeutic doses) are more effective than therapeutic doses of one antihistamine (2).

For unknown reasons, some patients get best results with one type of antihistamine, and other, similar patients prefer another kind. Unsatisfactory results with one type of antihistamine justify trying an antihistamine of a different chemical group (31).

Prolonged antihistamine use may lead to decreased response to that drug, but a substantial degree of tolerance to the antihistaminic effects does not generally occur. Switching to another type of antihistamine may be useful in patients who appear to develop refractoriness to an initially effective drug. However, there are data showing that the development of tolerance to hydroxizine was also associated with the development of cross-tolerance to the effects of five chemically unrelated antihistamines (1).

Therapeutic doses of all H_1-antagonists (Table 2) can cause side effects that are rarely serious, and most mild reactions may be relieved by a reduction in dosage or change to a different class, or they often disappear after a few days of continued use. However, there is marked variation in frequency and severity of side effects among individuals.

The most common side effect is sedation, which may interfere with activities requiring alertness and motor coordination. The new nonsedating antihistamines can avoid the sedation, which can range from mild drowsiness to deep sleep; these drugs are also devoid of anticholinergic effects, and their adverse effects can be avoided: dryness of the mouth and throat, blurred vision, palpitations, urinary retention or dysuria. Paradoxical central nervous system excitement (euphoria, nervousness, irritability, and insomnia) are sometimes observed, especially in children. Gastrointestinal disturbances (anorexia, nausea, diarrhea, or constipation) caused by antihistamines may be observed. However, increased appetite and weight gain have been noted in some children receiving anti-H_1-blockers (32).

Two nonsedating antihistamines have recently reached the market in the United States (terfenadine and astemizole), with others being developed for potential release in the near future (loratadine, cetirizine, azelastine, and mequitazine). The chemical structure for these agents are different from the classic H_1-blockers, which may account for their different side effect profile.

Table 2 Classification of Representative Classic Antihistamines (H_1-Blockers) Used in Children

Chemical Class	Usual Dosage
Alkylamines	
Brompheniramine	Oral: children 6–12 yr, 2 mg 4–6 hr (maximum, 12 mg daily); 2–6 yr, 1 mg 4–6 hr (maximum, 6 mg daily)
	Intramuscular, intravenous: children under 12 yr, 0.5 mg/kg daily divided into 3 or 4 doses
Chlorpheniramine	Oral: children under 12 yr, 0.35 mg/kg daily divided into 4 doses
Dexchlorpheniramine	Oral: children under 12 yr, 0.15 mg/kg daily divided into 4 doses
Triprolidine	Oral: children under 6 yr, 1.25 mg, tid or qid; under 6 yr, 0.3–0.6, mg tid or qid, depending on age
Ethanolamines	
Carbinoxamine	Oral: 0.2 mg/kg, tid or qid
Clemastine	Oral: children up to 1 yr 0.125 mg bid; 1–3 yr: 0.125–0.150 mg, bid; 3–6 yr, 0.250 mg, bid; 6–12 yr: 0.375 mg bid; over 12 yr, 0.750 mg, bid
Diphenhydramine	Oral: children under 12 yr, 5 mg/kg daily, in 4 divided doses
	Intramuscular, intravenous: 5 mg/kg daily in 4 divided doses (maximum 300 mg daily)
Doxylamine	Oral: 2 mg/kg daily divided in 4 doses
Ethylenediamines	
Tripelennamine	Oral: 5 mg/kg every 24 hr, in 4–6 divided doses
Phenothiazines	
Methdilazine	Oral: children over 3 yr, 4 mg, bid, tid, or qid
Promethazine	Oral: 25 mg at bedtime or 6.25–12.5 mg, tid
	Intramuscular: no more than 12.5 mg repeated in 2 hr if necessary
Trimeprazine	Oral: children 6 mo–3 yr, 3.75 mg daily divided into 3 doses; 3–12 yr, 7.5 mg daily divided into 3 doses
Piperazines	
Hydroxyzine	Oral: children under 6 yr, 50 mg daily divided into 3–4 doses; over 6 yr, 50–100 mg daily divided into 3–4 doses.

continued

Table 2 *Continued*

Chemical Class	Usual Dosage
Piperidines	
Azatadine	Oral: children 6–12 yr, 0.5 mg, bid
Cyproheptadine	Oral: children 2–6 yr, 2 mg, bid or tid (maximum 12 mg daily); 7–14 yr, 4 mg bid or tid daily (maximum 16 mg daily)
Diphenylpyraline	Children over 6 yr, 2 mg q 8 hr (maximum 6 mg daily); 2–6 yr, 1–2 mg q 8 hr (maximum 4 mg daily)
Miscellaneous nonsedating class	
Terfenadine	Oral: 4 mg/kg q 24 hr, in 2 divided doses
Astemizole	Oral: children 2–6 yr, 2 mg/10 kg once a day; children 6–12 yr, 5 mg once a day
Loratadine	Doses not established in children
Temelastine	Doses not established in children
Mequitazine	Oral: 0.25 mg/kg q 24 hr, in 2 divided doses
Cetirizine	
Mast Cell-Stabilizing Effect	
Ketotifen	Oral: 1 mg, bid
Azelastine	Oral: 2 mg, bid
Azatadine	Oral: children 6–12 yr, 0.5 mg, bid
Mequitazine	Oral: 0.25 mg/kg 8 24 hr, in 2 divided doses
Antihistamines (H_2-Blockers)	
Cimetidine	Oral or intravenous: 20–40 mg/kg q 24 hr, divided into 2–4 doses
Ranitidine	Doses not established in children

Terfenadine is rapidly absorbed from the gastrointestinal tract and produces peak plasma concentrations usually between 1 and 2 hr after drug administration. Its plasma half-life is 4.5 hr, and its elimination half-life is between 16 and 22 hr, making it ideal for administration every 12 hr. Astemizole is also readily and completely absorbed from the gastrointestinal tract. However, its excretion is very slow and its half-life is 11 days. Because of the rather long half-life, the recommended schedule for administration is once daily. This slow onset of action precludes the use of astemizole for acute situations, whereas it is best suited for chronic daily use. It has been suggested that terfenadine is similar in onset of action to the classic antihistamines and can be used in a similar fashion. Astemizole is recommended for prohylactic use given a few days before an exposure begins, or in high initial doses for symptom relief until adequate blood levels are established.

Both of the currently available nonsedating antihistamines are clinically as effective as the older more-established agents. Their major advantage is their lack of sedating potential, which may be a major factor in children who might otherwise have difficulties concentrating in school. The chief problem with them is the increase in cost over other antihistamines. Because of this significant difference, physicians need to consider all of the factors, such as efficacy, side effects, and cost, before prescribing a particular antihistamine.

Loratadine has been evaluated in both adults and children with allergic rhinitis. Although it is not currently on the market in the United States, numerous studies have been performed and it will soon be released. Like the other two antihistamines discussed above, loratadine has neither sedating nor anticholinergic side effects seen with the older antihistamine preparations. It has been successfully studied in both perennial and seasonal allergic rhinitis in adults and children. It will probably be released for once-a-day use in a dose of 5 or 10 mg for children. It has been demonstrated to have similar antihistaminic properties as chlortrimeton.

Another relatively nonsedating antihistamine that will probably soon be ready for approval is cetirizine. This medication has not be as extensively studied in children as yet. It has been shown in adult studies to have good antihistamine effects and nonsedating properties. Higher doses in some studies have shown some sedation. More work needs to be performed in children in the future.

III. DRUGS WITH MAST CELL-STABILIZING EFFECT

Cromolyn sodium, nedocromil, and azatadine were discussed in Section I.

A. Ketotifen

Ketotifen is a benzocycloheptathiophene derivative. Its mode of action is multifactorial, and the strong antianaphylactic activity does not appear to be due to its antihistaminic effects. On the basis of several animal models, the pharmacologic profile of ketotifen consists of the antagonism to histamine at the H_1-receptor, the functional antagonism of the effects of leukotrienes, the ability to block calcium channels, and the inhibition of mediator release in IgE-dependent reactions (7).

Oral dosing is very convenient in the management of allergic diseases, mainly in children. The metabolism of ketotifen in children is faster than in adults, and for maintaining the same blood levels, children need full adult doses. The recommended dosage is 1 mg twice a day, and patients will benefit from regular and long-term treatment. Ketotifen has a slow onset of action, and its initial evaluation for a clinical demonstration of efficacy should be done after 8–12 weeks of treatment (7).

Ketotifen was able to inhibit antigen-induced reactions in humans and also to decrease the nasal airway resistance measured by a direct rhinomanometry technique (33).

A double-blind, comparative study of ketotifen and clemastine in perennial allergic rhinitis showed that ketotifen was effective in controlling the symptoms of sneezing, rhinorrhea, and nasal obstruction, whereas clemastine did not change the nasal congestion, but controlled sneezing and nasal discharge (34). In a similar study in patients with seasonal allergic rhinitis to grass pollen, symptom scores and the nasal response to histamine were significantly reduced in the ketotifen-treated group after 6 weeks of therapy (35).

The efficacy of oral ketotifen was similar to a nasal spray of cromolyn sodium in the prophylactic treatment of pollen-induced nasal allergic manifestations (36).

A trial involving 107 patients, randomly allocated to either ketotifen, 1 mg or 2 mg, and long-acting chlorpheniramine, given twice daily, was carried for the duration of the hay fever season (3 months). The three drugs' regimens produced significantly better results than placebo and better results were recorded for ketotifen, 1 mg (37).

The administration of ketotifen before the pollen season, in a double-blind study involving 240 patients, showed an enhancement of its efficacy during the season, suggesting a prophylactic effect for the drug (38).

A retrospective study of 382 patients with allergic rhinitis showed that children responded better to ketotifen treatment. However, drug efficacy was better in pollen-induced than in house dust-induced rhinitis (39).

In children with perennial allergic rhinitis, a clinical comparison between the therapeutic effects of ketotifen, beclomethasone dipropionate, and cromolyn showed similar improvement to all treatments (40). A double-blind/multicenter study (162 patients) with perennial allergic rhinitis using terfenadine and ketotifen, showed similar therapeutic effects; side effects were significantly lower in the terfenadine-treated group (41).

Recently, ketotifen was given to 124 children with allergic diseases, aged 6 months to 15 years, for 12 weeks to investigate the clinical efficacy of the drug on the progress of "allergy march" (atopic dermatitis, asthma, and allergic rhinitis). Favorable results were obtained from the severity of rhinitis, suggesting that ketotifen can prevent the progress of allergy march (42).

The most frequent side effect of ketotifen is drowsiness. The tired feeling is most prominent in the first week of treatment and subsequently lessens (2). The association with oral antidiabetic drugs should be avoided because some cases of reversible thrombocytopenia have been observed. Other antihistamines should not be given concomitantly with ketotifen. Although antihistamines have a relatively large margin of safety, the addition of two medications, with similar central nervous system side effects, may produce significant sedation.

B. Mequitazine

Mequitazine is a phenothiazine derivative, nonsedating antihistamine of the H_1-blocker class. If has some degree of anticholinergic activity and mast cell-stabilizing properties. A recent study of the symptomatic treatment of seasonal allergic rhinitis showed mequitazine to be similar to loratadine, and both superior to placebo. Loratadine was superior at 3 days, whereas mequitazine was superior at 7 days (43).

IV. COMBINATIONS (ANTIHISTAMINES AND SYMPATHOMIMETICS)

Antihistamines (H_1-antagonists) have long been considered effective in relieving symptoms in allergic rhinitis, such as sneezing, itching, and rhinorrhea, but they are not useful in reducing nasal congestion (stuffiness). Oral decongestant medications are effective in shrinking turbinate size, thus reducing the nasal airway resistance (NAR). They also inhibit the rise in NAR following intranasal challenge with antigen and histamine (44).

The combination of oral antihistamines with oral decongestants is often used to better control allergic rhinitis patients and to counteract partially the drowsiness produced by the classic antihistamines (10). This information provides the rationale for the use of antihistamines and oral decongestants in single, fixed-dose combination preparations; several studies have demonstrated that the efficacy of these combinations in the management of allergic rhinitis is superior to the efficacy of either component alone (1). There are over 100 antihistamine and decongestant combinations available, a number of which contains anticholinergics (30,45). Table 3 lists some representative antihistamine and sympathomimetics combinations. A representative antihistamine–decongestant–parasympatholytic includes chlorpheniramine, phenylephrine, and methscopolamine.

The effect of an antihistamine–decongestant (chlorpheniramine and phenylpropanolamine) on nasal and eustachian tube functions following intranasal

Table 3 Representative Antihistamine and Sympathomimetic Combinations

Antihistamine class	Combinations

Alkylamines	Chlorpheniramine
	  Phenylepherine
	Triprolidine
	  Pseudoephedrine
	Brompheniramine
	  Pseudoephedrine
	Dexbrompheniramine
	  Pseudoephedrine

Ethanolamines	Carbinoxamine
	  Pseudoephedrine
	Clemastine
	  Phenylpropanolamine

Ethylenediamines	Pyrilamine
	  Pheniramine
	  Phenylpropanolamine
	Pyrilamine
	  Chlorpheniramine
	  Phenylephrine

Piperidines	Azatadine Pseudoephedrine

Nonsedating	Terfenadine
	  Pseudoephedrine
	Loratadine
	  Pseudoephedrine

pollen challenge was studied in subjects with documented ragweed allergic rhinitis (44). There was a significant improvement in nasal and eustachian tube functions, demonstrating a role for drug combinations in the treatment of allergic rhinitis.

There are several recent reports showing that drug combinations are safe and efficacious for treatment of seasonal allergic rhinitis: loratadine and pseudoephedrine (46), terfenadine and pseudoephedrine (47) and chlorpheniramine, pyrilamine, and phenylephrine (48).

Many of these combination preparations are used in the composition of cold remedy preparations. Because there are so many combination drugs (some as nonprescription) and because many children are cold and allergic rhinitis sufferers, pediatric dosage guidelines are important. An FDA advisory panel has tentatively recommended: for children 6–12 years old, one-half the adult dosage; 2–6 years, one-fourth the adult dosage; under 2 years, dosage to be determined by physician (6).

V. H_2-ANTIHISTAMINES

Several clinical trials have demonstrated that histamine antagonists reduce sneezing and nasal discharge, but not obstruction in allergic rhinitis. In the nose, H_1- and H_2-receptors, distributed throughout the resistance vessels are responsible for vasodilation in response to histamine. The effects of large doses of histamine are completely blocked only by a combination of H_1- and H_2-antagonists (2). The pretreatment of the nose with topical H_1 (chlorpheniramine) and H_2 (ranitidine) antagonists improved the response to topical histamine provocation (49). Combined oral histamine antagonists (H_1, diphenydramine and H_2, cimetidine) were significantly more effective in reducing the nasal resistive response to topical histamine than an H_1-antagonist alone (50). The additive effect of the H_1-antagonist (chlorpheniramine) to the H_2-antagonist (cimetidine) significantly reduced allergic symptoms and the need for concomitant medication in seasonal allergic rhinitis (51).

In a recent study, patients with allergic rhinitis were pretreated intranasally with an H_1-antagonist (levocabastine) or an H_2-antagonist (ranitidine), or a combination thereof, before a local allergen challenge. The allergen-induced sneezes and rhinorrhea were inhibited by the histamine antagonists. The increase in NAR was not affected, and the decrease in blood flow was blocked by both antagonists. These findings suggest that the H_1- and H_2-receptors are involved in the regulation of the tone of the resistance, but not the capacitance, vessels on the nasal mucosa in allergic rhinitis (52).

In another study, ten patients affected by allergic rhinitis were treated with the H_2-receptor antagonist, cimetidine, with a dosage of 3 mg/kg per day, administered intravenously, a total of 15 times. The remaining ten patients were treated intravenously with placebo. The cellular immune response was evaluated in vitro and the OKT4/OKT8 ratio after treatment showed a statistically significant decrease compared with initial values, expressing a relative increase in the OKT8 suppressor subpopulation. These results suggest that H_2-antagonists act in allergic rhinitis by modulating the activity of the T-suppressor lymphocytes, which are reduced in allergic patients. In rhinitis, the combined use of H_1- and H_2 antagonists in the treatment will require further investigations.

VI. OTHER TREATMENTS FOR ALLERGIC RHINITIS

A. Nonsteroidal Anti-Inflammatory Agents

Because medications such as aspirin and indomethacin prevent production of the prostaglandins by the cyclooxygenase pathway of arachidonic acid, a possible beneficial role for these agents in allergic diseases has been considered. Responses after intranasal challenge in pollen allergic patients were inhibited by aspirin (topical, oral), indomethacin (oral), and flurbiprofen (oral). The role of these medications in allergic rhinitis needs further evaluation (2). However, it should be remembered that aspirin and nonsteroidal anti-inflammatory agents sensitivity is not uncommon in patients with rhinitis and sinusitis, especially when there is an association with polyps and asthma.

B. β-Adrenergic Agonists

β-Adrenergic agonists are inhibitors of cell release of chemical mediators. Fenoterol (topical nasal spray) produced statistical improvement in patients with seasonal allergic rhinitis; the results were less impressive in patients with perennial allergic rhinitis. Because of the β-adrenergic-mediated nasal vasodilation, an increase in NAR was observed (2).

It was shown that theophylline reduces histamine release during pollen-induced rhinitis; there were significant reductions in both the physiological response to antigen challenge and the appearance of mediators in secretions after drug administration, compared with placebo (53).

β_2-Agonists and theophylline, widely used in the treatment of bronchial asthma, could offer some relief for some patients with respiratory allergy. However, because of the interaction of these drugs and nasal vasculature, more studies should be performed to find the true place of cyclic AMP increasers in the management of allergic rhinitis.

C. Water Vapor-Induced Nasal Hyperthermia

Previous studies with steam inhalation therapy demonstrated improvement of nasal patency. Recently, the treatment of seasonal allergic rhinitis with water vapor-induced nasal hyperthermia administered through a special high-flow nasal cannula, showed some symptomatic improvement (54). This topical treatment needs additional evaluations.

VII. SINUSITIS

The diagnosis of sinusitis in children remains controversial, particularly when the radiographical criteria are considered. Nevertheless, there is a good correlation between bacteria recovered and an abnormality found on sinus x-ray films (55). Maxillary sinus aspiration in children when sinusitis is suspected is not a routine procedure; however, the knowledge of the bacteriology in acute and chronic sinusitis is important in the choice of the appropriate antibiotic. In children with acute sinusitis the predominant organisms are *Streptococcus pneumoniae*, *Branhamella catarrhalis* and *Haemophilus influenzae*; in chronic sinusitis, in addition to the foregoing aerobes, anaerobes of the respiratory tract and *Streptococcus viridans* can be found (56). Probably the bacteriology of sinusitis may vary geographically; we found that in children with chronic sinusitis and with complete opacification of one or both maxillary sinus (x-ray findings), in 70% of the children submitted to a maxillary sinus aspiration, the only isolated organism was *S. pneumoniae* (57).

The treatment of acute sinusitis includes analgesics to relieve pain and discomfort; topical sympathomimetic vasoconstrictors may improve sinus drainage, but should be used for only a short period (3–5 days), to avoid rhinitis medicamentosa; oral administration of antibiotics for 2 weeks (amoxicillin, erythromycin, trimethoprim–sulfamethoxazole, cefaclor, amoxicillin–clavulanate potassium) (56).

The improvement in sinus drainage is vital in the management of chronic sinusitis. The medical therapy should include (1) repeated applications of a large volume of saline solution, from a pipette or a drop bottle, but correct administration is the most important point (3); (2) oral decongestants or antihistamines or combinations (antihistamines and sympathomimetics)—there is no supporting data on the value of these drugs in the treatment of sinusitis; (3) oral or topical corticosteroids; (4) antibiotics—the same used to treat acute sinusitis, but the antimicrobial therapy should be maintained for 3–4 weeks.

We treat our patients who have chronic sinusitis with repeated irrigations with saline, oral prednisone (1 mg/kg per day) for 1 week, followed by the topical use of beclomethasone (one puff in each nostril four times a day) for the next 3 weeks, and oral antibiotic for 4 weeks. Although the effectiveness of oral decongestants and oral and topical corticosteroids in the treatment of chronic sinusitis has not been adequately studied (56), our clinical impression is that the concomitant initial use of oral corticosteroids (followed by topical beclomethasone) is critical in decreasing the nasal inflammatory response associated with chronic sinusitis, increasing the effectiveness of the antimicrobial therapy.

The patient who fails to respond clinically to several 3- to 4-week courses of correct medical treatment, with continuous symptoms (nasal purulent drainage, persistent cough, and bronchial asthma that is difficult to control) may be a candidate for surgical treatment.

The resolution of repeated episodes of sinusitis depends on the management of the chronic inflammatory changes of the nasal mucosa in perennial allergic rhinitis. If the rhinitis is well controlled, with minimal nasal blockage, sinusitis probably will not be a major problem.

REFERENCES

1. Meltzer EO, Schatz M, Zeiger RS. Allergic and non-allergic rhinitis. In: Middleton E, Reed CE, Ellis EF, Adkinson NF, Yunginger JW, eds. Allergy—principles and practice, 3rd ed. St Louis: CV Mosby, 1988:1253–1289.
2. Meltzer EO, Schatz M. Pharmacotherapy of rhinitis—1987 and beyond. Immunol Allergy Clin North Am 1987; 7:57–91.
3. Mygynd N. Conventional medical treatment: "nasal allergy." Oxford: Scientific Publications, 1978:257–270.
4. Kaliner M, Eggleston P, Mathews KP. Rhinitis and asthma. JAMA 1987; 258:2851–2873.
5. Simons FER. Chronic rhinitis. Pediatr Clin North Am 1984; 31:801–819.
6. AMA Drug evaluations. Decongestant, cough and cold preparations. 5th ed. Chicago: American Medical Association, 1984:549–576.
7. Naspitz CK, Tinkelman DG. Therapeutic approaches to the treatment of chronic asthma. In: Tinkelman DG, Falliers CJ, Naspitz CK, eds. Childhood asthma—pathophysiology and treatment. New York: Marcel Dekker, 1987:249–280.
8. Schwartz HJ. The effect of cromolyn in nasal disease. ENT J 1986; 65:449–456.
9. Fradis M, Podoshin L, Gertner R. Treatment of perennial allergic rhinitis by sodium cromoglycate plus 0.025 per cent xylametazoline. J Laryngol Otol 1987; 101:667–672.
10. Norman PS. Allergic rhinitis. J Allergy Clin Immunol 1987; 75:531–545.
11. Schwartz HJ, Sher TH, Ellis LD. Efficacy of nedocromil sodium 1% nasal solution in the treatment of ragweed seasonal allergic rhinitis. J Allergy Clin Immunol 1987; 79:186.
12. Togias A, Proud D, Kagey-Sobotka A, Norman P, Lichtenstein L, Naclerio R. The effect of a topical tricyclic antihistamine on the response of the nasal mucosa to challenge with cold, dry air and histamine. J Allergy Clin Immunol 1987; 79:599–604.
13. Pecoud A, Zuber P, Kolly P. Effect of a new selective H_1 receptor antagonist (levocabastine) in a nasal and conjunctival provocation test. Int Arch Allergy Appl Immunol 1987; 82:541–543.
14. Turkeltaub PC, Norman PS, Crepea S. Treatment of ragweed hayfever with an

intranasal spray containing flunisolide: a new synthetic corticosteroid. J Allergy Immunol 1976:58:597.
15. Prahl P, Wilken-Jensen K, Mygind N. Beclomethasone diproprionate aerosol in treatment of hay fever in children. Arch Dis Child 1975; 50:875.
16. Norman PS, Winkenwerder WL, Agbayani AF, Migeon CJ. Adrenal function during the use of dexamethasone aerosols in the treatment of ragweed hayfever. J Allergy 1967; 40:57–61.
17. Kobayashi R, Tinkelman D, Reese M, Sykes S. Effectiveness of Beconase AQ in treating seasonal rhinitis in children ages 5 to 12 years [abstract]. J Allergy Clin Immunol 1987; 79:152.
18. Physician's Desk Reference 43rd ed. Oradell, NJ: Medical Economics, 1988:2103.
19. Orgel HA, Meltzer EO, Kemp JP, Welch MJ. Clinical, rhinomanometric, and cytologic evaluation of seasonal allergic rhinitis treated with beclomethasone dipropionate as aqueous nasal spray or pressurized aerosol. J Allergy Clin Immunol 1986:77:858–864.
20. Pakes GE, et al. Flunisolide: overview of its pharmacologic properties and therapeutic efficacy in rhinitis. Drugs 1980; 19:397.
21. Mygind N. Topical steroid treatment for allergic rhinitis and allied conditions. Clin Otolaryngol 1982; 7:343–347.
22. Pipkorn U, Rundrantz H, Lindqvist N. Budesonide—a new topical steroid. Rhinology 1980; 18:171.
23. Brattsand R, et al. Development of new glucocorticoids with a very high ratio between topical and systemic activities. Eur J Respir Dis Suppl 63 1982; 122:62.
24. Pipkorn U, Geterud A. A comparative trial testing budesonide and flunisolide nasal sprays in patients with seasonal allergic rhinitis. Ann Allerg 1984; 52:183.
25. Cauna N. Blood nerve supply of the nasal lining. In: Proctor DF, Anderson I, eds. The nose—upper airway physiology and the atmospheric environment. Amsterdam: Elsevier Biomedical, 1982:45–69.
26. Borum P. Intranasal ipratropium: inhibition of methacholine induced hypersecretion. Rhinology 1978; 16:225–233.
27. Borum P, Larsen FS, Mygind N. Nasal methacholine provocation and ipratropium therapy of perennial rhinitis. Acta Otolaryngol Suppl 1979; 360:35–39.
28. Von Haacke NP, Moore-Gillon V, Capel LH. Double-blind crossover trial of ipratropium and placebo in chronic rhinorrhea. Br Med J 1983; 287:1258–1259.
29. Flowers FR, Araujo OE, Nieves CH. Antihistamines. Int J Dermatol 1986; 25:224–231.
30. Crawford LV, Cohen RM. Therapy for allergic rhinitis. Comp Ther 1985; 11:60–69.
31. Mathews KP, Portnoy JM. Allergic rhinitis. In: Lichtenstein L, Fauci AS, eds. Current therapy in allergy, immunology and rheumatology. Toronto: BC Deker, 1985:1–5.
32. Popa V. The classic antihistamines (H_1 blockers) in respiratory medicine. Clin Chest Med 1986; 7:367–382.

33. Labus J, Hlinka V. Effect of ketotifen on nasal airways resistance in allergic rhinitis. Eur J Respir Dis Suppl 146 1986; 69:88.
34. Okuda M. Clinical investigation of ketotifen in perennial allergic rhinitis: a double-blind, comparative study of ketotifen and clemastine fumarate. Rhinology 1984; 22:171.
35. Blainey AD, Ollier S, Gould C, Davies RJ. Antihistamines in seasonal allergic rhinitis: a double-blind study of clemastine and ketotifen. Thorax 1983; 38:701.
36. Businco L, Bellioni P, Beniconi N, Bruno G, DiCicco C, Gorgiolu M, Corbetta G. Oral ketotifen versus disodium cromoglycate nasal spray for the prophylactic treatment of pollen-induced allergic manifestations. Curr Ther Res 1984; 35:239–246.
37. Wheatley D, Deering RB. Ketotifen in hayfever and allergic rhinitis. In: Wuthrich B, Jager L, eds. The prophylaxis of allergic rhinitis. Amsterdam: Excerpta Medica 1986:36–42.
38. Okuda M. Prophylactic effect of ketotifen on pollinosis. In: Wuthrich B, Jager L, eds. The prophylaxis of allergic rhinitis. Amsterdam: Excerpta Medica, 1986:28–35.
39. Fernandes M, Wong E, Oehling A. Retrospective study of ketotifen protective action in different allergopathies. Allergol Immunopathol 1987; 15:369–373.
40. Farri A, Lucisano P, Mora T. Clinical comparison between the therapeutic effect of ketotifen, beclomethasone dipropionate and disodium cromoglycate in childhood perennial rhinitis. Riv Ital Orl 1987; 7:447–450.
41. Saito Y, Baba S, Furuuchi I, Shimizu T. Double-blind comparative study of terfenadine vs ketotifen in perennial allergic rhinitis. J Allergy Clin Immunol 1987; 79:189.
42. Baba M, Kavai H, Matsui T, Kubogawa T. Clinical efficacy of ketotifen in children in the process of allergy march. NER Allergy Proc 1988; 9:354.
43. Skassa-Brociek W, Bousquet J, Montes F. Verdier M, Schwab D, Lherminier M, Michel FB. Double-blind placebo-controlled study of loratadine, mequitazine, and placebo in the symptomatic treatment of seasonal allergic rhinitis. J Allergy Clin Immunol 1988; 81:725–730.
44. Stillwagon PK, Doyle WJ, Fireman P. Effect of an antihistamine/decongestant on nasal and eustachian tube function following intranasal pollen challenge. Ann Allergy 1987; 58:442–446.
45. Conner BL, Georgitis JW. Practical diagnosis and treatment of allergic and nonallergic rhinitis. Primary Care 1987; 14:457–473.
46. Storms WW, Bodman SF, Nathan RA, Trochelman L, Greenstein S. SCH 434 (loratadine 5 mg plus pseudoephedrine 120 mg) versus components in the treatment of seasonal allergic rhinitis. J Allergy Clin Immunol 1988; 81:173.
47. Kurseja A, Riedelsheimer BR, Kohler M, Henauer S. Effectiveness of a terfenadine/pseudoephedrine combination in a nasal provocation test. NER Allergy Proc 1988; 9:367.
48. Weiler JM, Glassman JP. Double-blind, placebo controlled study of Rynatan to treat allergic rhinitis. J Allergy Clin Immunol 1988; 81:176.

49. Secher K, Kirkgaard J, Borum P. Significance of H_1 and H_2 receptors in the human nose: rationale for topical use of combined antihistamine preparations. J Allergy Clin Immunol 1982;70:211.
50. Havas TE, Cole P, Parker L, Oprysk D, Ayiomamitis A. The effects of combined H_1 and H_2 histamine antagonists in nasal airflow resistance induced by topical histamine provocation. J Allergy Clin Immunol 1986;78:856–860.
51. Carpenter GB, Bunker-Soler AL, Nelson HS. Evaluation of combined H_1 and H_2 receptor blocking agents in the treatment of seasonal allergic rhinitis. J Allergy Clin Immunol 1983;71:412.
52. Holmberg K, Bake B, Blychert LO, Pipkorn U. Topical treatment with H_1 and H_2 receptor antagonists and allergic rhinitis. NER Allergy Proc 1988;9:369.
53. Testa B, Misolella C, Costa F, Catalanotti PG, Benedetto N, Matera S. Histamine 2 antagonists in allergic rhinitis. Arch Otolaryngol Head Neck Surg 1986;112:432–434.
54. Grossman J, Ball MD, Ball R, Shulan D, Porcella J. Treatment of seasonal allergic rhinitis with water induced nasal hyperthermia. J Allergy Clin Immunol 1988;81:175.
55. Shapiro GG. Sinusitis in children. J Allergy Clin Immunol 1988;81:1025–1027.
56. Wald ER. Management of sinusitis in infants and children. Pediatr Infec Dis 1988;7:449–451.
57. Arruda L, Naspitz CK, Mimica I, Schoettler J, Almeida MF, Heiner DC. Abnormal maxillary sinus radiographs in children: do they represent bacterial infection? J Allergy Clin Immunol 1988;81:285.

5

Immunotherapy in Allergic Rhinitis

Ahmed A. Mohiuddin
National Jewish Center for Immunology and Respiratory Medicine, Denver, Colorado

Henry Milgrom
University of Colorado Health Sciences Center and National Jewish Center for Immunology and Respiratory Medicine, Denver, Colorado

I. INTRODUCTION

Immunotherapy is a term introduced by Norman et al. (1) in 1968 to describe the process of injecting slowly increasing doses of allergen into a sensitive individual to develop an increased tolerance to that particular allergen. The older terms, "hyposensitization" and "desensitization," are misleading for this form of therapy and should be reserved for the procedure used for the treatment of antibiotic or insulin sensitivity. Immunotherapy has been in use since 1911 (2), and a number of double-blind, placebo-controlled studies have proved its efficacy both in allergic rhinitis (Table 1) and in asthma (3–15). However, the mechanisms through which it works are not yet clearly understood. The importance of immunotherapy in the treatment of allergic disease has been diminished in recent years, with the introduction of much more effective pharmacologic agents. Its proper place in the therapeutic

Table 1 Double-Blind Studies of Immunotherapy in Patients with Allergic Rhinitis

Investigator and year reported	Antigen used	Technique	Treated patients	Controls	Results
Frankland and Augustin, 1954 (8)	Grass	Preseasonal	100 children and adults	100 children and adults	Treatment better than placebo
Johnstone, 1957 (9)	Ragweed	Perennial	58 children	14 children	"High-dose" treatment better than placebo
Lowell and Franklin, 1963	Ragweed	Perennial	84 children and adults	80 children and adults	Treatment better than placebo
Lowell and Franklin, 1965 (22)	Ragweed	Perennial	12 adults	12 adults	Treatment better than placebo
Fontana et al., 1966	Ragweed	Preseasonal	51 children	50 children	Treatment no better than placebo
Norman and Winkenwerder, 1968	Ragweed antigen E	Preseasonal	29	27	Treatment better than placebo
Lichtenstein, 1968	Ragweed antigen E	Preseasonal	18	18	Treated patients demonstrated fewer symptoms than placebo patients
Sadan et al. 1969	Ragweed	Preseasonal	18	17	Treatment better than placebo
Pence et al., 1976	Mountain cedar	Perennial	17 adults	15 adults	Treatment better than placebo

hierarchy is after the institution of allergen avoidance and aggressive medical therapy. In this chapter, we will present evidence for the effectiveness of immunotherapy and the proposed mechanisms through which it works, and we will offer some guidelines on its practical use.

II. HISTORICAL PERSPECTIVE

John Bostock was the first physician to give a precise and accurate clinical description of hay fever in a paper delivered in 1819 before the Royal Medical and Chirurgical Society of London (16). Bostock did not concur with the popular belief of the time that the "affluvium" from new hay was a factor in the pathogenesis of hay fever. Nine years after his first description, he described 18 additional cases and proposed the term "Catarrhus Aestivus" (summer catarrh) for this malady. He felt firmly that sunshine and heat were extremely important factors in its pathogenesis. Two of his contemporaries, Wilhaim Gordan and Phillip Phoebus, argued against this theory. They felt that the aroma and probably the pollen from grasses and flowers were the most important factors in causing symptoms of hay fever. It remained for Charles Harrison Blackley (17), however, in 1871, to furnish actual proof that pollen caused hay fever. By doing experiments on himself, he not only showed that most kinds of pollen could give rise to symptoms of hay fever, but he also described, for the first time, a positive skin test to pollen. In 1903, W. P. Dunbar confirmed the original findings of Blackley. He used an ophthalmic test, first described by Blackley, and an intranasal instillation test to identify the offending pollen and to determine, to some extent, the degree of the patient's sensitivity. He also showed that the injection of the "pollen toxin" gives rise in animals to the production of an "antitoxin" having the specific power of neutralizing the "toxin."

Immunotherapy for inhalant allergy was first employed by Noon, an English surgeon, in 1911 (2). He treated hay fever patients with grass pollen extracts and was able to correlate the subjective clinical improvement of his patients with changes in the dilutions of allergen extracts required to elicit the ophthalmic test (Fig. 1). Immunotherapy was soon introduced into America and, in 1915 Cooke (18) reported the first study in the United States on the successful treatment of hay fever by active immunization. Subsequently, he reported (19) on the presence, in the blood of treated patients, of a substance that could inhibit the passive transfer of allergic antibody described by Prausnitz and Kustner (20). He called this substance "blocking antibody." He noted, however, that there was not a constant relationship between the presence of this blocking antibody in the serum and relief of symptoms. He also observed that

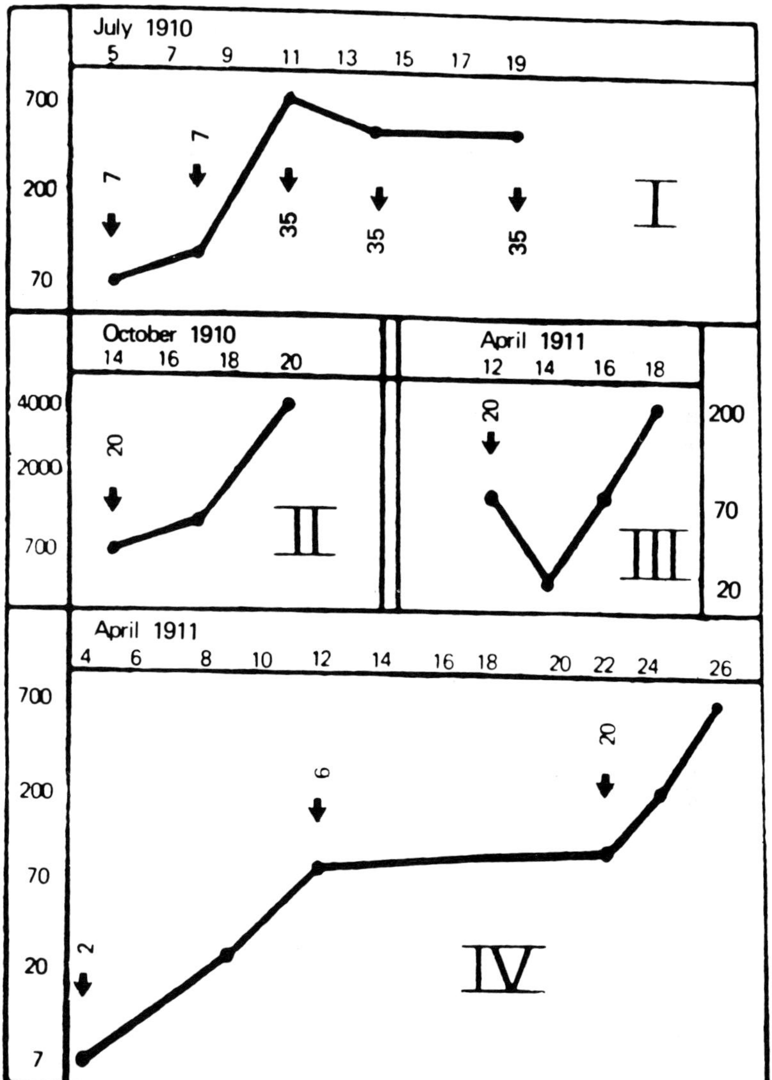

Figure 1 The numbers at the sides denote the resistance of the patient, given in terms of the strength of pollen extract, one drop of which was sufficient to excite a conjunctival reaction. The arrows indicate subcutaneous inoculations of pollen extract, quantitites given in the units described in the text; I and II refer to one patient at different periods of treatment; III shows the response obtained after about a month's treatment in another case; and IV the early stages of treatment. [From (2).]

immunotherapy did not uniformly decrease skin reactivity. In 1940, Loveless (21) showed that the blocking antibody is different from the reaginic ("allergic") antibody in its heat stability at 56 °C and its failure to bind to human skin. Bruun (3) noted, in 1949, that "the literature contains few, if any, unquestionable control examinations." He conducted the first controlled study of immunotherapy in 100 asthmatics sensitive to house dust and showed a significant improvement in treated subjects. Since then, double-blind studies have established immunotherapy as an effective mode of therapy in patients with hay fever (see Table 1).

III. EFFICACY OF IMMUNOTHERAPY

In 1954, Frankland and Augustin (8) reported the first placebo-controlled study of immunotherapy in hay fever. They studied 200 patients with hay fever and grass pollen sensitivity and showed that 79% of patients who received immunotherapy with grass pollen extracts improved, compared with 39% of those on placebo injections. Similar results were reported by Lowell and Franklin (22) in patients with ragweed hay fever. Comparable results can be expected in properly selected patients treated with currently available immunotherapy regimens.

The study by Lowell and Franklin (22) demonstrated the specificity of immunotherapy. The subjects, who had multiple allergic sensitivities, were started on an immunotherapy regimen with appropriate allergens. However, some ragweed-sensitive subjects received ragweed extract in their immunotherapy, whereas others did not. Symptoms in ragweed season were significantly less severe in the subjects who received the ragweed extract. This proved that, in patients with ragweed sensitivity, immunotherapy with other allergens does not reduce symptoms. This finding was later confirmed by Norman and coworkers, (23) who studied a group of patients with hay fever who were sensitive to both ragweed and grass pollen. One group of patients was started on a preseasonal course of immunotherapy with ragweed extract, whereas the control group received placebo injections. No difference was noted in the symptoms reported by both groups during the grass-pollinating season, but the treated group had significantly fewer symptoms during the ragweed season. In a series of elegant studies (1,24,25) this group from Johns Hopkins firmly established the role of immunotherapy in hay fever. In the study presented in Figure 2, daily symptom scores of all patients allergic to ragweed correlated well with ragweed pollen counts, but the scores reported by 22 patients treated with antigen E, the main allergen of ragweed, were consistently lower than those of 18 patients given placebo injections. Blinded physician evaluations also favored

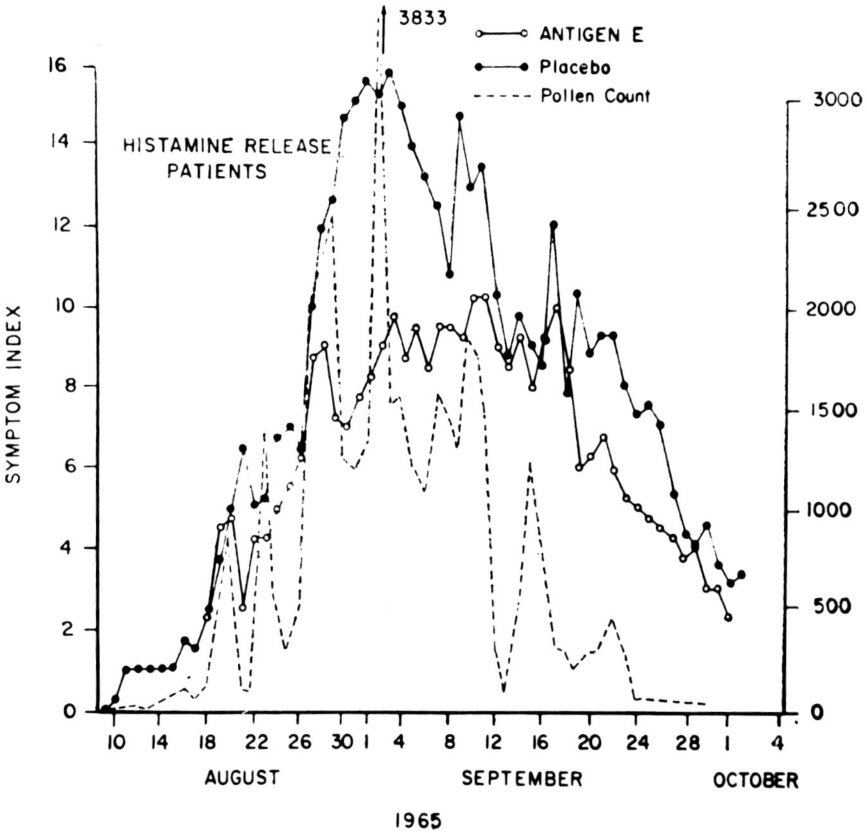

Figure 2 Daily symptom scores correlate with ragweed pollen counts. Symptom scores are significantly lower in the group treated with antigen E extract. [From Lichtenstein, et al. (21).]

the treatment group. Immunotherapy with antigen E showed comparable efficacy to whole ragweed extracts, and both were superior to placebo.

The efficacy of immunotherapy clearly depends on the dosage administered. Figure 3 shows how the severity of symptoms decreased in proportion to the increase in the cumulative dosage of immunotherapy with both antigen E and whole ragweed extract. The importance of dosage is also borne out by the total lack of efficacy of the low-dose Rinkel form of immunotherapy. In this form of immunotherapy, the "optimal dose" determined by skin-test titration,

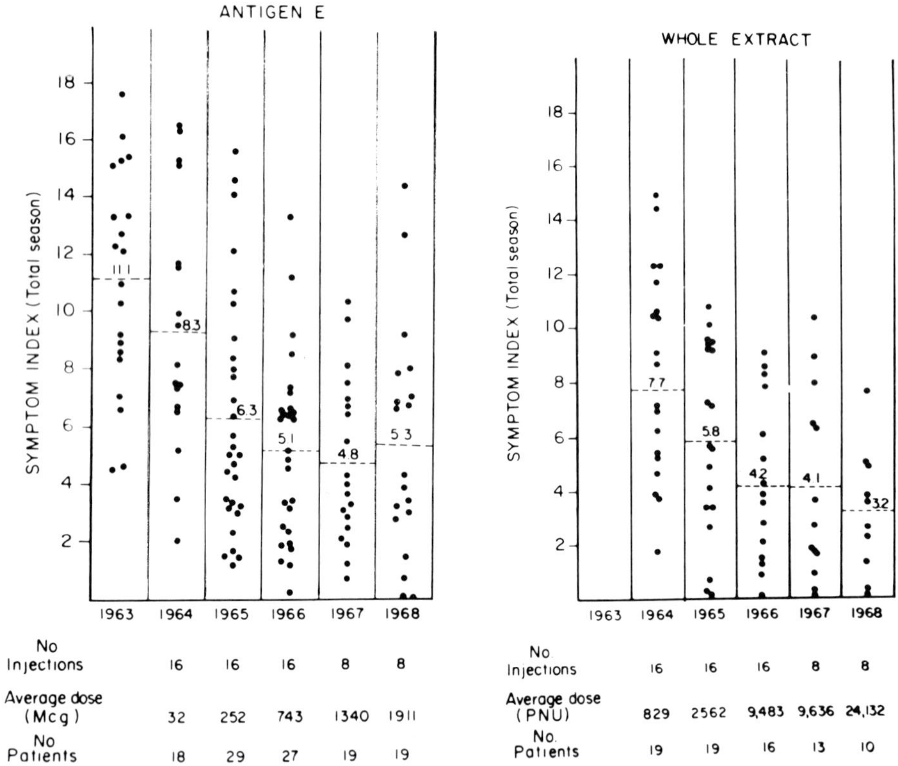

Figure 3 Individual average daily symptom indexes in patients receiving antigen E (left) and whole ragweed extract injections (right). [From Norman, et al. (25).]

is on the average 1000–10,000 times lower than the maximum dose given in the course of standard immunotherapy. Van Metre and associates (26) showed clearly that the low-dose Rinkel method of immunotherapy was no different from placebo, and inferior to the "current standard" method in controlling symptoms of hay fever, in inducing the rise in antiragweed IgG levels and in diminishing the seasonal rise in antiragweed IgE levels (Fig. 4).

There is evidence that immunotherapy is effective in the treatment of asthma (3–15), and one study has suggested that immunotherapy of patients with allergic rhinitis prevents the later onset of asthma (9)

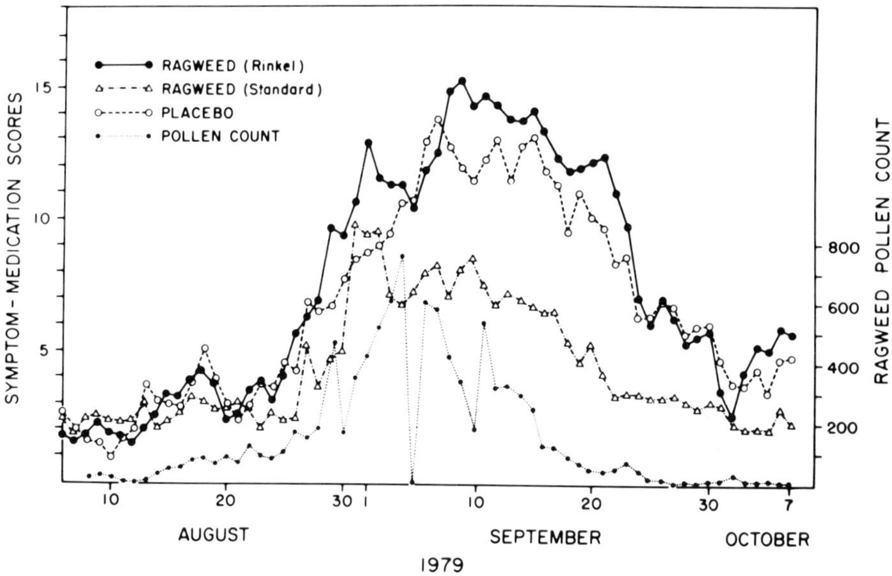

Figure 4 Comparison of low-dose (Rinkel) and high-dose immunotherapy. Rinkel IT is no better than placebo. Standard IT caused significantly lower symptom scores. [From Van Metre (26).]

IV. MECHANISMS OF IMMUNOTHERAPY

Properly carried out immunotherapy results in clinical improvement in most patients with allergic rhinitis. A satisfactory clinical response usually depends on the administration of adequate doses of high-quality, well-characterized allergen extracts to patients whose clinical histories and allergy testing prove that they are sensitive to those allergens (26). The basic principles are those of Noon (2), whose regimen was initiated with minute doses of allergen administered at intervals of 3–4 days and progressed to high doses of allergen administered 10–14 days apart. Noon monitored the progress of immunotherapy by instilling dilutions of allergen extracts into the patient's eye and observing the ensuing conjunctival reactions (see Fig. 1). More recent investigation into the mechanisms of immunotherapy has identified other immunological changes that occur in patients in the course of treatment (Table 2).

Table 2 Immunological Changes Occurring During Immunotherapy

Reduction in allergen specific IgE
Reduction in seasonal rise in IgE
Suppression of the late-phase allergic response
Development of anti-idiotypic antibodies
Generation of suppressor T cells
Reduction in mediator release

A. Reduction in Allergen-Specific Immunoglobulin E

Passive transfer studies conducted in the 1930s at Roosevelt Hospital in New York showed that specific immunotherapy led to a reduction in the titers of allergic antibody (27,28). Later work has shown that in the course of immunotherapy IgE antibody specific for the injected allergens first increases significantly and, later, gradually declines (Fig. 5). This response is highly variable, and it does not reflect the clinical efficacy of immunotherapy. Another, perhaps more reliable finding seen with immunotherapy, is the blunting of the expected seasonal rise of IgE that is seen in sensitive individuals. This occurs even in the absence of a fall in specific IgE (29). The magnitude of the reduction of the IgE levels and its failure to manifest a seasonal rise, however, are not sufficient to explain the success of immunotherapy.

B. Elevation of Allergen-Specific Immunoglobulin G and Immunoglobulin A

Cooke (19,27), in 1922, described the blocking antibody, a serum factor that inhibited the Prausnitz–Kustner (PK) reaction (the passive transfer of reaginic antibody). High titers of blocking antibody, which may appear in the course of immunotherapy (see Fig. 5), correlate with a reduction in allergic symptoms (30). Perhaps a better reflection of the success of immunotherapy has been found in the ratio between the blocking antibody and specific IgE (31). Allergen-specific IgA and IgG have been reported in the nasal secretions of patients undergoing immunotherapy (32), suggesting the importance of the production of local immunity. However, studies on the passive administration of the blocking antibody to volunteers have yielded conflicting results for its clinical benefits (33,34). It has been questioned, therefore, whether allergen-specific IgG present in circulation can play a protective function in allergic reactions localized in the skin or the mucosa (35). Hence, attention has been

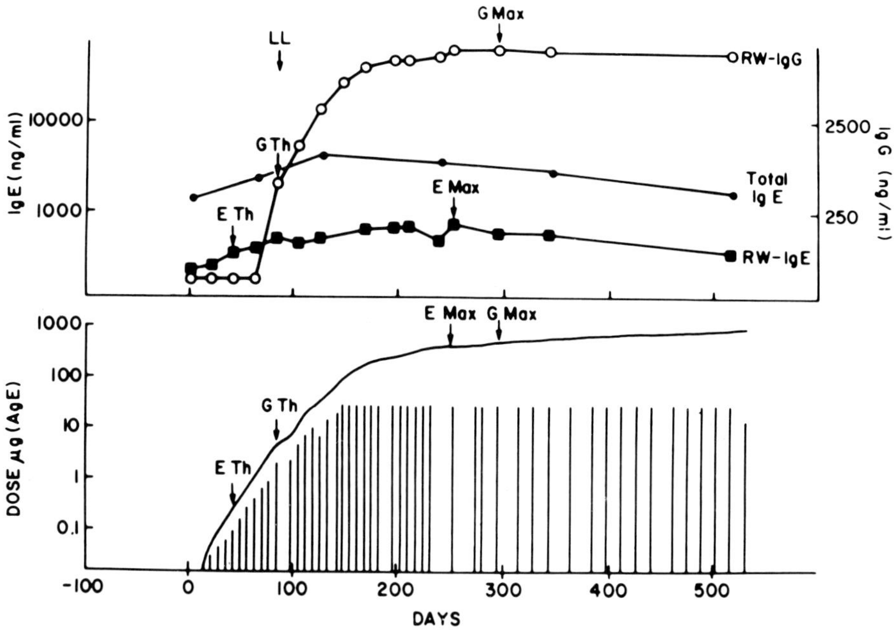

Figure 5 Profile of a typical patient illustrating the dose regimens for immunotherapy and the IgE and IgG antibody response. Plotted are the relationships between time expressed in days, individual and cumulative doses of RW pollen extract expressed in nanograms of antigen E (AgE), and serum levels of RW-IgE, RW-IgG. Top panel: RW-IgE, RW-IgG, total IgE data. LL, large local reaction, Bottom panel: Progressive cumulative dose (line) over respective single doses (bars) over time in days. (From Creticos et al. J Allergy Clin Immunol 1984; 73:97.)

focused recently on IgG_4 because antibodies of this subclass, which appear in the course of immunotherapy (36,37), are cytotropic for mast cells and may interfere with the bridging of cell-bound IgE antigen (35).

C. Modification of the Late-Phase Allergic Response

After exposure to an antigen, an allergic individual may manifest an immediate classic allergic reaction, which occurs within minutes. It is brought about by the release of mast cell mediators and is characterized by smooth-muscle contraction, vascular leakage, mucus secretion, and pruritus. Two to eight hours later some individuals experience a late-phase reaction, characterized by cellular infiltration with eosinophils and neutrophils, fibrin deposition, and tissue destruction (38). The late-phase reaction has been observed in the skin (39,40), the lung (41,42), and the nose (43). It has been suggested that it resembles clinical disease more closely than the immediate response (44).

Allergen-specific IgG appears to play an important role in blunting the late-phase reaction. This has been especially well documented in the rabbit model of the late asthmatic response (45). In some patients, the late-phase cutaneous response is suppressed in the course of immunotherapy, and there is a strong inverse relationship between the levels of antigen-specific IgG and the incidence of late-phase reactions (46).

D. Immunoglobulin E Regulation by Anti-idiotypes

In the early 1970s, Jerne formulated the concept of the regulation of immunoglobulin production by an idiotype–anti-idiotype network. He proposed that the variable region of an antibody molecule, or its combining site, functions also as an antigen, termed *idiotype*, against which anti-idiotypic antibody molecules can be made (47). Several years later Blaser and deWeck showed that this concept is valid for the control of IgE production in mice (48). They demonstrated, in several systems, that the production of specific IgE is suppressed by anti-idiotypic antibodies. More recently, it has been shown that auto–anti-idiotypic antibodies are generated in the serum of allergic patients in the course of immunotherapy (49–51). Thus, the reduction in specific IgE during immunotherapy may be the result of suppression by auto–anti-idiotype antibodies generated by the repeated administration of antigen.

E. Generation of Suppressor T Cells

Atopic individuals have reduced numbers of suppressor T cells (52). This deficiency can be corrected in the course of immunotherapy (53–55). Rocklin and colleagues (53) showed that the mononuclear cells of patients who received immunotherapy with ragweed specifically suppress the proliferative response to ragweed. Later studies showed that immunotherapy results in an increase in specific suppressor T cells (54), which have the ability to suppress the production of specific IgE in vitro (55).

F. Mediator Release

The release of histamine in vitro from the basophils of some allergic patients is markedly reduced by immunotherapy (56,57). This observation was extended to a patient model in an elegant series of experiments employing nasal challenges with antigen. In allergic subjects, nasal antigen challenge led to sneezing and rhinorrhea and to the appearance of mast cell and basophil mediators in the nasal secretions (58). Results of nasal challenge with ragweed, conducted in 12 patients treated with high-dose ragweed immunotherapy for 3–5 years, were compared with those of 26 untreated patients (Fig. 6). The immunized group had a diminished response to antigen, as demonstrated by (1) a requirement for much higher pollen doses to trigger sneezing or mediator release, (2) fewer responders at any dose, (3) smaller quantities of mediators released (59).

V. PURPOSE

There is good evidence now that appropriate use of immunotherapy will increase a patient's tolerance to specific allergens. However, it does not eliminate symptoms or the requirement for medication. These limitations of immunotherapy should be clearly understood by both physicians and patients before immunotherapy is started. The purpose of immunotherapy is to reduce symptoms and, possibly, medication use in patients whose disease is not controlled by allergen avoidance and appropriate medical therapy.

VI. INDICATIONS

Immunotherapy requires a long-term commitment on the part of both the physician and the patient. Therefore, careful patient selection is a prerequisite for success. It is imperative that the patient have symptoms upon exposure to the specific allergen. Such a history is quite easily elicited when the patient develops symptoms immediately after every occasional exposure to an allergen. Exacerbation of symptoms during particular months of the year implicates those grasses, trees, and weeds that are pollinating during those months. However, there is considerable overlap in pollination seasons, and a number of species of the flora may be pollinating at the same time. This may make it difficult to implicate a particular allergen as the main cause of symptoms. In patients with perennial symptoms and multiple sensitivities, a clear-cut history is not present. Training the patient to keep accurate symptom–medication scores and correlating them to known exposures to airborne allergens can be very helpful in such situations.

Late-phase responses to allergens may occur in the absence of an immediate response (60). Patients with sensitivity to animals may experience no clear-cut exacerbations, even upon intimate contact. Nevertheless, their chronic symptoms may in part, be due to an ongoing late-phase response to their animal

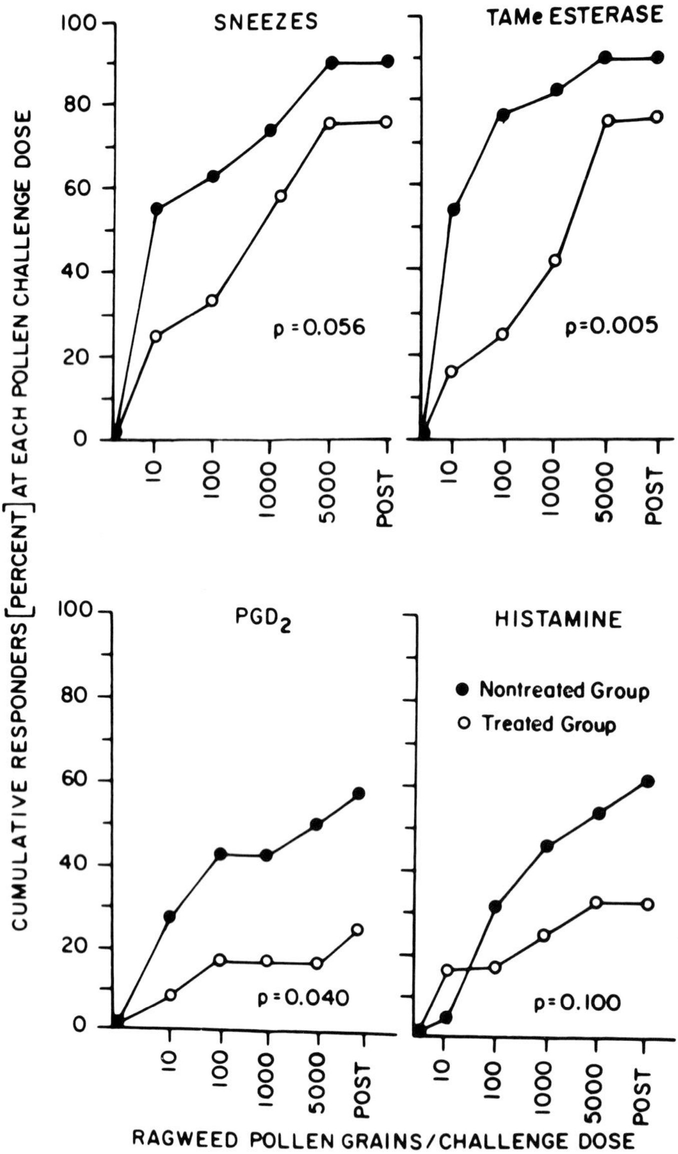

Figure 6 Comparison of nontreated (n = 26) (solid circles) and treated (n = 12) (open circles) groups of patients based on cumulative percentage of patients sneezing or demonstrating mediator release at each respective pollen challenge dose. Statistical comparison made on threshold dose of pollen required to provoke significant response: TAME, tosyl-L-arginine methyl esterase; PGD, prostaglandin D_2. [From Creticos et al. (59).]

exposure. Selected allergen challenges can be helpful in evaluating these patients.

The second requirement for starting patients on an immunotherapy regimen is the demonstration in the patient of IgE specific to the particular airborne allergen suspected by history. This may be done either by skin tests or by Radioallergosorbent tests (RAST). Prick skin testing is the preferred method for evaluating patients for immunotherapy. Clinical sensitivity correlates with positive skin tests to high dilutions (i.e., low concentrations) of the allergen extract (61,62). However, not all positive skin tests are indicative of clinical sensitivity, and a positive skin test to an allergen, without a supporting history, is not an indication for immunotherapy with that antigen.

Once it has been determined which airborne allergens are responsible for the patient's symptoms, it is imperative that avoidance measures be attempted first. This may occasionally be easy if a pet to which the patient is sensitive can be removed from the environment. It is well known that different pollens peak at different clock hours of the day, ragweed peaking in the morning hours, and grasses in the evening (63,64). This knowledge may be helpful for patients to take avoidance measures or use prophylactic medications. Immunotherapy is not indicated if decreased exposure and optimal medical therapy result in a significant reduction or amelioration of symptoms.

VII. CONTRAINDICATIONS

A. Absolute Contraindications

Immunotherapy should not be administered to patients with malignancies, serious immunopathological conditions, or severe psychological disorders, or to patients receiving β-blockers (15). Because epinephrine is the most important drug in the treatment of anaphylactic shock, a contraindication to its use in patients with cardiac disease, labile hypertension, or hyperthyroidism, may be considered a contraindication to starting immunotherapy. Nevertheless, immunotherapy may be undertaken cautiously in these patients when they present with life-threatening reactions following Hymenoptera stings (65).

B. Relative Contraindications

Although immunotherapy is effective in young children, it is generally not recommended for patients under 5 years of age (65). Immunotherapy seems to be safe during pregnancy, but concern for the safety of the fetus compels the clinician to exercise special caution. Hence, it is recommended that if a pregnant women is receiving maintenance immunotherapy, it be continued, albeit at a slightly lower dosage. If she is on an increasing dosage schedule, either conservative increments or no increases in the dose are recommended. It is not recommended that airborne allergen immunotherapy be started during pregnancy. A recent controlled study of 121 pregnancies in 90 women receiving immunotherapy showed no increase in fetal deaths, prematurity, congenital malformations, or maternal complications (66).

VIII. STANDARDIZATION OF EXTRACTS

Noon defined a *pollen unit* as 1×10^{-6} the quantity of protein that could be extracted from 1 g of pollen. Subsequently, the allergen content of an extract came to be expressed in terms of weight per volume (w/v). This defines the weight of allergen extracted by a given volume of fluid. For example, a 1:10 w/v extract denotes the quantity of allergen extracted from 1 g of pollen by 10 ml of the extracting fluid. Another method is to measure the precipitable protein in an extract, and to express it in protein nitrogen units (PNU) per milliliter (1 PNU = 0.00001 mg of protein nitrogen). These methods make it is possible to define extracts by their concentration, but not by allergen content. A consequence of this deficiency has been the marked variability in the antigenic potency of commercial extracts. Thousand-fold differences in potency among extracts comparable in weight/volume or PNU have been reported (67,68).

The amount of allergen administered in the course of immunotherapy is an important determinant of the success of this form of treatment (see Fig. 3). Hence, the International Union of Immunological Societies set out several years ago to provide the impetus and direction for standardization of major allergens. Currently, international reference standards endorsed by the World Health Organization (WHO) exist for short ragweed, timothy grass, and birch pollen, and for *Dermatophagoides pteronyssinus*. *Alternaria tenuis*, bermuda grass, rye grass, and cat and dog are in various stages of acceptance, and several other preparations are expected for later submission.

The new WHO reference preparations have been assigned the value of 100,000 international units (IU). The potency of other extracts can be compared with those standards by direct skin tests, histamine release assays, or by RAST inhibition (68). Two in vivo methods based on skin test titrations are in use. One method, in favor in the Scandinavian countries, compares the size of the wheal generated in a prick test by the test extract to that generated by 10 mg/ml histamine solution. The allergen concentration that causes a wheal equal in size is assigned one histamine equivalent prick (HEP) unit, which is equal to 1000 biologic units per millileter (BU/ml) (69). The second method, which is advocated by the Bureau of Biologics of the United States Food and

Drug Administration (FDA) uses standards expressed in arbitrary allergy units (AU). Potency of commercial extracts can be compared with that of standard preparations by RAST inhibition or by an intradermal assay. The latter compares skin tests obtained with threefold dilutions of the standard and of the test extract, and establishes a best-fit linear regression line for four dilutions of both extracts (70). Several pollen extracts are standardized in this manner. For some extracts, such as ragweed and cat, for which a major allergen has been characterized, standard sera are available to measure the major allergen by radial immunodiffusion. An extract labeled 1:10 w/v must contain at least 35 units of major allegen per milliliter. A unit equals approximately 1 μg of allergen (70).

The emergence of hybridoma technology and the production of monoclonal antibodies (71) have made it possible to develop reference standards that allow absolute quantification of allergens. The application of monoclonal antibodies to allergen standardization was proposed in the 1980s (72–74). The repertoire of monoclonal antibodies to inhalant antigens that is being developed will soon make this a realistic possibility (75). Monoclonal antibodies can be used to identify specific antigenic sites on allergen molecules, to investigate the epitope specificity of IgE, and to study idiotypic regulation of the IgE response. They can also be used to measure the content of major allergens in an extract. Immunoassays employing a monoclonal antibody are more reliable and more easily reproducible than methods for measuring allergens based on skin testing, which is inherently variable; RAST inhibition, which depends on the composition of pooled human sera, and radioimmunoassays and immunoelectrophoretic techniques, which use heterogeneous antisera that must be replaced from time to time (75). Through the use of techniques based on application of monoclonal antibodies, manufacturers of extracts for immunotherapy will be able to adhere to the same standards of activity that are now expected in the production of other pharmaceutic agents. Studies evaluating efficacy of immunotherapy will be conducted with extracts of known potency, and the selection of patients for studies and for treatment will be based on more precise understanding of their allergic susceptibility.

IX. PRACTICAL ASPECTS OF IMMUNOTHERAPY

A. Selection of Patients

The best candidates for immunotherapy are patients whose rhinitis is triggered by multiple allergens that are present in the environment for all or most of the year and that are difficult to avoid. Patients with multiple pollen sensitivities may have more severe symptoms because of the priming effect of some pollen species exaggerating the effects of others. All patients who are being considered for immunotherapy must have evidence of IgE sensitization to the suspected allergens. Allergen avoidance and medical therapy should be tried first before committing patients to immunotherapy.

B. Selection of Allergens

Allergen extracts should be selected on the basis of a clinical history and the demonstration of specific IgE to the particular allergens by skin tests or RAST. Skin testing should be done with individual allergens, rather than mixtures. Up to ten individual allergen extracts may be used in a single bottle for immunotherapy. The use of pooled allergens should be avoided because it may lead to inclusion of irrelevant materials and to excessive dilution of the final mixture.

1. House Dust and House Dust Mite Extracts

House dust extracts contain many household allergens including house dust mites, human dander, animal danders from household pets and pests, household insect debris, molds, and pollen. One concern with housedust extracts is the presence of household chemicals that may not have been removed by the extraction process. Other concerns for the use of the house dust extract for skin testing and immunotherapy involve their content of human dander and of bacterial endotoxin. Consequently, the FDA has recommended that all housedusts extracts be removed from distribution (76).

In the absence of household pets, house dust mites appear to be the major allergenic components of house dust. Mites were identified in Europe as a cause of asthma more than 50 years ago. There are more than 50,000 species of mites (77), but only a few seem to be related to clinical sensitivity. Studies in Holland pointed to *Dermatophagoides pteronyssinus* as the dominant species responsible for sensitivity to housedust. However, in areas in which the relative humidity and temperature are low for substantial portions of the year, *D. farinae* assumes the dominant role (78). A closely related mite, *Euroglyphus maynei*, may also be associated with clinical sensitivity (79). Mite feces appear to be the major source of allergens (80). More than ten different antigens have been identified, the major one designated *Der p* I (81). Studies of *D. farinae* extracts have shown two to four major antigens, some of which share antigenic determinants with *D. pteronyssinus* (82). There is good evidence for the efficacy of immunotherapy with housedust mites (12,15).

2. *Tree, Grass, and Weed Allergens*

The airborne allergens of pollinating plants constitute the most readily identifiable source of clinical sensitivity. Several major allergens responsible for clinical sensitivity have been identified and studied extensively. Good evidence exists for the efficacy of immunotherapy for at least some species (ragweed, grass, and birch; 1,83,84). Knowledge of pollination times and of cross-reactivity of aeroallergens is essential for determining clinical sensitivity and for deciding on the composition of the immunotherapy.

3. *Cat Extracts*

It has been estimated that over 24 million American homes have cats. Nine to forty-one percent of allergic patients may have positive immediate skin test reactions to cat extract (85). Sensitive individuals are notoriously resistant to removing their pets from their environments. There are also some situations in which indirect contact with cat allergens leads to clinical symptoms in highly sensitive individuals. Finally, there may be work-related exposures that are impossible to avoid. Immunotherapy with cat extracts may be indicated in these circumstances. Major sources of allergen are cat pelts, saliva, and urine. The major allergen in cat pelts, cat allergen 1 (*Fel d* I; 86), is present in substantial amounts in the salivary glands and the sebaceous glands of the pelts. Cat urine does not contain *Fel d* I. Evidence exists for the efficacy of immunotherapy with cat extracts (87).

4. *Dog Extracts*

Dog dander, saliva, and urine, all contain allergens (88). There may be no unique breed-specific antigens, and individual dogs from the same species may even exhibit different antigens (89). Immunotherapy with dog allergens may be efficacious (90).

5. *Insect Extracts*

Cockroach-derived aeroallergens have received increasing attention in recent years as a potential source of sensitivity affecting especially inner-city dwellers. About half of the patients who live in large urban areas exhibit positive skin tests and elevated cockroach-specific IgE (91). The major species of cockroach seem to have both unique and shared antigens. Two major allergens have been identified in cockroach extracts (92). Other insects are being studied. There now is no evidence that immunotherapy with insect-derived airborne allergens is beneficial.

6. *Mold Allergens*

The production of respiratory symptoms by exposure to airborne fungi has been known since Blackley described it in the 1870s. More recently, bronchial challenges with fungal extracts have been shown to produce both the immediate and the late asthmatic response in sensitive individuals (93,94). Fungal spores are present much more abundantly in the atmospohere than is pollen and, moreover, are present in the air throughout the year. Therefore, they may be a cause for perennial symptoms, sometimes with "seasonal" exacerbations during summer and fall. Sensitization of humans with airborne fungi is difficult to estimate. Studies differ greatly on the frequency of positive skin tests to fungi (95,96). The role of fungi in causing actual respiratory symptoms is also controversial. Studies have shown no better than 50% correlation between positive skin tests and clinical symptoms (97). The allergens of fungi have been extremely difficult to standardize and study; therefore, their clinical relevance is difficult to assess. In some situations, selected nasal or bronchial challenges may establish a cause-and-effect relationship (98). Immunotherapy for mold sensitivity is wrought with problems, and there are few controlled trials to document its efficacy. In one study, immunotherapy with cladosporium extract was shown to be clinically efficacious in 22 adult asthmatics (99). In other studies conducted in a few patients, immunotherapy with alternaria extracts was shown to decrease the late asthmatic response (100) and bronchial hyperresponsiveness (14). On the other hand, side effects of mold immunotherapy have been reported to be high (101, 102). These problems make mold immunotherapy a poor therapeutic option at this time.

X. ADMINISTRATION OF IMMUNOTHERAPY

At each visit, a decision must be made whether or not the patient should receive immunotherapy and at what dose. The dose should be modified, based on a history of local or systemic reactions to the previous injections, recent or ongoing infection, or exacerbation of respiratory symptoms. In the latter case, an attempt should be made to correlate the onset of respiratory symptoms with the injections to determine if a late-phase response is occurring. Patients who have an elevated temperature, a generalized rash, or evidence of viral infection should not be given immunotherapy because they may be at increased risk of adverse reactions. Caution should also be exercised in patients whose steroid dose is being reduced.

The vial and the proper dosage are checked carefully before the injection is given. Epinephrine and resuscitation equipment should be readily available.

A physician capable of administering cardiopulmonary resuscitation should be in attendance.

A. Storage of Extracts

Extracts lose their potency when stored at room temperature (103), even intermittently during the time immunotherapy is given in an allergy office. Exposure to room temperature for 13 h/week resulted in no loss of potency at the end of 3 months, but in a significant loss after 12 months. Ten percent glycerin and 0.03% human serum albumin are both acceptable as preservatives. Phenosaline alone is not an adequate preservative. Fifty percent glycerine is excellent, but it causes unacceptable local reactions in some patients and should not be used in dilutions of extracts for injection. ϵ-Aminocaproic acid, an inhibitor of proteolytic enzymes, has been shown to be effective in preserving antigenic activity in concentrations suitable for injection (104). Freeze-dried extracts retain their potency for at least 3 years when refrigerated (4 °C) or frozen (−9 °C). Dilute extracts lose potency more rapidly than concentrated ones.

B. Method of Injection

The injection of the extract should be given using a 1-ml tuberculin syringe so that the volume of the extract can be measured precisely. It is given subcutaneously, usually over the triceps area. Aspiration should be done before the injection to ensure that the needle is not in a blood vessel. The injection site should not be massaged to avoid unduly rapid absorption of the allergen. A record should be made of the date of the injection, the dose given, and the size of the cutaneous reaction. The presence of side effects should be assessed before the patient leaves the office. The patient should stay in the office for 30 min after receiving the allergen extract.

C. Dosage

In the preparation of mixes for immunotherapy fewer than ten 1-ml aliquots of 1:10 w/v allergen extracts are used. Diluent is added to make up the final volume of 10 ml, so that the final concentration of each stock extract or mixture of cross-reacting extracts is 1:100 w/v. This is serially diluted tenfold to give extract concentrations of 1:1000 w/v, 1:10,000 w/v, 1:100,000 w/v, and 1:1 million w/v. Most patients can be started with 0.05 ml of the 1:100,000 w/v concentration. Patients who have been determined to be exquisitely sensitive may be started with the higher dilution of 1:1 million w/v. The doses are then increased according to the schedule shown in Table 3.

Table 3 Immunotherapy Schedule[a]

Vial 5 1:1,000,000 w/v (ml)	Vial 4 1:100,000 w/v (ml)	Vial 3 1:10,000 w/v (ml)	Vial 2 1:100 w/v (ml)	Vial 1 1:100 w/v (ml)
0.05	0.05	0.05	0.05	0.05
0.10	0.10	0.10	0.07	0.07
0.20	0.20	0.20	0.10	0.10
0.40	0.40	0.40	0.15	0.15
			0.25	0.20
			0.35	0.30
			0.50	0.40
				0.50

[a]The injections are started with the most dilute vial, usually no. 4 (1:100,000 w/v). The doses are progressively increased to the highest dose 0.5 ml of vial no. 1 (1:100 w/v). This is the maintenance dose.

Immunotherapy is initially given once or twice a week. Once the highest dose is attained (usually after 20–25 injections) the frequency may be decreased to once every 3–4 weeks. Fresh extracts should be prepared every year to maintain potency. When a newly made extract is started, the dose of immunotherapy should be decreased by at least one-half.

D. Grading and Management of Reactions

1. Local Reactions

1. Negative (swelling up to 20 mm; i.e., nickel size): progress according to schedule.
2. A (swelling 20–25 mm; i.e., nickel to quarter size): repeat the same dose.
3. B (swelling greater than 25 mm; i.e., quarter size): return to the last dose that caused a negative reaction.
4. C (swelling persisting more than 12 hr): decrease dose by one-half and increase cautiously.
5. Large local reactions may be treated with antihistamines and local application of ice.

2. *Systemic Reactions*

Symptoms include those of the disorder for which immunotherapy is being given and, also, can include generalized itching, urticaria, faintness, flushing, perspiration, nausea, vomiting, pallor, cyanosis, a "thick" throat, tightness of the chest, and frank collapse.

1. Mild systemic reactions (mild asthma, mild rhinitis): Reduce dosage to one-quarter of the dose that produced the symptoms. If the lower dose is well tolerated, increase dosage cautiously to tolerance.
2. Moderate to severe reactions
   a. *Treat as a medical emergency.*
   b. Place tourniquet above injection site.
   c. Inject 0.01 ml/kg to a maximum of 0.3 ml aqueous epinephrine 1:1000, subcutaneously into the arm that was not used for allergen injection. Epinephrine may be repeated at 15 to 20-minute intervals, as needed.
   d. Inject an additional 0.1 ml of epinephrine into the site of allergen injection to retard allergen absorption.
   e. Intravenous fluids and pressors may be required for the treatment of shock.
   f. Oxygen may be needed for hypoxia.
   g. Cardiopulmonary resuscitation may rarely be required for respiratory or cardiac arrest.

If a moderate to severe systemic reaction occurs, the dose of immunotherapy is reduced to one quarter of the last dosage that caused no reaction and repeated three times before increasing the dose according to schedule.

E. Missed Doses

A. If a patient who is on weekly increasing doses misses the scheduled injection by
   1. One to two weeks, increase according to schedule
   2. Three to four weeks, repeat the last dose
   3. Five to seven weeks, reduce by one dose on the injection schedule for each week over 4 weeks
   4. More than 7 weeks, restart from the beginning
B. If a patient who has been receiving monthly injections
   1. Misses an injection by 6 weeks or fewer, repeat maintenance dose

2. Misses an injection by 6–10 weeks, reduce dose by one-half and increase according to schedule

F. Refill Extract Prescriptions

New extracts should be made every year to assure potency. The first dose from a refilled prescription vial should be one-half the last dose given. The doses are then increased according to schedule.

G. Duration of Immunotherapy

It is important to reassess patients who are receiving immunotherapy periodically to determine if it is helping. This should be done at least once a year. The following guidelines are suggested (adapted from Malling; 65).

A. Subjective evaluation
   1. Symptom scores
   2. Medication scores
   3. Documentation of days off school or work
   4. Number of days hospitalized
B. Objective evaluation
   1. Physicial examination

   In an occasional patient, the following may be indicated:

   2. Skin tests
   3. Allergen-specific IgE and IgG levels in the blood
   4. Methacholine or specific allergen challenges

If, after 2 years of immunotherapy, it is clear that there is no improvement in the patient's symptoms, it should be discontinued. However, the presence of a sensitizing pet at home, noncompliance with medications, or inappropriate immunotherapy may be the reasons for failure to respond. In addition, some patients may have acquired new sensitivities. These possibilities should be investigated before discontinuing immunotherapy.

Three to five years of perennial immunotherapy may be sufficient for most patients. However, this duration is purely arbitrary, and the decision to stop should be based on assessment of the individual patient. Some of the patients who stop immunotherapy after this period continue to do well. However, others relapse (105) and need to restart their treatment.

XI. UNTOWARD REACTIONS TO IMMUNOTHERAPY

Many patients receiving immunotherapy experience significant local or systemic reactions at some point in the course of treatment (106). In one study, 4% of 26,645 injections were associated with local reactions and 0.3% with systemic reactions (106). In another study, which followed 150,000 injections administered over a 6-month period, 0.1% of the injections led to systemic reactions (107). The usual prevalence of systemic reactions per patient course is reported to be between 7 and 29% (108). Systemic reactions are more likely to occur during the early months of immunotherapy when allergen dosage is being progressively increased. They may also occur when a new vial of extract is started. The risk of systemic reactions to immunotherapy is increased in patients who have had a previous systemic reaction to immunotherapy, patients who are highly sensitive, and patients who are receiving β-blockers concomitantly. Natural pollen exposure during season may also increase the risk for systemic reactions to immunotherapy. Other causes of systemic reactions are errors in dosage, use of the wrong extracts, and inadvertent intravenous injection.

The Committee on Allergen Standardization of the American Academy of Allergy and Immunology (109) obtained information on 46 fatalities associated with immunotherapy or skin testing over a 40-year period. Complete data were available on 24 fatalities that occurred after immunotherapy. Errors in administration accounted for three deaths. Ten fatalities occurred during seasonal exacerbation of the patient's disease, among whom, four were symptomatic at the time of the injection and two were receiving β-blockers. Previous reactions to immunotherapy had occurred in four patients. Three fatalities occurred in children. One child had suffered a respiratory failure 2 months before the fatal event. One received an incorrect dose of allergen extract. The third had had a previous reaction to immunotherapy, following which, immunotherapy with a new extract, obtained from a different manufacturer, had been instituted.

Most life-threatening reactions occur within 20–30 min of allergen injection (109); however, adverse reactions may occur several hours later (110–113). The most common manifestation of the late reaction is urticaria (112,113). Respiratory symptoms (wheezing or stridor) were reported in 27% of these reactions. In all cases, respiratory symptoms were present within 60 min of the injection (112,113).

Some concerns have been expressed about the development of autoimmune disease as a result of long-term antigen stimulation in the course of immunotherapy (114). However, several studies (115–117) have shown no increase in the frequency of autoimmune or lymphoproliferative disorders and no evidence of immune complex formation or complement activation in patients on long-term immunotherapy.

Immunotherapy is associated with a small risk of potentially life-threatening complications. This must be considered before immunotherapy is offered to patients.

XII. FORMS OF IMMUNOTHERAPY

Two forms of immunotherapy, perennial and preseasonal, are used. A third form, coseasonal immunotherapy, has not yielded satisfactory results and is no longer used. In preseasonal therapy, the allergen injections are started 3–4 months before the onset of the particular pollen season. This form of immunotherapy is useful in the absence of multiple pollen sensitivities. The goal is to reach the maximum dose by the beginning of the season. Therapy is discontinued at this point until the following year. Perennial immunotherapy seems to be the best method. In this form of immunotherapy, patients are placed on a year-round maintenance schedule once the dosage has been progressively built up. This form of therapy allows the patient to tolerate a higher cumulative dose of injected allergen, resulting in greater clinical protection. The total number of injections eventually may be smaller than with preseasonal therapy. Perennial immunotherapy may be started during the pollen season, except in the exceptionally sensitive patient, when it may be advisable to wait until the pollinating season is over. The maintenance dose may be slightly reduced during pollinating season, especially in very sensitive patients.

Rush immunotherapy was described originally by Freeman (118) in hay fever patients. He gave the injections every 1½ to 2 hr throughout a 14-hr day, each dose being 10–20% higher than the last one. Maintenance dose was reached in about 2 days. In a comparison with standard immunotherapy, Bousquet and associates showed the "rush" protocol to be clinically more efficacious (119). There was no increased frequency of mild reactions with the rush protocol, and no severe systemic reactions occurred. Although not routinely used, this form of immunotherapy occasionally may find use.

XIII. MODIFIED EXTRACTS

Despite their documented efficacy and years of use, current forms of immunotherapy continue to present problems. The prolonged course, with its time commitment and expense, makes it unattractive to many patients. The risk of adverse reactions, both local and systemic, has not been eliminated; therefore, investigators have sought to modify conventional extracts.

A. Emulsions of Aqueous Extracts in Mineral Oil

The first attempts at modifying conventional extracts were designed to slow down the release of allergens from the injected site. Loveless used a water-in-oil emulsion of the aqueous extract of ragweed in a double-blind study of immunotherapy and reported improvement in 90% of the subjects, compared with 45% receiving placebo (120). A later study by Norman and co-workers, however, did not support this conclusion (121). Late local reactions, including sterile abscesses; have occurred with this form of therapy, and mineral oil has produced sarcomas in mice (122). Therefore, this method has been abandoned.

B. Alum-Precipitated Extracts

Another way of slowing absorption of injected extract is to precipitate it with aluminum hydroxide (alum). Norman et al. (123) reported similar efficacy and fewer systemic reactions when they compared alum precipitated extracts with conventional aqueous extracts. Moreover, they were able to give the equivalent dose of the crude ragweed pollen in approximately half the number of injections. Immunological responses to the two types of extracts, measured by histamine release from isolated washed leukocytes, were similar. A slightly higher frequency of more severe local reactions was noted, however. This latter observation has been confirmed by other studies (124,125). A number of these extracts are now available on the market. One drawback of using alum-precipitated extracts is that they are not available in dilute concentrations. Therefore, using more than a few allergens in a single injection is not possible.

C. Alum-Precipitated Pyridine Extracts

In an attempt to improve on alum-precipitated extracts, extraction with pyridine was added as a step before the actual alum precipitation (126). The initial report suggested that such extracts were comparably efficacious and resulted in fewer systemic reactions than aqueous extracts. However, a subsequent report did not support this conclusion (127). The pyridine extraction process apparently denatures some proteins, most notably *Amb I* (antigen E of ragweed). However, efficacy has been shown for grass extracts (30), and these may be used for immunotherapy.

D. Reducing Allergenicity of Extracts

Several attempts have been made to reduce the allergenicity of extracts while, at the same time, ensuring their immunogenicity. Of the following such extracts, polymerized extracts seem to hold the most promise.

1. Purified Allergens

One of the first attempts to achieve this goal was to remove "minor" antigens from extracts because these could potentially be responsible for the side effects seen. A clinical study (128), however, failed to show increased efficacy of a purified ragweed extract, when compared with whole extract, although the average number of systemic reactions was reduced from 1.6 per patient receiving whole extract, to 0.4 per patient receiving the purified extract (128). The purification process is prohibitively expensive. Moreover, some of the "impurities" may be clinically relevant allergens, and their removal may not be desirable.

2. Allergoids

Treatment of extracts with formalin produces allergoids. A long-term study comparing ragweed allergoid and conventional ragweed extract showed that patients treated with the allergoid could receive higher doses of allergen. The mean symptom scores were somewhat lower in this group, although there was no difference in the overall changes in specific IgE and IgG (129). In another study, 5 of 17 patients receiving allergoids developed systemic reactions, while 8 of 20 receiving conventional extracts had systemic reactions (130). Interestingly, none of these eight patients required epinephrine for their systemic reactions, whereas three of the five in the allergoid group did.

3. Photoinactivated Allergens

Irradiation of allergens with ultraviolet light was attempted in Europe (131) to cleave the allergenic determinant of the protein—the lysine sugar conjugation. A reduction of allergenicity was demonstrated by diminished skin reactivity in atopic patients and in monkeys studied by passive transfer of sensitizing antibody. Although this was shown for extracts such as house dust allergen, kapok, feather, and human dander, ultraviolet irradiation of grass pollen allergens caused only a partial reduction of allergenicity.

4. Gluteraldehyde-Treated, Tyrosine-Absorbed Allergens

Another attempt at reducing the allergenicity of allergens was to treat grass pollen extracts with glutaraldehyde and, then, to absorb them on tyrosine (132).

The incidence of systemic reactions was dramatically reduced, permitting the number of injections to be reduced as well, without impairment of clinical effectiveness. However, in a later double-blind study, 62% of the 238 subjects receiving the modified extract reported late local reactions, including two patients who reported delayed onset of generalized urticarial reactions (133).

5. *Polymerized Allergens*

A slightly different approach has been to polymerize allergens with gluteraldehyde into large molecules between 200 and 20,000 kDa. It was reasoned that (1) these large molecules would diffuse more slowly through tissues, (2) the lower molecular concentrations of the large polymers would lead to a decreased ability to bridge IgE molecules, (3) some antigenic determinants would be "concealed" within the polymeric structure and, thus, be unavailable to attach to IgE on cells. Studies have shown that this form of immunotherapy is clinically effective (134,135). Significantly fewer injections were required than with conventional immunotherapy. There were few local reactions and no systemic reactions. Increases in specific IgG antibodies were 12- to 40-fold. Studies so far have shown effectiveness for ragweed (134,135), grass (136), and tree pollens (137). However, these extracts are not available for clinical use.

E. Induction of Tolerance by Stimulation of Suppressor T Cells

Attempts have been made to induce specific tolerance in humans by using extracts that have been treated with urea, polyethylene glycol (PEG), D-glutamic acid, and D-lysine. These compounds have fostered specific unresponsiveness in several animal models, including higher species such as dogs and monkeys (35). Treatment of antigen E with urea, and injection of this extract into mice causes suppression of specific IgE production (138). A clinical trial of such an extract, however, failed to produce improvement in hay fever symptoms, although some patients had some suppression of the seasonal rise of IgE antibodies to ragweed (139). Conjugation of antigen with PEG and D-glutamic acid and D-lysine has activated antigen-specific suppressor cells in animals (140,141). Clinical trials with such extracts produced rises in specific IgG as the predominant immunological change, with an initial increase in specific IgE, followed by a blunting of the seasonal increase in specific IgE, thus mimicking the results of immunotherapy with conventional extracts (142,143).

XIV. CONCLUSION

Immunotherapy, as it is practiced today, owes its origin to a hypothesis about its mode of action, which was based on the understanding of the neutralization of bacterial toxins. This hypothesis was wrong, but immunotherapy has survived for almost 80 years because, initially, clinical observations and, later, double-blind studies have supported its efficacy. As mechanisms of immunotherapy become better understood, new approaches based on experimental evidence will be developed. These approaches hold the promise of greater safety, efficacy and convenience, fewer injections, and lower cost. These factors, along with the fact that of all therapeutic alternatives only immunotherapy addresses the underlying immune disorder, hold out the possibility that immunotherapy will still be practiced in some form 80 years from now.

REFERENCES

1. Norman, PS, Winkenwerder WL, Lichtenstein LM, Tignall J. Immunotherapy of hay fever with ragweed antigen E: comparisons with whole pollen extract and placebos. J Allergy 1968; 42:93–108.
2. Noon L. Prophylactic innoculation against hay fever. Lancet 1911; 1:1572–1573.
3. Bruun E. Control examination of the specific desensitization in asthma. Acta Allergol 1949; 2:122–128.
4. Aas K. Hyposensitization in housedust allergy asthma. Acta Paediatr Scand 1971; 60:264–268.
5. Bruce CA, Norman PS, Rosenthal RR, et al. The role of ragweed pollen in autumnal asthma. J Allergy Clin Immunol 1977; 59:449–459.
6. D'Souza MF, Pepys J. Wells ID, et al. Hyposensitization with *Dermatophagoides pteronyssinus* in housedust allergy: a controlled study of clinical and immunological effects. Clin Allergy 1973; 3:177–179.
7. Forgacs P, Swan AV. Treatment of house dust allergy: a report from the Research Committee of the British Tuberculosis Association. Br Med J 1968; 3:774.
8. Frankland AW, Augustin R. Prophylaxis of summer hay-fever and asthma: a controlled trial comparing crude grass-pollen extracts with the isolated main protein component. Lancet 1954; 1:1055–1057.
9. Johnstone DE. Study of the role of antigen dosage in the treatment of pollinosis and pollen asthma. Am J Dis Child 1957; 94:1–5.
10. Johnstone DE, Crump L. Value of hyposensitization therapy for perennial asthma in children. Pediatrics 1961; 27:39–44.
11. Johnstone DE, Dutton A. The value of hyposensitization therapy for bronchial asthma in children: a 14 year old study. Pediatrics 1968; 42:793–802.
12. Smith AP. Hyposensitization with *Dermatophagoides pteronyssinus* antigen: trial in asthma induced by house dust. Br Med J 1971; 4:204–206.

13. Taylor WW, Ohman JL, Lowell FC. Immunotherapy in cat-induced asthma: double-blind trial with evaluation of bronchial responses to cat allergen and histamine. J Allergy Clin Immunol 1978; 61:283–287.
14. Tuchinda M, Chai H. Effect of immunotherapy in chronic asthmatic children. J Allergy Clin Immunol 1973; 51:131–138.
15. Warner JO, Price JF, Soothill JF, et al. Controlled trial of hyposensitization to *Dermatophagoides pteronyssinus* in children with asthma. Lancet 1978; 2:912–915.
16. Unger L, Harris MC. Stepping stones in allergy. Ann Allergy 1974; 32:266–278.
17. Taylor G, Walker J. Charles Harrison Blackley 1820–1900. Clin Allergy 1973; 3:103–108.
18. Cooke RA. The treatment of hay fever by active immunization. Laryngoscope 1915; 25:108–112.
19. Cooke RA, Barnard JH, Hebard S, et al. Serologic evidence of immunity with coexisting sensitization in a type of human allergy (hay fever). J Exp Med 1935; 62:733–750.
20. Prausnitz C, Kustner H. Studien uber Ueberempfindlichkeit. Zentralbl Bakteriol Abt I Orig 1921; 86:160.
21. Loveless MH. Immunological studies in pollonosis: presence of 2 antibodies related to same pollen-antigen in serum of treated hay-fever patients. J Immunol 1940,38:25–50.
22. Lowell FC, Franklin W. A double blind study of the effectiveness and specificity of injection therapy in ragweed hay fever. N Engl J Med 1965; 273:675–679.
23. Norman PS, Lichtenstein LM, Tignall J. The clinical and immunologic specificity of immunotherapy. J Allergy Clin Immunol 1978; 61:370–377.
24. Lichtenstein LM, Norman PS, Winkenwerder WI. Clinical and in vitro studies on the role of immunotherapy in ragweed by hay fever. Am J Med 1968; 44:514–524.
25. Norman PS, Winkenwerder WL, Lichtenstein LM. Maintenance immunotherapy in ragweed hay fever. J Allergy 1971; 47:273–282.
26. Van Metre TE Jr, Adkinson NF Jr, Amodio FZ, et al. A comparative study of the effectiveness of the Rinkel method and the current standard method of immunotherapy for ragweed pollen hay fever. J Allergy Clin Immunol 1980; 66:500–513.
27. Cooke RA. Studies in specific hypersensitiveness IX. On the phenomenon of hyposensitization (the clinically lessened sensitiveness of allergy). J Immunol 1922; 7:219–241.
28. Sherman WB, Stull A, Cooke RA. Serologic changes in hay fever cases treated over period of years. J Allergy 1940; 11:225–244.
29. Levy DA, Lichtenstein LM, Goldstein EO, et al. Immunologic and cellular changes accompanying the therapy of pollen allergy. J Clin Invest 1971; 50:360–369.
30. Starr MS, Weinstock M. Studies in pollen allergy III. The relationship between

blocking antibody levels and symptomatic relief following hyposensitisation with allpyral in hay fever subjects. Int Arch Allergy Appl Immunol 1970; 38:514–521.
31. Zeiss CR, Metzger WJ, Levitz D. Quantitative relationships between IgE antibody and blocking antibodies specific for antigen E in patients given immunotherapy with ragweed antigen E. Clin Exp Immunol 1977; 28:250–255.
32. Platts-Mills TAE, von Maur RK, Ishizaka K, et al. IgA and IgG anti-ragweed antibodies in nasal secretions. J Clin Invest 1976; 57:1041–1050.
33. Connell JT, Klein DE. Protective effect of nasal sprays containing blocking antibody in hay fever [Abstract]. J Allergy 1970; 45:115.
34. Gleich GJ, Yunginger JW. Ragweed hay fever: treatment by local passive administration of IgG antibody. Clin Allergy 1975; 5:79–87.
35. deWeck AL. New approaches to desensitization in IgE-mediated allergy. Clin Immunol Allergy 1985; 5:1–11.
36. Aalberse RC, van der Gaag R, van Leeuwen J. Serologic aspects of IgG_4 antibodies I. Prolonged immunization results in an IgG_4-restricted response. J Immunol 1983; 130:722–726.
37. van der Giessen M, Homan WL, van Kernebeek G, et al. Subclass typing of IgG antibodies formed by grass pollen-allergic patients during immunotherapy. Int Arch Allergy Appl Immunol 1976; 50:625–640.
38. Kaliner M, Lemanske R. Inflammatory responses to mast cell granules. Fed Proc 1984; 43:2846–2851.
39. Dolovich J, Hargreave FE, Chalmers R, et al. Late cutaneous allergic responses in isolated IgE-dependent reactions. J Allergy Clin Immunol 1973; 52:38–46.
40. Solley GO, Gleich GJ, Jordon RE, et al. The late phase of the immediate wheal and flare skin reaction: its dependence upon IgE antibodies. J Clin Invest 1976; 52:38–46.
41. Pepys J, Hutchcroft BJ. Broncial provocation tests in etiologic diagnosis and analysis of asthma. Am Rev Respir Dis 1975; 112:829–859.
42. Robertson DG, Kerigan AT, Hargreave FE, et al. Late asthmatic responses induced by ragweed pollen allergen. J Allergy Clin Immunol 1974; 54:244–254.
43. Naclerio RM, Proud D, Togias AG, et al. Inflammatory mediators in late allergen-induced rhinitis. N Engl J Med 1985; 313:65–70.
44. Gleich GJ. The late phase of the immunoglobulin E-mediated reaction: a link between anaphylaxis and common allergic disease? J Allergy Clin Immunol 1982; 70:160–169.
45. Behrens B, Clark R, Marsh W, et al. Modulation of the late asthmatic response by antigen-specific immunoglobulin G in an animal model. Am Rev Respir Dis 1984; 130:1134–1139.
46. Pienkowski M, Norman PS, Lichtenstein LM. Suppression of late phase skin reactions by immunotherapy with ragweed extract. J Allergy Clin Immunol 1985; 76:729–734.
47. Jerne NK. The generative grammar of the immune system. Science 1985; 229:1057–1059.

48. Blaser K, deWeck AL. Regulation of the IgE antibody response by anti-idiotype network. Prog Allergy 1982; 32:203–227.
49. Malley A, Dresser DW. Anti-idiotype regulation of timothy grass pollen IgE antibody formation I. In vivo induction of suppressor T cells. Immunology 1982; 46:653–659.
50. Bose R, Marsh DG, Duchateau J, et al. Demonstration of auto–anti-idiotypic antibody cross reacting with public idiotypic determinants in the serum of rye-sensitive allergic patients. J Immunol 1984; 135:2474.
51. Castracane JJ, Rocklin RE. Detection of human auto-anti-idiotypic antibodies (Ab2). I. Isolation and characterization of Ab2 in the serum of a ragweed immunotherapy-treated patient. Int Arch Allergy Appl Immunol 1988; 86:288–294.
52. Canonica GW, Mingari MC, Milioli G, et al. Imbalances of T cell subpopulations in patients with atopic diseases and effect of specific immunotherapy. J Immunol 1979; 123:2669–2671.
53. Rocklin RE, Sheffer AL, Greineder DK, et al. Generation of antigen-specific suppressor cells during allergy desensitization. N Engl J Med 1980; 302:1213–1219.
54. Nagaya H. Induction of antigen-specific suppressor cells in patients with hay fever receiving immunotherapy. J Allergy Clin Immunol 1985; 75:388–394.
55. Tamir R, Castracane JM, Rocklin RE. Generation of suppressor cells in atopic patients during immunotherapy that modulate IgE synthesis. J Allergy Clin Immunol 1987; 79:591–598.
56. Lichtenstein LM, Norman PS, Winkenwerder WL, et al. In vitro studies of human ragweed allergy: changes in cellular and humoral activity associated with specific desensitization. J Clin Invest 1966; 45:1126–1136.
57. Melam HL, Pruzansky JJ, Patterson R. Correlations between clinical symptoms, leukocyte sensitivity, antigen-binding capacity and Prausuitz–Kustner activity in the longitudinal sutdy of ragweed pollinosis. J Allergy 1970; 46:292–299.
58. Naclerio RM, Meier HL, Kagey-Sobotka A, et al. Mediator release after nasal challenge with allergen. Am Rev Respir Dis 1983; 128:597–602.
59. Creticos PS, Adkinson NF Jr, Kagey-Sobotka A, et al. Nasal challenge with ragweed pollen in hay fever patients. Effect of immunotherapy. J Clin Invest 1985; 76:2247–2253.
60. Robertson DG, Kerigan AT, Hargreave FE et al. Late asthmatic responses induced by ragweed pollen antigen. J Allergy Clin Immunol 1974; 54:244–254.
61. Norman PS, Lichtenstein LM, Ishizaka K. Diagnostic tests in ragweed hay fever. A comparison of direct skin tests, IgE antibody measurements, and basophil histamine release. J Allergy Clin Immunol 173; 52:210–224.
62. Connell JT, Sherman WB. Hay fever symptoms related to immunological findings. Ann Allergy 1967; 25:239–250.
63. Durham OC. Coopertive studies in ragweed pollen incidence: atmospheric data from 22 cities. J Allergy 1929; 1:12–21.

64. Hyde HA, Williams AJ. Studies of atmospheric pollen: diurnal variation in the incidence of grass pollinosis. New Physol 1945; 44:83–93.
65. Malling HJ. Immunotherapy: position paper. Eur Acad Allergol Clin Immun 1988; 43:1–33.
66. Metzger WJ, Turner E, Patterson R. The safety of immunotherapy during pregnancy. J Allergy Clin Immunol 1978; 61:268–272.
67. Baer H, Godfrey H, Maloney CJ, et al. The potency and antigen content of commercially prepared ragweed extracts. J Allergy 1970; 45:347–354.
68. Gleich GJ, Larson JB, Jones RT, et al. Measurement of the potency of allergenic extracts by their inhibitory capacities in the radioallergosorbent test. J Allergy Clin Immunol 1974; 53:158–169.
69. Aas K, Beckman A, Belin L, et al. Standardization of allergen extracts with appropriate methods. Allergy 1978; 33:130–137.
70. Creticos PS, Norman PS. Why are standardized extracts necessary? Clin Rev Allergy 1986; 4:355–361.
71. Kohler G, Milstein C. Continuous cultures of fused cells secreting antibody (with) predefined specificity. Nature 1975; 256:495–497.
72. Krilis S, Blado GA, Basten A. Standardization of allergens: lectins and monoclonal antibodies as primary standards for house dust mite allergen. Int Arch Allergy Immunol 1981; 66:252–258.
73. Baldo BA. Standardization of allergens. Examination of existing procedures and the likely impact of new techniques on the quality control of extracts. Allergy 1983; 38:535–546.
74. Krilis S, Baldo BA, Raison RL, et al. Standardization of antigen E in ragweed pollen extracts using a monoclonal antibody based enzyme immunoassay. J Allergy Clin Immunol 1983; 71:261–265.
75. Chapman MD. Allergen specific monoclonal antibodies: new tools for the management of allergic disease. Allergy 1988; 43:7–14.
76. Allergenic Products Advisory Committee. Allergenic products advisory committee recommends category II classification for housedust extracts. [News and Notes]. Am Acad Allergy Immunol 1986; Winter:13.
77. Solomon WR, Mathews KR. Aerobiology and inhalant allergen. In: Middleton E Jr, Reed CE, Ellis EF, et al., eds. *Allergy: principles and practice*. St Louis, CV Mosby, 1988:312–372.
78. van Bronswijk JE, Sinha RH. Pyroglyphid mites (acari) and house dust allergy. J Allergy 1971; 47:31.
79. Collins-Williams, C, Hung F, Brenner K. House dust mite and mite allergy. Ann Allergy 1976; 37:12.
80. Tovey ER, Chapman MD, Platts-Mills TAE. Mite faeces are a major source of house dust allergens. Nature 1981; 289:592–593.
81. Krilis S, Baldo BA, Basten A. Antigens and allergens from the common house dust mite *Dermatophagoides pteronyssinus*. II. Identification of the major IgE binding antigens by crossed radioimmunoelectrophoresis. J Allergy Clin Immunol 1984; 74:142–146.

82. LeMao J, Dandeu JP, Rabillon J, et al. Comparison of antigenic and allergenic composition of two partially purified extracts from *Dermatophagoides farinae* and *Dermatophagoides pteronyssinus* mite cultures. J Allergy Clin Immunol 1983; 71:588–596.
83. Osterballe O. Immunotherapy with grass pollen major allergens. Clinical results from a prospective 3-year double blind study. Allergy 1982; 37:379–388.
84. Viander M, Koivikko A. The seasonal symptoms of hyposensitized and untreated hay fever patients in relation to birch pollen counts: correlations with nasal sensitivity, prick tests and RAST. Clin Allergy 1978; 8:387–396.
85. Rynes SE. Critical analysis of animal dander reactions. J Allergy 1937; 8:470–474.
86. IUIS Subcommittee for Allergen Nomenclature. Allergen nomenclature. Bull WHO 1986; 64:767.
87. Ohman JL, Findlay SR, Leitermann KM. IT in cat-induced asthma. Double blind trial with evaluation of in vivo and in vitro responses. J Allergy Clin Immunol 1984; 74:230–239.
88. Viander M, Valovista E, Vanto T, et al. Cross reactivity of cat and dog allergen extracts. Int Arch Allergy Appl Immunol 1983; 71:252–260.
89. Blands J, Lowenstein H, Weeke B. Characterization of extract of dog hair and dandruff from six different dog breeds by quantitative immunoelectrophoresis: identification of allergens by crossed radioimmunoelectrophoresis (CRIE). Acta Allergol 1977; 32:147–169.
90. Bucus J, Breborg S, Einarsson R, et al. Immunotherapy with dog and cat allergen preparations in dog-sensitive and cat-sensitive asthmatics. Ann Allergy 1989; 62:355–361.
91. Kang B. Study on cockroach antigen as a probable causative agent in bronchial asthma. J Allergy Clin Immunol 1976; 58:357–365.
92. Kemp B, Vallody D, Homburger H, et al. Cockroach cause of allergic asthma: its specificity and immunologic profile. J Allergy Clin Immunol 1979; 63:80–86.
93. Itkin IH, Dennis M. Bronchial hypersensitivity to extract of *Candida albicans*. J Allergy 1966; 37:187–194.
94. Pepys J. Hypersensitivity diseases of the lungs due to fungi and organic dusts. Mongr Allergy 1969; 4:147.
95. Hilsby J. Allergy to molds in Sweden: a botanical and clinical study. Acta Allergol 1949; 11:57.
96. Pennington ES. Study of the incidence of air-borne molds and of skin sensitivity to molds. South Med J 1940; 33:931–939.
97. Ordman D. The regional aspects of respiratory allergy in South Africa. S Afr Med J 1964; 38:369–372.
98. Lehrer SB, Aukurst l, Salvaggio JE. Respiratory allergy induced by fungi. Clin Chest Med 1983; 4:23–41.
99. Malling HJ, Dreborg S, Weeke B. Diagnosis and immunotherapy of mould allergy V. Clinical efficacy and side effects of immunotherapy with *Cladosporium herbarum*. Allergy 1986; 41:507–519.

100. Metzger WJ, Donnelly A, Richerson HB. Modification of the late asthmatic responses (LAR) during immunotherapy for alternaria-induced asthma [Abstract]. J Allergy Clin Immunol 1983; 71:119.
101. Kaad PH, Ostergaard PA. The hazard of mould hyposensitization in children with asthma. Clin Allergy 1982; 12:317–320.
102. Osergaard RA, Kaad PH, Kristensen T. A prospective study on the safety of immunotherapy in children with severe asthma. Allergy 1986; 41:588–593.
103. Nelson HS. The effect of preservatives and conditions of storage on the potency of allergy extracts. J Allergy Clin Immunol 1981; 67:64–69.
104. Van Hoeyveld EM, Lejoly M, Walravens MJ, et al. Analysis of the stabilizing effect of epsilon amino caproic acid by electrophorectic techniques and immunoblotting. J Allergy Clin Immunol 1989; 83:601–609.
105. Patterson R, Lieberman P, Irons J et al. Immunotherapy. In: Middleton E, Reed CE, Ellis EF, eds. Allergy: principles and practice. 1978; 2:1119–1142.
106. Nelson BL, Dupont LA, Reid MJ. Prospective survey of local and systemic reactions to immunotherapy with pollen extracts. Ann Allergy 1986; 56:331–334.
107. Vervloet D, Khairallah E, Arnaud A, et al. A prospective national study of the safety of immunotherapy. Clin Allergy 1980; 10:59–64.
108. Levy DA. Hazards and adverse reactions associated with the administration of allergenic extracts. In: Brede HD, Going H, eds. Regulatory Control and Standardization of Allergenic Extracts. New York: Gustav Fischer Verlag, 1980:179.
109. Lockey RF, Benedict LM, Turkletaub PC, Burkantz SC. Fatalities from immunotherapy and skin testing. J Allergy Clin Immunol 1987; 79:660–677.
110. Fizley KD. The continuous method of hay fever treatment. J Allergy 1931; 2:39.
111. Levine ML. Systemic reactions to immunotherapy [Abstract]. J Allergy Clin Immunol 1979; 63:209.
112. Greenberg MA, Kaufman CR, Gonzalez GE. Late and immediate systemic allergic reactions to inhalant allergen immunotherapy. J Allergy Clin Immunol 1986; 77:865–870.
113. Greenberg MA, Kaufman CR, Gonzalez GE, et al. Late system-allergic reactions to inhalant allergen immunotherapy. J Allergy Clin Immunol 1988; 82:287–290.
114. Phanuphak P, Kohler P. Onset of polyarteritis nodosa during allergic hyposensitization treatment. Am J Med 1980; 68:479–485.
115. Stein MR, Brown GL, Lima JE, et al. A laboratory evaluation of immune complexes in patients on inhalant immunotherapy. J Allergy Clin Immunol 1978; 62:211–216.
116. Levinson AI, Summers RJ, Lawley TJ, et al. Evaluation of the adverse effects of long term hyposensitization. J Allergy Clin Immunol 1978; 62:109–114.
117. Katelaris CH, Walls RS. A study of possible ill effects from prolonged immunotherapy in the treatment of allergic diseases. Ann Allergy 1984; 53:257–261.
118. Freeman F. Rush innoculation. Lancet 1930; 1:744.
119. Bousquet J, Guerin B, Dotte A, et al. Comparison between rush immunotherapy

with a standarized allergen and an alum adjuved pyridine extract material in grass pollen allergy. Clin Allergy 1985; 15:179–193.
120. Loveless MH. Respository immunization in pollen allergy. J Immunol 1957; 79:68–79.
121. Norman PS, Winkenwerder WL, D'Luboff BC. Controlled evaluations of repository therapy in ragweed hay fever. J Allergy 1967; 39:82–92.
122. Factsheet. Carcinogenic potential of mineral oil. Washington, DC: US Department of Health, Education and Welfare, Food and Drug Administration, 1967.
123. Norman PS, Winkenwerder WL, Lichtenstein LM. Trials of alum-precipitated pollen extracts in the treatment of hay fever. J Allergy Clin Immunol 1972; 50:31–44.
124. Rudolph R, Staud RT, Kunkel G, et al. Semi-depot hyposensitization in severe hay fever: its clinical effectiveness and the therapeutic problems. (A four year study using intranasal challenge testing to monitor success.) Allergol Immunopathol 1978; 6:133–152.
125. Frost L, Johansen P, Pedersen S, et al. Persistent subcutaneous nodules in children hyposensitized with aluminum-containing allergen extracts. Allergy 1985; 40:368–372.
126. Fuchs AM, Strauss MB. The clinical evaluation and the preparation and standardization of suspensions of a new water-insoluble whole ragweed pollen complex. J Allergy 1959; 30:66–82.
127. Reisman RE, Arbesman CE. Clinical studies of two new ragweed preparations: "purified" delta and allpyral. Int Arch Allergy 1965; 28:353–365.
128. Lichtenstein LM, Norman PS, Winkenwerder W. A single year of immunotherapy for ragweed hay fever: immunologic and clinical studies. Ann Intern Med 1971; 75:663–671.
129. Norman PS, Marsh DG, Lichtenstein LM. Long term immunotherapy with ragweed allergen and allergoid [Abstract]. J Allergy Clin Immunol 1979; 63:167.
130. Norman PS, Lichtenstein LM, Kagey-Sobotka A, et al. Controlled evaluation of allergoid in the immunotherapy of ragweed hay fever. J Allergy Clin Immunol 1982; 70:248–260.
131. Berrens L, Henocq E, Radermecker M. Photo-inactivated allergen I. Preparation, physiochemical and biological properties. Clin Allergy 1973; 3:449–459.
132. Johansson SG, Miller AC, Mullan N, et al. Glutaraldehyde–pollen–tyrosine: clinical and immunological studies. Clin Allergy 1974; 4:255–263.
133. Metzger WJ, Dorminey HC, Richerson HB, et al. Clinical and immunologic evaluation of glutaraldehyde-modified tyrosine-absorbed short ragweed extract. A double blind, placebo controlled trial. J Allergy Clin Immunol 1981; 68:442–448.
134. Hendrix SG, Patterson R, Zeiss CP, et al. A mutli-institutional trial of polymerized whole ragweed for immunotherapy of ragweed allergy. J Allergy Clin Immunol 1980; 66:486.
135. Grammer LC, Zeiss CR, Suszko IM, et al. A double-blind, placebo-controlled

trial of polymerized whole ragweed for immunotherapy of ragweed allergy. J Allergy Clin Immunol 1982; 69:494–499.

136. Grammer LC, Shaughnessy MA, Suszko IM, et al. A double-blind histamine placebo-controlled trial of polymerized grass for immunotherapy of grass allergy. J Allergy Clin Immunol 1983; 72:448–453.

137. Patterson R, Suszko IM, Grammer LC. Polymerization of individual species of tree pollen allergens. Int Arch Allergy 1984; 73:1–4.

138. Ishizaka K, Okudaira H, King TP. Immunogenic properties of modified antigen E II. Ability of urea-denatured antigen and alpha-polypeptide chain to prime T-cells specific for antigen E. J Immunol 1975; 114:110–115.

139. Norman PS, Ishizaka K, Lichtenstein LM, Adkinson NF Jr. Treatment of hay fever with urea-denatured antigen E. J Allergy Clin Immunol 1980; 66:336–341.

140. Lee W-Y, Sehon AH. Abrogation of reaginic antibodies with modified proteins. Nature 1977; 267:618–619.

141. Liu F, Katz DH. Immunological tolerance to allergenic protein determinants: a therapeutic approach for selective inhibition of IgE antibody production. Proc Natl Acad Sci USA 1979; 76:1430.

142. Juniper EF, O'Connor J, Roberts RS, et al. A two year study of Pegalgen (a polyethylene glycol modified ragweed extract) in ragweed rhinoconjunctivitis [Abstract]. J Allergy Clin Immunol 1983; 71:119.

143. Norman PS, King TP, Alexander JF Jr, et al. Immunologic responses to conjugates of antigen E in patients with ragweed hay fever. J Allergy Clin Immunol 1984; 73:782–789.

6

The Nose

Brian K. Flowers and Robert M. Naclerio
The Johns Hopkins University School of Medicine, Baltimore, Maryland

I. INTRODUCTION

As a major portal for air between the internal and external environments, the human nose developed into an efficient air-conditioning organ. Control of temperature, humidification, and filtration of particulate matter from inspired air represent its major functions. The latter property led to the development of local immunological functions, which serve as a first-defense system against inspired pathogens. Olfaction, although less important to humans than to lower mammals, warns of environmental hazards, complements the perception of taste, and enhances social interactions. Despite these varied homeostatic and protective functions, the clinical manifestations of nasal diseases are primarily congestion, rhinorrhea, and sneezing.

Because an understanding of nasal structure and function is essential to the physician treating allergic rhinitis and other diseases of the upper airways, this chapter begins by describing basic nasal embryology, anatomy, and physiology. Next, the pathophysiology of allergic rhinitis is presented as a preclude to a discussion of its evaluation and treatment. Finally, complications of allergic rhinitis will be presented. This chapter provides a concise overview of the nose in health and disease.

II. EMBRYOLOGY OF THE UPPER RESPIRATORY SYSTEM

The embryological development of the fetal face recapitulates the stages of evolution of water-breathing vertebrates to air-breathing mammals. In primitive fish, the nasal organ exists only as blind sacs, the sole function of which is olfaction. In more developmentally advanced fish, such as the shark, a channel connecting each olfactory pit and the mouth occurs, permitting sampling of water before entering the mouth. The development of the human nasal cavity reiterates these evolutionary stages (1).

During the fourth week of human development, the formation of the nasal cavities begins with the appearance of a pair of ectodermal thickenings located on each side of the frontal prominence, just above the stomodeum (Fig. 1), known as the olfactory, or nasal, placodes. During the fifth week of development, these placodes descend, forming the floor of the nasal pits. Each pit is surrounded by a U-shaped elevation, with its opening located caudally at the stomodeum. The medial and lateral aspects of the nasal placodes are the medial and lateral nasal processes, respectively. The large frontal process separates the two nasal pits and, with its underlying mesenchyme, forms a broad primitive nasal septum. At this stage of development, with the nasal cavities completely separated from the oral cavity, the human fetus resembles primitive fish (1).

As the nasal pits deepen and approach the ectoderm of the oral cavity, the bucconasal membrane is formed. Simultaneously, the paired lateral maxillary processes move medially, fusing with the lateral nasal process. The nasal pits move medially, overshadowing the intervening frontal process. The result is paired external nares with the cavities posteriorly covered by the thin bucconasal membrane. During the seventh week, the bucconasal membrane ruptures, yielding two openings into the anterior part of the oral cavity, the primitive choanae (Fig. 2C). This arrangement, the nares opening into the anterior oral cavity, parallels that seen in some sharks and in amphibians (1,2).

The primary palate, which becomes the medial palatine process toward the close of the second month, is a triangular area in the midline formed by the mesenchyme deep to the union of the medial nasal and frontal processes (see Fig. 2A). The base of this triangle lies posterior to the developing upper jaw, whereas the apex lies between the two bucconasal membranes. Continuous with this primary palate is the nasal septum located above and slightly dorsally. The medial palatine process forms the anteromedial portion of the definitive secondary palate. The lateral palatine processes, deep to the maxillary processes, form the remainder of the secondary palate. The lateral palatine processes, appearing along the sides of the oral cavity, extend inferomedially to lie at either side of the tongue. As the tongue descends during the seventh week, the lateral palatine processes migrate upward and medially, fusing with each other in the midline, and with the medial palantine process anteriorly (Fig.

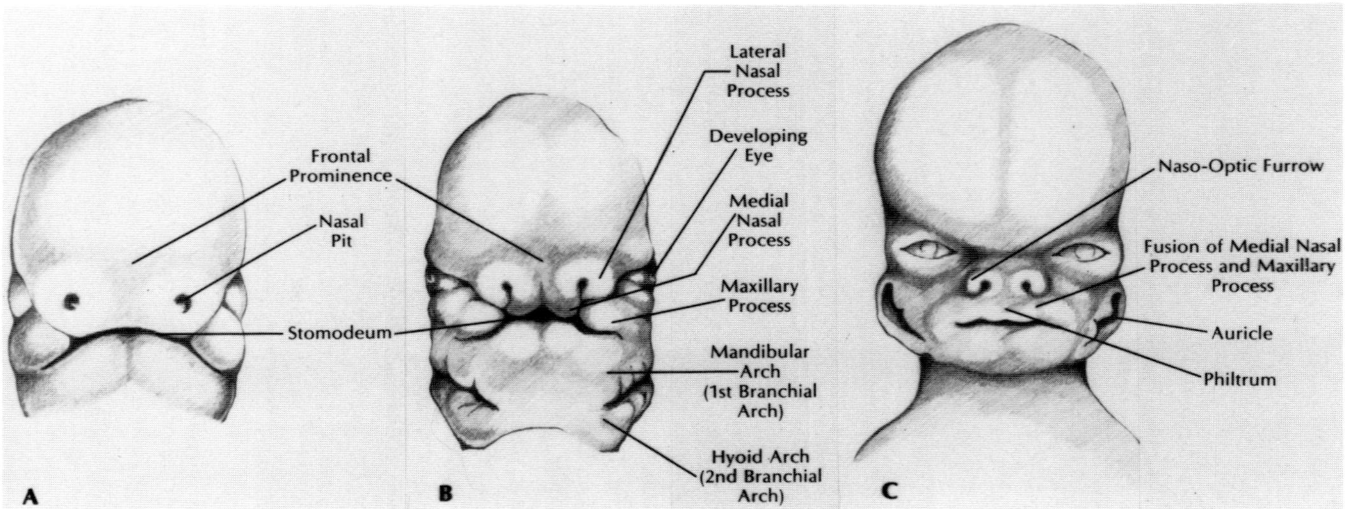

Figure 1 Frontal view, showing development of the fetal face at (A) 4–5 weeks, (B) 5–6 weeks, and (C) 7–8 weeks.

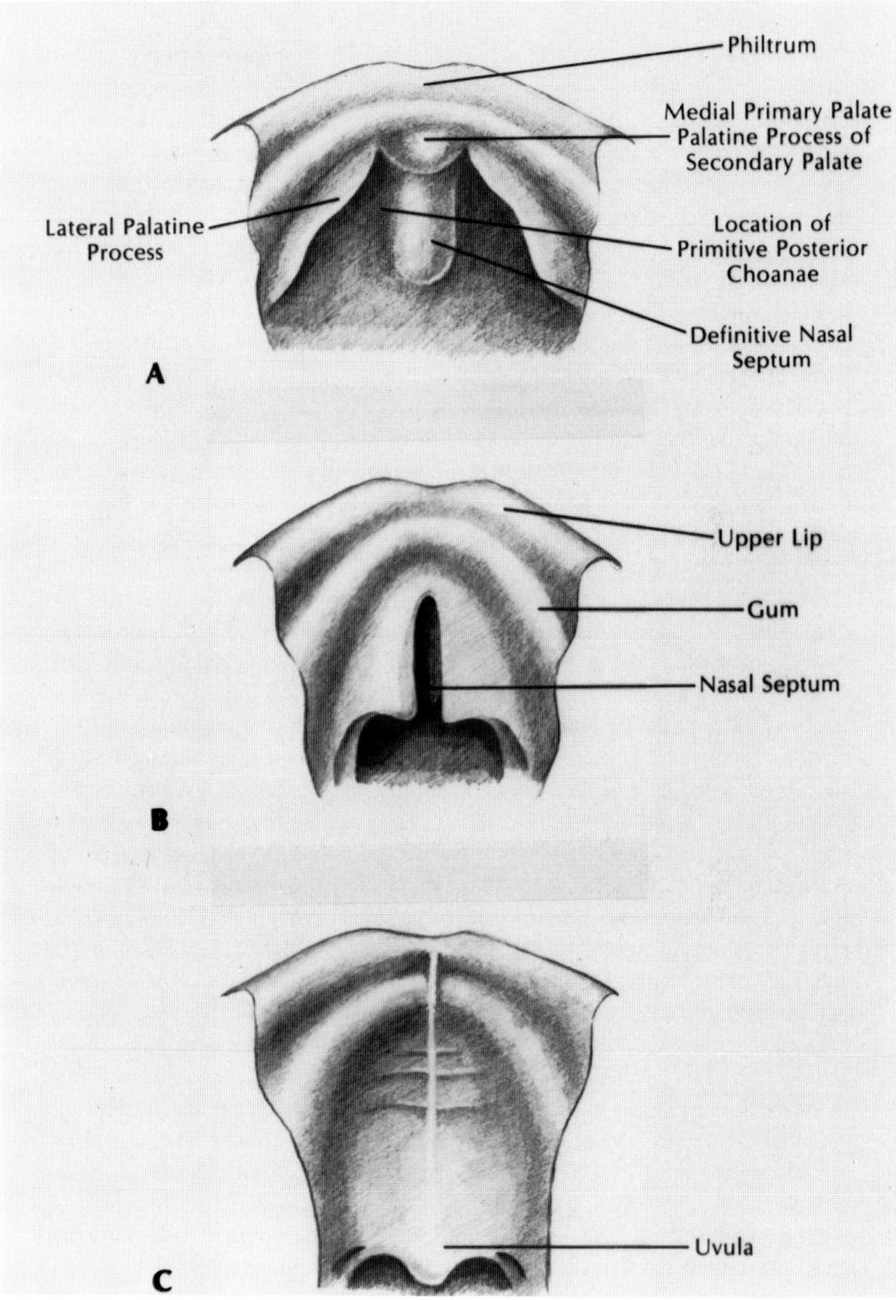

Figure 2 Ventral view, showing development of the secondary palate at (A) 6–7 weeks, (B) 7–8 weeks, and (C) 8–9 weeks. Note that the lateral palatine processes fuse in the midline in an anteposterior direction as the nasal septum fuses with the palate in the dorsal midline.

2B). Simultaneously, the nasal septum grows toward the cephalic face of the secondary palate in a posterior direction. Thus, by the end of the 11th week, the separation of the right and left nasal chambers from each other and from the oral cavity is complete.

The nasal conchae, or turbinates, scroll-like outcroppings from the lateral aspect of the mature nasal cavities, first appear as linear outgrowths of the lining epithelium (2). Cartilage initially supports the fetal conchae, but later ossifies to form the thin turbinate bones. The inferior turbinate, the largest, forms first. Above the inferior turbinate, a series of five ethmoidal turbinates develop each one smaller than the one below. The inferiormost of these forms the middle concha, and the second and third merge to form the superior concha. The upper two ethmoidal turbinates generally undergo regression, but occasionally remain as a supreme concha. The turbinates greatly increase the surface area of the nasal cavities.

Given the complicated development of the nasal structures, congenital abnormalities of nasal development are surprisingly rare. In the pediatric patient with nasal symptoms, particularly nasal obstruction, a few disorders of development should be considered. Choanal atresia is believed to result from failure of the bucconasal membrane to disintegrate during the fourth week of fetal life (3). It may be unilateral or bilateral and either membranous (10%) or bony (90%) (4). Unilateral choanal atresia, the most common form, may remain asymptomatic beyond the neonatal period. The patient usually has persistent unilateral nasal discharge. In the obligate nose-breathing neonate with unilateral choanal atresia, however, obstruction of the contralateral nasal cavity from an upper respiratory infection may cause respiratory distress. Complete bilateral choanal atresia, in contrast, presents as a respiratory emergency at birth. Initial management necessitates an oropharyngeal airway, with definitive surgical management deferred to a later date. Less common causes of congenital obstruction are also seen. Dermoid cysts and sinuses of the nose, usually present as enlarging masses in the midline of the nasal dorsum, cause nasal obstruction (5). Nasal encephaloceles are extrusions of meningeal-lined brain matter that communicate freely with the intracranial ventricular system and subarachnoid space. Most encephaloceles present externally, although 30% are intranasal, and 10% both intra- and extranasal (4). Nasal gliomas also present with nasal obstruction. Similarly to the encephalocele, development of a glioma results from faulty closure of the anterior neuropore. They often arise from the lateral nasal wall and may be confused with nasal polyps (6).

Malformations of the nasal structure occur. Complete or partial nasal agenesis, clefts, and facial dysostosis have been reported and are typically seen in combination with a cleft lip (6). The cleft lip–nose deformity is characterized by the triad of nasal tip deformity, dorsal displacement of the nasal dome, and buckling of the alar cartilage (4). Although these are quite devastating to the patient and family, they usually do not present a diagnostic dilemma to the physician.

III. ANATOMY AND PHYSIOLOGY

A. External Nose

The external nose is a pyramidal structure with its base at the facial skeleton and its apex projecting anteriorly (Fig. 3). The two nasal bones at the superior portion of the base articulate medially with one another, superiorly with the frontal bone, and laterally with the frontal processes of the maxilla. Inferiorly, the apex of the nose is formed by two pairs of nasal cartilages. The upper lateral nasal cartilages attach to the nasal bones and extend caudally. They articulate with one another in the midline and provide the shape of the middle third of the external nose. The lower lateral (alar) cartilages, shaped as an inverted U with a medial and a lateral crus, are located in the inferior portion

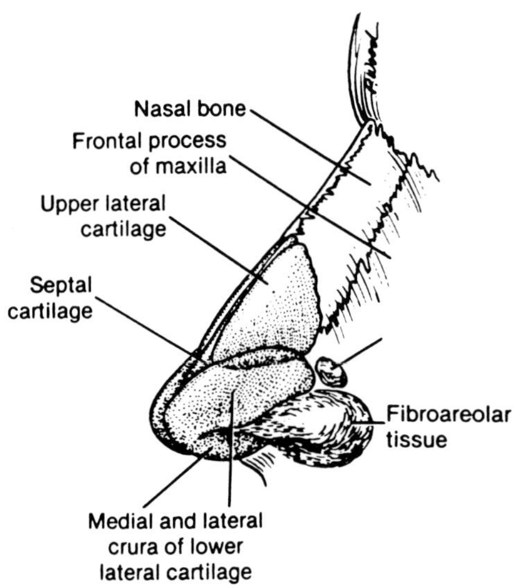

Figure 3 Lateral view of the nasal skeleton. (Adapted from Graney DO, Anatomy. In Cummings CW, Frederickson JM, Krause CJ, Schuller DE, eds. *Otolaryngology–head and neck surgery*. St. Louis CV Mosby, 1986:513–526.)

of the external nose. The two medial crura articulate in the midline, forming the columella. The lateral crus gives structure to the alae of the nose and maintains the patency of the nasal vestibule (7).

Small muscle groups contribute to the shape and function of the external nose (Fig. 4). The procerus extends from the frontalis muscle to the nasal bones and elevates the skin over the dorsum of the nose. The nasalis muscle extends lateral from the alae and functions to depress the nares. The anterior and posterior dilator naris, the depressor septi, and the levator labii superioris alaeque nasi all function to dilate the nostrils, decreasing nasal resistance (8).

B. Vestibule

Air enters each nasal cavity through the vestibule. The vestibule differs from the remainder of the nasal cavity in that it is lined by stratified squamous epithelium, its innervation and blood supply enter from the surrounding face,

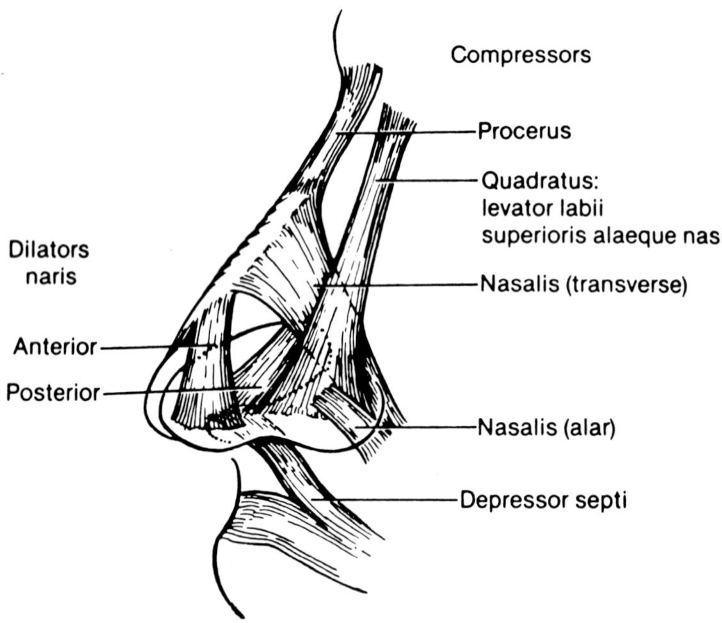

Figure 4 The muscles of the external nose. (Adapted from Graney DO. Anatomy. In Cummings CW, Frederickson JM, Krause CJ, and Schuller DE, eds. *Otolaryngology—head and neck surgery*. St. Louis CV Mosby, 1986:513–526.)

and it contains hairs known as vibrissae. The vibrissae, which are associated with sebaceous glands, but are devoid of erector pili muscles, function to filter out large particulate matter (9). The ducts that carry the serous secretions of the anterior nasal glands enter near the junction of the squamous and columnar epithelium. Forced inspiration, as in sniffing, atomizes these secretions (10).

The most important aspect of the vestibule is the nasal valve, which causes approximately half of the total resistance to inspired airflow from ambient air to alveolus (11). Its structure arises from the butterfly-shaped lower lateral cartilages. Contraction of the dilator nares muscle, innervated by the facial nerve, increases the cross-sectional area (8), permitting increased airflow. Strohl (12) found a rhythmic increase in tone of this muscle just before the onset of inspiration. The structure of the nasal valve directs inspiratory air upward past the middle turbinate, where air reaches its greatest velocity before curving in a horizontal direction through the main part of the nasal cavity (Fig. 5) (13). With maximum inspiratory effort, airflow plateaus when transnasal pressures exceed approximately 10 cm H_2 (14). To achieve flows greater than 20–30 1/min, individuals switch to oronasal breathing.

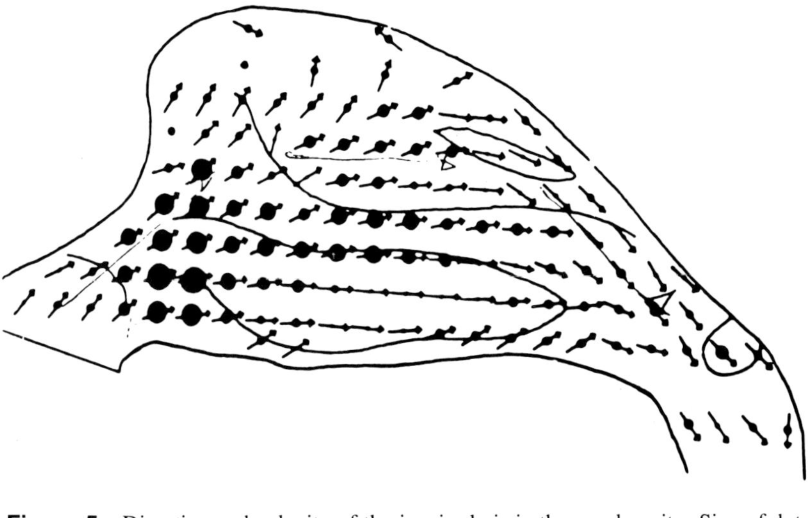

Figure 5 Direction and velocity of the inspired air in the nasal cavity. Size of dots indicates relative velocity. (From Proctor DF, Andersen IB. *The nose—upper airway physiology and the atmospheric environment*. Amsterdam Elsevier Biomedical, 1982.)

C. Septum

The nasal septum consists of an anterior cartilaginous portion formed by the quadrilateral cartilage and a posterior bony portion formed by the vomer and perpendicular plate of the ethmoid. The septum divides the nasal cavity into two separate compartments, increasing the total mucosal surface area. Additionally, the cartilaginous portion provides support for the nasal tip.

Structural deviations of the septum alter the pattern of airflow. Likewise, weakening of the cartilage, such as occurs following a septal abscess, lessens support to the nasal tip and the nasal valve, thus compromising airflow (15).

D. Turbinates

The lateral nasal wall projects three, and occasionally four, turbinates into the nasal cavity: the inferior, middle, superior, and supreme turbinates (Fig. 6). The inferior and middle turbinates are of the most functional significance. Each consists of a bony structure, usually lined with pseudostratified columnar epithelium, similar to that lining the tracheobronchial tree (16). The turbinates

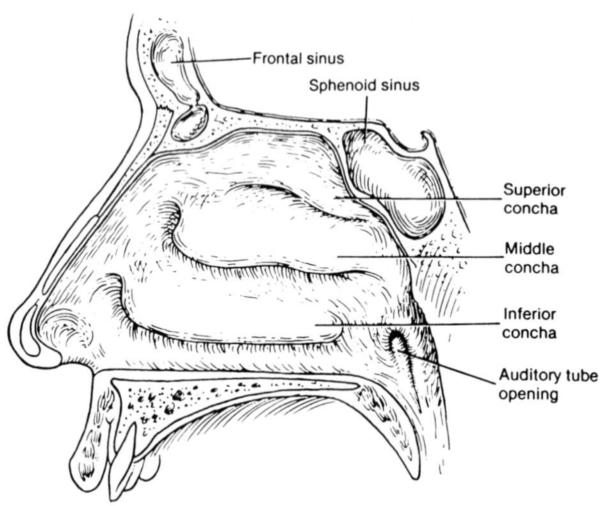

Figure 6 View of the lateral wall of the nasal cavity. (Adapted from Graney DO. *Anatomy*. In Cummings CW, Frederickson JM, Krause CJ, Schuller DE, eds. *Otolaryngology—head and neck surgery*. St Louis. CV Mosby, 1986:513–526).

increase the mucosal surface of the nasal cavity to approximately 100–200 cm^2 (13).

In health, the total nasal airway resistance remains relatively constant, but the airflow of each nasal cavity varies in a reciprocal fashion, (i.e., as the flow in one nasal cavity increases, the flow in the other decreases). This alteration in airflow reflects changes in vascular engorgement of the turbinates and is known as the nasal cycle, first reported by a German rhinologist, Kayser, in the late 19th century (17). It occurs in 80% of normal volunteers (8,19). The reason for this cycling is unknown.

E. Histology

The nasal mucosa (Fig. 7) consists of a subepithelial and submucosal layer covered by pseudostratified columnar epithelium containing goblet cells, nonciliated columnar cells with microvilli, and, occasionally, intraepithelial mast cells (20). The cilia, 5-μm cellular projections, are composed of a shaft covered with the cell membrane (Fig. 8). The shaft, or axoneme, primarily consists of microtubules arranged as nine peripheral doublets surrounding two central singlets. Nexin links connect adjacent pairs of doublets, and each doublet is connected to the central tubules by spokes. Each doublet has two dynein arms, which contain the ATPase, providing the energy of motion (21). The epithelial goblet cells produce apocrine-type secretions that contribute to the mucous blanket (22). The epithelial cells themselves provide both a protective barrier and produce inflammatory substances (23) and the secretory portion of IgA (24).

The submucosa, or lamina propria, is separated from the epithelial layer by a basement membrane and contains primarily nerves, blood vessels, and tuboalveolar glands. During inflammatory reactions, circulating cells enter the interstitium of the submucosa. However, unlike the gut and bronchial mucosa, the nasal mucosa does not routinely contain lymphoid aggregates (25). The B and T cells found in the nasal mucosa arrive from the bloodstream after generation in the palatine, lingual, and nasopalatine tonsils. The tonsils thus function similarly to the lymphoid aggregates in the bronchi and gut.

F. Mucus

A mucous blanket, 10–15 μm deep, covers the entire nasal cavity (26). It consists of a sol and a gel phase, with the gel phase being closest to the air. The mucus traps particles and gases, effectively filtering and removing nearly 100% of particles larger than 4 μm in diameter (27–30). Water-soluble gases, such as formaldehyde and carbon dioxide, dissolve in the mucus (31–33). Besides filtration, the mucous layer provides water for humidification.

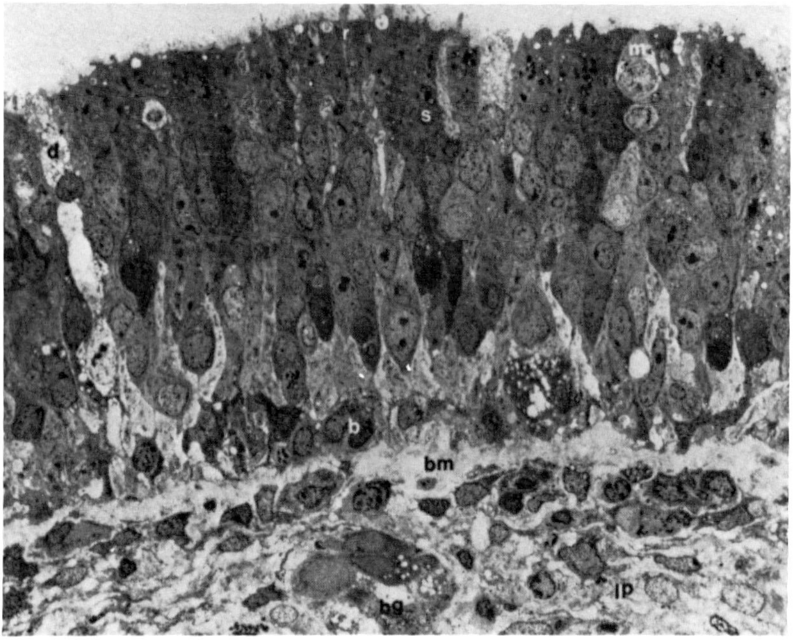

Figure 7 High-power (original magnification × 1500, toluidine blue stain) light photomicrograph of nasal respiratory epithelia showing goblet cell (G), ciliate cell (C), intermediate cell (I) and basal cell (B). [From Jafek BW (20).]

Estimates of daily nasal mucous production range from 0.1 to 0.3 mg/kg per day (34). Part of the nasal secretions comes from the approximately 40,000 tuboalveolar glands in the submucosa. Here, serous glands predominate over the mucous glands by 8:1 (22). One of the glandular products is mucin, a unique glycoprotein of extremely large size (2.3×10^6 Da). A polypeptide backbone constitutes 10–20% of its total structure, with the rest of the molecule containing oligosaccharide side chains (35,36). The interaction of these side chains with water, 95% of mucus by weight, produces a matrix, which gives mucus its negative charge and its ability to lubricate and protect mucosal surfaces. Although large, mucin represents only a small portion of the total protein content of mucus (37,38). Other components of mucus include immunoglobulins of the IgA (39,40), IgG (40), and IgE (41) classes, histamine (42), albumin (43) bacteria (44), lactoferrin (40), lysozyme (45), ions (46), and cells (47).

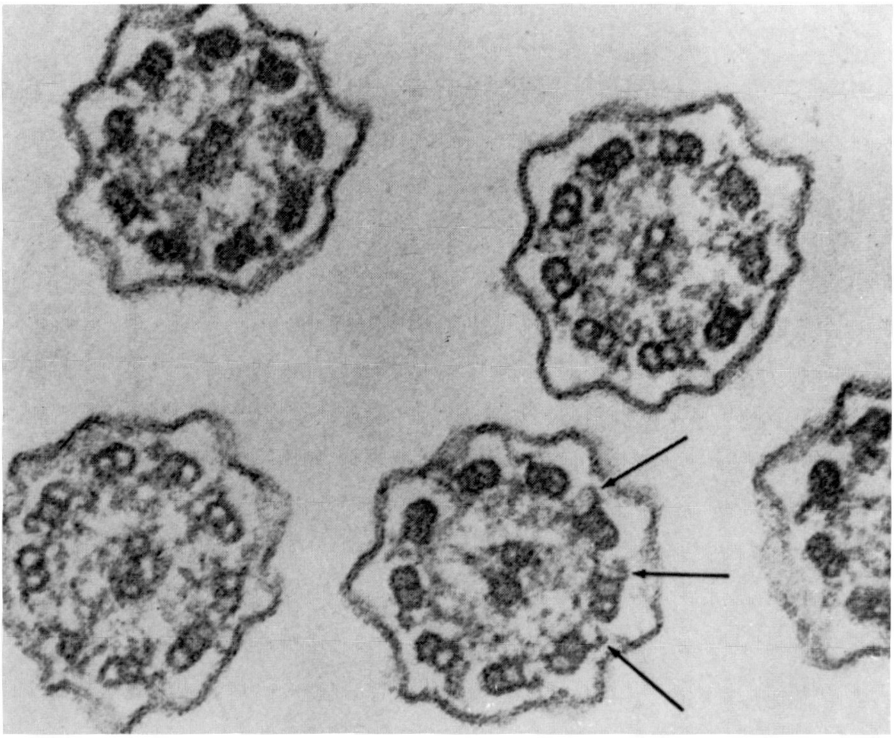

Figure 8 High-power electron micrograph of respiratory cilia (original magnification × 145,300). Radial spokes connect the A microtubules to the central sheet. Dynein arms (arrows) project from the A microtubule. [From Jafek BW (20).]

G. Mucociliary Transport

Mucus and the ciliated epithelial cells function together in mucociliary transport. Mucus and its contents move toward the nasopharynx, except from the anterior inferior turbinate, where transport is anteriorly. Anderson and colleagues showed that cilia transported radiolabeled particles an average of 6 mm/min, with a range of 1–20 (48). Thus, it takes about 10–20 min to clear inhaled particles from the nasal cavity (Fig. 9). Clearance of mucus can be aided by sniffing, sneezing, and nose blowing (49).

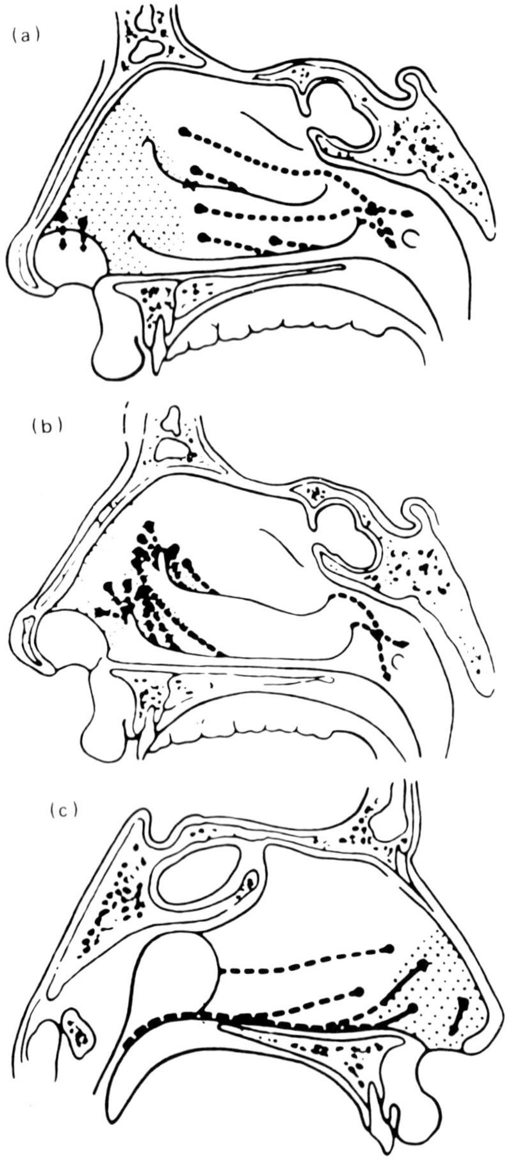

Figure 9 Pattern of mucociliary transport in the nose. (a) The course of the lateral wall ciliated are (clear area) and most anterior aspect of the nasal cavity. (b) The course from the lateral wall nonciliated area (stippled area). (c) The course of transport on the nasal septum. (From Hilding AC *Arch Environ Health* 1963;6:61–73.)

Cilia move in a characteristic manner. During the recovery phase, they bend and move in the sol layer. During the effector stroke they straighten, contacting the gel phase, thus moving the mucus in only one direction (Fig. 10; 50). Videofluoroscopic techniques can be used to study cilia beat frequency (approximately 1000 beats/min) and motion (21). This dynamic evaluation provides the functional counterpart to structural abnormalities seen ultrastructurally. Besides congenital structural abnormalities, such as with Kartagener's syndrome, in which the cilia are deficient in the number of outer dynein arms (51), mucociliary transport can be altered alter viral infections (52). Disorders of ciliary movement present clinically with pooled secretions on the floor of the nasal cavity.

The composition of mucus also affects the rate of mucociliary transport (53,54). Pharmacologic agents can likewise alter the composition of mucus and affect clearance. Guafenesin decreases the viscosity of respiratory secretions, thereby conceptually, providing more effective clearing of secretions, both by mucociliary transport and sneezing (55). Similarly, circulating iodide stimulates nasal glands to produce a low-viscosity, water secretion that increases the beat frequency of mucosal cilia (56). The efficacy in humans of potassium iodide and guafenesin has not been proved in controlled studies. Anticholinergic agents increase the viscosity of secretions, thereby decreasing clearance (57).

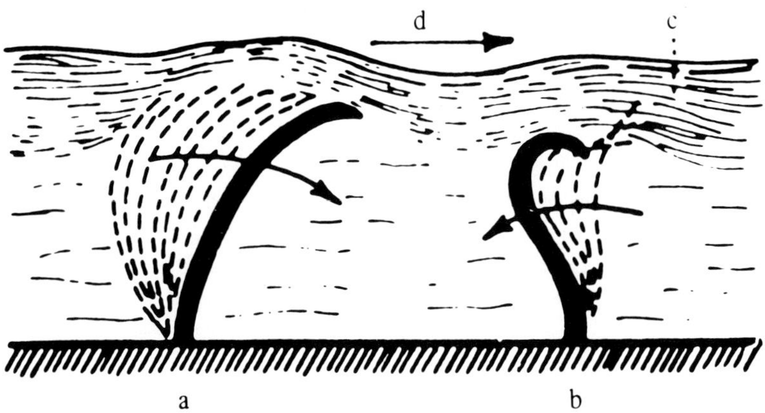

Figure 10 Schematic drawing of the movement of a cilium through (a) the effector stroke and (b), the recovery stroke. The mucous blanket (c) thus moves in only one direction (d). (From Proetz AW (50).]

Mucociliary transport functions over a wide range of environmental conditions. In normal subjects, the nose can change inspired air from 9% to nearly 100% relative humidity by the time it reaches the nasopharynx. Despite the water loss encountered by breathing air at 9% relative humidity for 72 hr, normal individuals show no change in mucociliary clearance, partly because heat and water are conserved when warm, moist air condenses as it moves past a cooling gradient during expiration (58).

H. Nasal Vasculature

Both the internal and external carotid circulations contribute to the arterial supply of the nasal cavity (9). The anterior and posterior ethmoidal arteries, branches of the ophthalmic artery, enter the nose after passing through the orbit and the lamina papyracea. The sphenopalatine artery, a terminal branch of the external carotid artery, enters the nose through the posterior lateral inferior wall. These vessels anastamose with branches of the facial artery in the cartilaginous septum of the vestibule. This area is the most common site of epistaxis (59). The veins of the nasal cavity run adjacent to the arteries and drain into the pterygoid and ophthalamic venous plexi, with some of the venous drainage subsequently passing intracranially into the cavernous sinus (9).

The arteries supplying the subepithelial and glandular zones arise from the perichondrial and periosteal arteries. They ascend toward the surface, giving branches to the cavernous plexi before forming a subepithelial network of fenestrated capillaries (60). The fenestrations face the respiratory surface and are believed by Cauna to be the major source of fluid for humidification (61).

Alteration in blood flow into the cavernous sinusoids of the inferior turbinate, middle turbinate, and the septum regulates nasal airflow (9). The tone of the vessels in the arteriovenous anastomosis and venous drainage regulate the amount of blood in this valveless plexus. Changes in the size of the cavernous sinusoids also occur with recumbency (62), with elevated levels of inspired carbon dioxide (63), and with changes in inspired temperature (64,65). Vascular engorgement within the sinusoids presents clinically as nasal congestion.

Pharmacologic studies suggest the presence of α, β, cholinergic, histamine, and hormone receptors on blood vessels. α-Adrenergic agents cause vasoconstriction in both the arteries and the cavernous plexus (66,67). Phentolamine, an α-adrenergic antagonist, blocks α-induced vasoconstriction (68). Nasal administration of β-agonists causes vasodilatation and some increase in watery secretions (66). Parasympathomimetics, such as methacholine induce water secretions and vasodilatation (69). Ipratropium, an anticholinergic, completely blocks the watery secretions induced by methacholine, but not the vasodilatation (70). Histamine, administered topically, causes vasodilatation, an increase in vascular permeability, an increase in glandular secretion, and sneezing or a tickling sensation (71). Premedication with H_1-antagonists blocks the symptoms associated with histamine stimulation, with the exception of nasal congestion, which appears to be partially blocked by the addition of an H_2-antagonist (72). The nasal vasculature appears to be four times more sensitive to circulating epinephrine than the heart (73). Changes in the levels of circulating hormones during pregnancy can cause rhinitis, which clears postpartum (74). Sexual excitement (34), hypothyroidism (75), and emotional stress (76) also affect the nasal vasculature. The physiological role of adrenergic and cholinergic agents in the normal control of nasal secretions is not certain.

I. Nervous System

Neuronal control plays a major role in the local regulation of airflow, blood flow, and glandular secretion. Reflexes originating within the nose have distal effects (e.g., sneezing). After irritation of a sensory receptor (to date, only mechanical and pain receptors have been identified in the nasal mucosa (77), the sneeze propagates one or more spasmodic inspirations. The glottis and velopharyngeal aperture close, allowing an increase in lower airway pressure. These structures suddenly open, allowing a blast of air to escape through the nose and mouth, in an attempt to clear the nasal passage (78). This reflex occurs with viral infection (79), irritants (80), exposure to allergens (42) and, in some individuals, after exposure to bright light (81). The latter exemplifies afferent sensory innervation into the nasal cavity.

Neuronal stimulation originating within the nose can affect function elsewhere. Mucosal irritation can initiate the submersion reflex, marked by apnea, glottic closure, bradycardia, and vasoconstriction (80,82,83), in an attempt to protect the heart and brain by redistributing blood flow to these vital organs (84). In contrast, cooling of the skin causes nasal vasoconstriction (64).

A nasopulmonary reflex has been hypothesized to explain a relationship between events occurring in the upper and lower airways. Sercer suggested the existence of such a reflex after he observed that blowing air into one nostril induced expansion of the ipsilateral thorax (85). In another study (86), bronchoconstriction occurred in individuals who had silica dust blown into their nose and, in one subject who had previously undergone a unilateral trigeminal nerve resection, bronchoconstriction occurred only when dust was blown through the neurologically intact side (87). Other investigators, however, have been unable to confirm nasopulmonary reflex (88,89).

Fibers of the parasympathetic and sympathetic nervous systems enter the nose through the sphenopalatine foramina. The parasympathetic fibers originate in the superior salivary nucleus of the midbrain and then travel with the fibers of the seventh cranial nerve. At the geniculate ganglion in the temporal bone, these fibers separate to form the greater superficial petrosal nerve. These fibers traverse the floor of the anterior cranial fossa and the pterygomaxillary space and synapse in the sphenopalatine ganglion. From this point, parasympathetic fibers distribute to mucosal and submucosal appendages through the vidian nerve (90,91). Stimulation of the parasympathetic nerves induces both glandular secretions and vasodilatation, effects that occur after nasal challenge with cholinergic agents (70). Sympathetic fibers originate in the hypothalamus. These fibers synapse in the superior cervical ganglion and then travel with the carotid plexus until they join the parasympathetic fibers in the vidian nerve (92). The sympathetic fibers, in contrast with the parasympathetic do not synapse in the sphenopalatine ganglion. Stimulation of the sympathetic system causes vasoconstriction with a concomitant decrease in nasal airway resistance (93). Exercise stimulates the sympathetic system, causing an increase in nasal airflow, which can be blocked by an anesthetic injection into the superior cervical ganglion (94). Reserpine, an antihypertensive agent that blocks sympathetic innervation, induces nasal congestion (95).

In addition to the classic cholinergic and adrenergic innervation, the nerve supply to the nose also consists of a nonadrenergic, noncholinergic (NANC) system. The NANC nerves, first described in the gastrointestinal tract, have subsequently been found in the lung and upper respiratory system (96). The neurotransmitters of the NANC system may be neuropeptides, such as vasoactive intestinal peptide (VIP), substance P, neurokinins, and calcitonin gene-related peptide. An increase in VIP immunoreactive nerves has been reported in the nasal mucosa of patients with vasomotor rhinitis (97,98). Although the pathophysiological role of this system is unclear, further understanding should lead to therapeutic advances.

J. Olfaction

The roof of the nasal cavity and the area extending inferiorly for 8–10 mm along the septum and lateral nasal wall is the olfactory area. Sniffing brings air into this part of the nasal cavity. The olfactory epithelium contains bipolar neurons from the first cranial nerve, the most peripheral portion of the central nervous system (20). Little is known of the mechanisms of differentiation and recognition. In recent years, odorant-binding proteins have been identified, which act as specific receptors for odorant molecules (99). These binding proteins help transport the lipophilic odorant molecule through the hydrophilic mucus to the olfactory epithelium (100). Although better developed in lower mammals, humans use the sense of smell to perceive taste, to warn of impending hazards, and for social interactions.

K. Lymphatics

Lymphatics from the two vestibuli drain toward the external nose, whereas those of the nasal fossae drain toward the nasopharynx. Two main collecting trunks, one in the olfactory region that communicates with the subarachnoid space, and one parallel to this system located inferiorly, compose the main source of drainage. The trunks flow above and below the eustachian tube orifice. Their first eschulean lymph nodes are the lateral retropharyngeal nodes, which cannot be palpated (101). This pattern explains the rare observation of lymphodenopathy with isolated rhinitis and sinusitis.

IV. PATHOPHYSIOLOGY OF THE ALLERGIC NASAL RESPONSE

In an effort to recreate his symptoms of allergic rhinitis, Blackley, in the 19th century, inhaled pollen grains. This recognition of pollen as the cause of the signs and symptoms of allergic rhinitis—sneezing, nasal congestion, and conjunctival itching (102)—was the first major understanding of the pathophysiology of this disease. Since that time, a number of laboratories have developed increasingly sophisticated means for studying allergic rhinitis in vivo (42,103–105).

The next major contribution was the discovery of IgE (106). Immunoglobulin E antibodies attach to the surface of mast cells. Upon exposure to antigen, the IgE antibodies cross-link, activating these cells to release a host of inflammatory mediators (107). Within minutes after challenge of an allergic individual with antigen, increases are detected in the levels of histamine (42), kinins (43), plasma and glandular kallikrein (108,109), mast cell tryptase (108,110), prostaglandin D_2 (PGD_2) (42), leukotriene C_4 (LTC_4) (111,112), leukotriene B_4 (LTB_4) (112,113), and major basic protein (MBP) (114) (Fig. 11). Concurrently, patients note rhinorrhea, congestion and nasal itching, and experience sneezing.

Because the immediate anaphylactic release of mediators from mast cells does not entirely explain the clinical disease, investigators have attempted to understand the inflammatory events occurring hours after mast cell activation. Following the early reaction, symptoms and the levels of mediators detected

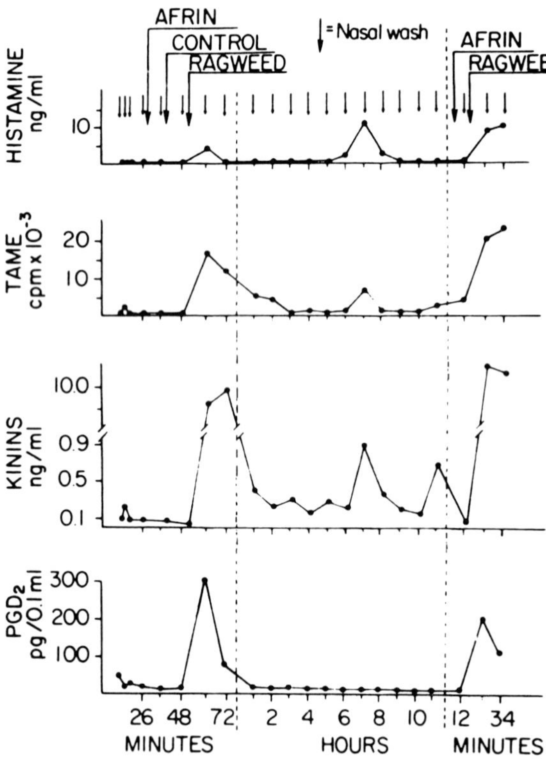

Figure 11 An example of mediator release by an allergic individual after nasal challenge with ragweed extract. In this example, the patient was challenged with a second dose of antigen 11 hr after the initial challenge. Large arrows represent administration of medication or challenge. Vertical lines represent nasal lavages. TAME represents TAME-esterarse activity. [From Naclerio RM, et al; (115).]

in nasal lavage fluid subside, and the patients enter a clinically quiescent phase. In some individuals, symptoms spontaneously recur 3–11 hr after the initial challenge, with a concomitant increase of mediators (115). This response, known as the late-phase response, has been the subject of intense study. Late responses follow antigen challenge of the skin (116), lung (117,118) and eye (119).

In a study of 55 patients with ragweed hay fever and positive intradermal skin tests, 93% had an early response and 44% had a late response to ragweed pollen (12). The late-phase response was associated with an increase in the levels of histamine, tosyl arginine methyl ester (TAME)-esterase activity (enzymes capable of generating kinins), albumin, kinins, LTC_4, LTB_4, and MBP (113–115,121). Kinin levels during the late-phase response were elevated over controls, but tended to be significantly lower than those during the immediate response (115), whereas MBP levels were much higher in the late-phase response than in the early response (114). Most striking, however, was the increase in the level of histamine, without an increase in PGD_2, during the late response (see Fig. 11). Mast cells, not basophils, generate PGD_2 (122). These facts suggest that mast cells were activated in the early response, whereas basophils release histamine in the late response.

Alcian blue-positive cells, approximately 1% of the total cells, significantly increased in both percentage and in total number during the late-phase response, compared with the prechallenge numbers. By morphological criteria, at least 68% of these cells are basophils (47), and their number correlates with histamine levels in the late-phase response. Pretreatment with topical steroids blocked increase in alcian blue cells and the late increase in histamine (47). These observations support the role of the basophil as the source of histamine in the late-phase response.

"Basophilic cells" are present in nasal secretions obtained during symptomatic seasonal pollen exposure (123,124). The origin of these cells, either mast cells or basophils, and their function remain obscure. Ultrastructural (125) and light microscopic (125–127) studies of the basophilic cells in allergic secretions suggest that most of these cells are identical with blood basophils. In contrast, nasal mucosal scrapings (126–128) and biopsies (127,129) detect preponderantly mast cells. Ultrastructural studies, furthermore, suggest two distinct subpopulations of mast cells: one located in the epithelium and one located deeper, in the lamina propria (130). The clinical severity of allergic rhinitis correlates positively with the number of epithelial mast cells (124,128). Subjects without allergies, on the other hand, have no, or significantly fewer, basophilic cells in the nasal secretions and significantly fewer mast cells in the mucosa (126,127). An increase in epithelial mast cell numbers after exposure to antigen in vivo and during the natural pollinosis season has been reported (128). Pipkorn and Enerback (129), however, found a migration of tissue-bound mast cells, from the mucosal connective tissue stroma to the mucosal surface, with no change in the total number of these cells. The shift in location could make subjects more sensitive to subsequent exposure.

A number of eosinophil characteristics indicate a significant participation of this cell type in allergic rhinitis. Eosinophils increase in nasal secretions after antigen provocation, initially within 1–2 hr, reaching a peak in 4–6 hr

(47). Systemic or localized tissue eosinophilia occurs hours after immediate hypersensitivity reactions in the skin (131), lung (132), and nasal mucosa (133). The increase of MBP, the primary constituent of eosinophil granules, in the nasal late-phase response to antigen challenge, concordant with an increase in the number of eosinophils (134), indicates that these cells are activated and play a role in the pathogenesis of this response. Furthermore, the decrease in the number of eosinophils in the late-phase response after topical and systemic steroid treatment (47,114), accompanied by a decrease in symptoms, suggests a role of this cell in the late phase. Although the precise role of the eosinophil in the late-phase response is unclear, one might hypothesize that damage to the mucosa or basement membrane by MBP (135) allows increased presentation of antigen to submucosal cells.

Eosinophils and basophils are not the only cells to increase in number during late-phase reactions. Neutrophils and mononuclear cells also increase, but their precise role is less well characterized.

The existence of a priming response, an augmented response to a second antigen challenge given hours after an initial antigen challenge, may better model the repetitive challenges that occur during the allergy season. Connell (136) challenged ragweed-sensitive subjects with ragweed pollen on 4 successive days and found that the dose of pollen necessary to create symptoms decreased over fivefold by the fourth day. He subsequently found that this increased responsiveness was not antigen-specific, was a transient phenomenon, and occurred with environmental exposure during the natural pollen season (105). Other studies (137,138) confirm the work of Connell. Associated with increased clinical sensitivity are increased levels of histamine, TAME-esterase activity, and kinins (138). This increase in mediators could result, at least in part, from the stimulation of additional target cells arriving as part of an inflammatory cell influx. Activation of basophils, for example, would be expected to result in increased levels of histamine. Interestingly, PGD_2 levels increase only on the third of 3 days of successive challenge, whereas other mediators increase from the second day. Because basophils do not release PGD_2 (122), the lack of increase of this mediator further supports the possibility that basopohils are responsible for the augmentation in histamine release. The increase in PGD_2 on the third challenge day may reflect the migration of a subpopulation of mast cells to the nasal mucosa, as is seen during the natural pollen season (129). Release of MBP after activation of eosinophils indirectly or directly by low-affinity IgE receptors (139) may also have an effect on the rechallenge reaction. Another potential, and not mutually exclusive, explanation of priming is increased reactivity of end organs (i.e., an equivalent amount of mediator release induces greater symptomatology). The latter could explain the increase in nonspecific reactivity often described by patients during seasonal exposure.

In summary, after antigen stimulation, mediators are released from tissue mast cells in allergic individuals. It appears that the nasal reaction to antigen challenge does not end with the early response, dominated by mast cell activation. Basophils, eosinophils, and other cells are recruited to the nasal mucosa, where they contribute to the late-phase and priming response. In the treatment of allergic rhinitis, therapies that prevent the influx and activation of these cells are most efficacious.

V. EVALUATION OF ALLERGIC RHINITIS IN THE PEDIATRIC POPULATION

A. History

A careful history is essential. Begin by defining the onset of illness, with particular emphasis on the temporal relationship to life events (e.g., change in school or locale, acquiring a pet, trauma). Were other symptoms, such as wheezing or urticaria, present during the initial presentation? Define current symptoms as to the characteristic of secretions (clear versus purulent), the presence or absence of pain, itching or sneezing (very characteristic of atopic disease), degree of airflow obstruction, duration of symptoms, exacerbating factors (irritants and cold air), and seasonal patterns. Inquiry into the sense of smell aids in determining the degree of airflow obstruction. Severe nasal obstruction decreases the sense of smell, which is usually perceived as a loss of taste. Ocular symptoms associated with allergic rhinitis include conjunctival itching, tearing, injection and edema of the eyelids and periorbital area. Questions should be directed at disturbances of sleep. Snoring frequently is seen with nasal obstruction, but apnic episodes may be a sign of sleep apnea and its sequelae. Children may also be noted to have paroxysmal nocturnal coughing spells and to awaken in the morning complaining of sore throat and fatigue. Halitosis as a complaint by the parent may indicate infection. The history should detail previous treatments. Patients easily discuss prescription medications used, but infrequently mention over-the-counter preparations, such as aspirin or topical medications. A family history of allergic diathesis as well as details of the environmental history (type of home heating, presence of humidification, chemical exposures) are important components of the initial history.

B. Physical Examination

A complete ear, nose, and throat examination is essential for all patients complaining of nasal symptoms. Examination of the ears may show unilateral or bilateral otitis media with effusion. Although this disorder may be associated with allergic rhinitis (140), it is most frequently associated with infection. Tenderness over the sinuses may reflect an underlying infection, whereas numbness raises suspicion of a tumor. The nasal examination begins with the external face. Perennial nasal obstruction, whether mechanical or functional in origin, may present with a black or blue discoloration beneath the lower eyelids, related to chronic periorbital edema secondary to venous stasis (141). Chronic nasal obstruction is thought to cause underdevelopment of the zygoma, nasal processes, and maxillary sinuses, resulting in the flattened "adenoid facies" (142). The classicially described "allergic salute," in which the patient attempts to relieve nasal itching and obstruction by pushing the nasal tip upward with the palm of the hand may, after a period of years, result in a transverse groove at the proximal nasal tip (143). Structural deviations or asymmetry should raise suspicion of trauma or congenital deformities.

After examining the external nares, use a nasal speculum to examine the anterior third of the nasal cavity. Although classic descriptions of the nasal mucosa exist in textbooks, personal experience has found no consistent physical finding to rule in allergic rhinitis. Rather, the examination rules out other potential causes of similar nasal symptoms. Unilateral signs, particularly purulent drainage, should raise suspicion about foreign bodies. Pooling of secretions under the inferior turbinate hints at immotile cilia syndrome.

Applying a topical decongestant permits better visualization of the deeper portions of the nasal cavity. Lateral to the anterior portion of the middle turbinates lie the openings to the frontal, maxillary, and anterior ethmoidal sinuses. Nasal polyps usually originate in this area. A slow or absent response to a decongestant indicates a hyperplastic nasal mucosa. In children, the contribution of the adenoids to nasal obstruction must be appreciated. Most children over 5 years of age will permit an endoscopic examination of view the nasopharynx. Rarely, a unilateral choanal atresia may be noted. Examination of the oral cavity may reveal a high arched, V-shaped palate with poor dental occlusion related to chronic mouth breathing. Posterior cervical lymphadenopathy may signal adenoiditis, whereas tonsillar infections relate to jugular digastric lymph nodes.

C. Diagnostic Tests

Diagnostic tests confirm the diagnosis of allergy or rule out other causes in the differential diagnoses. Skin testing with suspected allergens and in vitro testing of a patient's serum for specific IgE antibodies are widely employed. A thoughtful plan takes into account the likely possibilities based on a thorough history, as opposed to the routine ordering of all possible antigens. Positive results must always be viewed in association with the history.

Historically, the most widely used method of identifying the specific offending allergen in a patient with allergic rhinitis is by skin testing. The basic principle of the test is that sensitized (i.e., containing IgE antibodies against specific allergens) mast cells in the patient's skin release histamine and other mediators in response to a dilute solution of the relevant allergen. A positive result, marked by a localized wheal-and-flare reaction, tests several components of the allergic response: IgE, mast cell releasibility, metabolism of mediators, and end-organ sensitivity. As with any test, there are advantages and disadvantages. The skin test is the most sensitive means of making a diagnosis, is inexpensive, gives an immediate answer, and is not affected by levels of specific IgG or total IgE. On the other hand, children do not always tolerate the multiple needle punctures, and the skin test may be affected by dermatological conditions or systemic drug administration. Besides being the historical gold standard, skin testing correlates best with seasonal disease (144,145).

In vitro measurements of IgE antibodies to document allergy occurred soon after its discovery in the 1960s. Measurement of total serum IgE in a patient with allergic disease provides relatively little information (146). Extremely low levels tend to exclude allergic disease, whereas extremely high levels indicate a hyper-IgE syndrome. The development of the radioallergosorbent test (RAST), enabled the quantification of allergen-specific IgE antibodies in a patient's serum (147). A highly significant correlation exists between RAST scores and the results of skin testing (148). The RAST, however, measures only one component of the allergic diathesis (i.e., specific IgE). It detects IgE antibodies to pollens, molds, animal dander, insect venoms, drugs, and foods. In comparison with skin testing, RAST is more expensive, takes more time to obtain results, and is less sensitive, but it eliminates some of the disadvantages of skin tests. In particular, it requires only one venipuncture. As with skin testing, screen patients only for allergens considered to be potentially relevant by clinical history. The indiscriminate ordering of multiple tests not only increases the cost to the patient, but also increases the likelihood of obtaining a false-positive result.

Since the introduction of the RAST test into clinical practice, a number of other in vitro tests have been developed to measure specific IgE. The multiple allergosorbent test (MAST) measures total and specific IgE for multiple antigens using autoradiography and densitometry (149). The LAST, or latex allergosorbent test, utilizes antigen-coated latex particles to bind specific IgE. The bound IgE is subsequently digested by pepsin, and agglutination by latex-bound antihuman Fc is quantitiated (150). Monoclonal anti-IgE and binding of a fluorescent substrate characterize the FAST, or fluorescent allergosorbent test (151). Although each of these tests is purported to have advantages over the traditional RAST, none has been shown to be more sensitive than traditional in vivo testing.

When evaluating infants and small children, remember that the synthesis of specific IgE antibodies requires prior exposure. For instance, pollens remain airborne only for short periods each year. A 1-year-old child has experienced only several months of pollen exposure; hence, pollens rarely cause problems in children under 5 years of age. In contrast, perennial allergens, such as foods, pets, and dust, present more prolonged exposure.

Whereas skin testing and in vitro measurement confirm the diagnosis of allergic rhinitis, other miscellaneous tests may help. Nasal smears can identify eosinophils, pointing to an allergic problem or nonallergic rhinitis with eosinophilia syndrome (NARES). Pulmonary function testing detects asthma. Sinus radiographs evaluate for the presence of infection. Plain sinus radiographs in children under 2 years of age are extremely difficult to interpret. Computed tomography (CAT) scans, and possibly magnetic resonance imaging (MRI) scans, are more definitive (152). A complete blood cell count (CBC) and quantitative immunoglobulins, particularly IgA levels and IgG subclasses, in children may indicate confounding immunological defects.

D. Differential Diagnosis

Infections, foreign bodies, neoplasms, drug reactions, anatomical abnormalities, congenital abnormalities, and nonallergic and allergic rhinitis must all be considered in the differential diagnosis of a child presenting with nasal congestion or rhinorrhea. Upper respiratory infections are the entity most frequently confused with allergic rhinitis, and patients with allergic rhinitis often present to the physician complaining of a persistent cold. Clear rhinorrhea and itching favors a diagnosis of allergic rhinitis.

Mechanical nasal obstruction, whether from a foreign body, nasal polyps, choanal atresia, or nasopharyngeal tumor, can also be confused with allergic rhinitis. Unilateral, foul-smelling rhinorrhea in a child suggests the presence of a nasal foreign body. Nasal polyps are rare in younger children, but, if found, usually indicate the presence of cystic fibrosis (153). Unilateral choanal atresia may be unrecognized at birth. An angiofibroma is the most common nasopharyngeal tumor of childhood, occurring only in pubescent males (154). Lymphoma, rhabdomyosarcoma, and primary nasopharyngeal carcinoma are all much rarer (155). A careful history, followed by physical examination, possibly including endoscopy, will detect these problems. However, a delay in diagnosis of a child with one of these disorders can be devastating.

Rhinitis medicamentosa results from prolonged use of intranasal vasoconstrictor nasal sprays (156). The nasal mucosa becomes less responsive to these agents with continued use, requiring larger and more frequent doses to achieve the desired decongestion. Treatment is discontinuation of the medication and determination of the initiating event. Topical, and even oral, corticosteroid preparations appear to help until the mucosal tolerance subsides—usually within 2 weeks.

The NARES syndrome is a poorly understood entity, easily confused with allergic rhinitis (157). It is characterized by pale, edematous nasal mucosa, with the occurrence of eosinophilia in the nasal secretions. It is seen much more frequently in adults than in children.

The term vasomotor rhinitis has been applied to the condition of chronic nasal obstruction and rhinorrhea of unknown etiology (158). Patients generally complain of profuse, watery nasal discharge or of a minimal, thick nasal secretion. Sneezing may occur, but patients generally have no complaint of nasal itch and no history of atopy. Nonspecific irritants, such as smoke, particulate matter, strong odors, and temperature changes have been noted to exacerbate symptoms. Adults are much more frequently affected than children. Eosinophilia in the secretions of patients with vasomotor rhinitis is rarely seen. The presumed cause is an imbalance in the autonomic innervation of the nasal mucosa, although experimental support for this theory is lacking (159,160).

VI. THERAPEUTIC OPTIONS

A. Avoidance

The elimination of offending agents from the patient's environment provides the potential for cure (see Chaps. 2 and 3). Most perennial allergens are encountered in the home. The bedroom or nursery should be made free of clutter. Feather pillows or comforters, stuffed animals, fabric-covered furniture, and thick carpeting should be avoided. Dust mite, a major component of dust (161), feed on human epithelial scales and organic debris. They prefer humid environments, so avoid rug shampooing. Washing bedding in hot water kills them. Mattresses and pillows should be vacuumed twice a week or encased in protective linings. Mold, another perennial allergen, can be reduced in the home by cleaning and dehumidifying the basement. Removing house plants from the bedroom decreases mold exposure. Pets may be the direct cause of the problem or may act indirectly by carrying pollens into the home on their coats.

The use of electrostatic precipitators and high-energy particulate adsorbent (HEPA) filters is controversial (162). These devices precipitate airborne particles, but the aerodynamics of most antigens cause them to settle quickly from the air, limiting the effectiveness of the devices. Disturbing the reservoir of particles, as in sitting on a sofa, causes them to become airborne in the immediate environment. Twice weekly vacuuming of all carpets, sofas, and other furnishings is more helpful than electrostatic air cleaning in decreasing this reservoir. Furthermore, some electrostatic precipitators produce ozone, which may itself be an irritant (163).

Seasonal allergies can be problematic both inside the home and outdoors. Air conditioners in cars and homes reduce pollen exposure. Outdoor activities, such as grass cutting, picnics, and camping trips are best avoided during appropriate seasons.

B. Pharmacotherpay

1. Antihistamines and Decongestants

Antihistamines are the most utilized agents in the treatment of allergic rhinitis (see Chap. 4). They function by competitively antagonizing the H_1 effects of histamine. However, they have additional properties that may contribute to their therapeutic effects or be responsible for adverse side effects. They show greatest efficacy in the relief of sneezing, itching, and rhinorrhea (164). Symptoms of seasonal allergic rhinitis are more likely to respond to antihistamines than those of perennial rhinitis. There are several different classes of antihistamines (Table 1) that differ in chemical structure, action, and side effects. The loss of efficacy with continued usage of one class of antihistamine is frequently described by patients. Switching to another class often alleviates this problem. Side effects also vary with class. Many patients use over the counter preparations containing antihistamines; therefore, it is important to ascertain this history to avoid prescribing a medicine that previously failed or caused unacceptable side effects. The long clinical experience with these medications makes them a safe choice for prolonged treatment.

Although rarely dangerous, the side effects of antihistamines can be bothersome. Many patients report sedation (165). Administration of these medicines at bedtime reduces this problem, whereas their long half-life leads to daytime efficacy. The use of nonsedating antihistamines provides another alternative. Terfenadine, a nonsedating antihistamine, is widely used in the United States. In clinical trials it has been found to be as potent as chlorpheniramine, but caused no more sedation than placebo (166). However, it is expensive, when compared with generically available antihistamines. Astemizole, another

Table 1 H_1 Antihistamines

Drug	Dosage
Ethanolamines	
Diphenhydramine	< 12 yr: 1.25 mg/kg qid
(Benadryl, Caladryl)	> yr: 25–50 mg tid–qid
Carbinoxamine	< 12 yr: 0.2 mg/kg tid–qid
(Clistin)	> 12 yr: 4–8 mg tid–qid
Clemastine	< 12 yr: not recommended
(Tavist)	> 12 yr: 1.34 mg bid–qid
Ethylenediamines	
Tripelennamine (PBZ)	< 12 yr: 5 mg/kg/24 hr, divided into 4–6 doses
	>12 yr: 25–50 mg qid
Pyrilamine	< 12 yr: not recommended
	> 12 yr: 75–200 mg daily in 3–4 divided doses
Alkylamines	
Chlorpheniramine	< 12 yr: 0.35 mg/kg, divided into 4 doses
(Chlor-Trimeton, Teldrin)	> 12 yr: 2–4 mg tid-qid
	7 yr: 8 mg bid (timed-release)
Brompheniramine	2–6 yr: 1 mg q. 4–6 hr (elixer)
(Dimetane)	6–12 yr: 2 mg q. 4–6 hr (elixer) or 18–12 mg (timed-release)
	> 12 yr: 4 mg q 4–6 hr (tablets, elixer) or 8 mg tid (timed-release)
Dexchlorpheniramine	<12 yr: 0.15 mg/kg daily, divided qid
(Polaramine)	> 12 yr: 1–2 mg tid–qid to 4–6 mg bid
Dimethindene	< 6 yr: not recommended
(Triten)	> 6 yr: 2.5 mg daily to bid
Triprolidene	< 6 yr: 0.3 mg to 0.6 mg tid–qid
(Actidil)	> 6 yr: 1.25 mg tid–qid
Phenothiazines	
Methdilazine	> 3 yr: 4 mg bid–qid
(Tacaryl)	
Promethazine	> 12 yr: 25 mg q hs or 6.25–12.5 mg tid
(Phenergan)	
Trimeprazine	6 mo–3 yr: 1.25 mg tid
(Temaril)	3–12 yr: 2.5 mg tid
Miscellaneous	
Azatadine	Dosage in children not established
(Optimine)	

(continued)

Table 1 *Continued*

Drug	Dosage
Cyproheptadine (Periactin)	2–6 yr: 2 mg bid–tid 7–14 yr: 4 mg bid–tid
Diphenylpyraline (Diafen, Hispril)	2–6 yr: 1–2 mg tid (max. 4 mg/day) > 6 yr: 2 mg tid
Hydroxyzine (Atarax, Vistaril)	< 6 yr: 50 mg/day, divided tid–qid > 6 yr: 50–100 mg/day, divided tid-qid
Terfenadine (Seldane)	< 12 yr: dosage not established > 12 yr: 1 tablet bid

nonsedating antihistamine, was recently approved for use in the United States. The half-life of this drug is extremely long (167). All antihistamines have gastrointestinal side effects, including anorexia, nausea, vomiting, constipation, and diarrhea, which may occur in any age group. Administration with meals may reduce some of these symptoms. In the pediatric population, toxic doses of antihistamines may cause excitation, halluncinations, ataxia, muscular twitching, fever, convulsions, and death (168). A number of antihistamines are approved for use in the pediatric age groups (see Table 1).

Because antihistamines have limited efficacy in the treatment of nasal congestion, they are frequently combined with systemic and topical decongestants (Table 2). Both oral and topical decongestants decrease mucosal congestion by constriction of the small blood vessels supplying the nasal mucosa. Pseudoephedrine hydrochloride and phenylpropanolamine are the two oral decongestant medications most commonly used. Side effects of oral administration result from central nervous system and cardiovascular stimulation and include tachycardia, increased blood pressure, irritability, nervousness, and vomiting (169).

Topical decongestant sprays or drops are more effective in achieving nasal decongestion than their oral counterparts and lack the side effects associated with oral administration (156,170). Xylometazoline hydrochloride (Otrivin), for example, has an onset of action within minutes and a 10-hr duration of action (170). The main disadvantage of these medications, however, is the development of rhinitis medicamentosa with prolonged use (156). Consequently, topical decongestants are recommended for only a few days. In the young child, nasal drops should be instilled with the patient supine and the head turned to one side. The drops are then placed into the dependent nostril and the position maintained for 1 minute. Nasal sprays are administered with the head

Table 2 Selected Antihistamine–Decongestant Preparations

Name	Drug Content	Dosages
Rynatan (Syrup and Tablets)	Phenylephrine (25 mg/tablet, or 5 mg/5 ml syrup) Chlorpheniramine (8 mg/tablet, or 2 mg/5 ml syrup) Pyrilamine (25 mg/tablet, or 12.5 mg/5 ml syrup)	< 2 yr: individualize 2–6 yr: ½ to 1 tsp syrup bid > 6 yr: 1-2 tsp syrup bid > 12 yr: 1-2 tablets bid
Tavist-O (tablets)	Clemastine (134 mg) Phenylpropanolamine (75 mg)	< 12 yr: not recommended > 12 yr: 1 tablet bid
Rondec (oral drops, syrup and tablets)	Carbinoxamine (2 mg/ml drops, or 4 mg/5 ml syrup, or 4 mg/tablet Pseudoephedrine (25 mg/ml drops, or 60 mg/5 ml syrup, or 60 mg/tablet	1–3 yr: not recommended 3–6 mo: 0.5 ml drops qid 6–9 mo: 0.75 ml drops qid 9–18 mo: 1 ml drops qid 18 mo–6 yr: ½ tsp syrup qid >6 yr: 1 tsp syrup or 1 tablet qid
Triaminic (oral drops, Juvelets and tablets)	Pheniramine (10 mg/ml drops, or 25 mg/Juvelet and 25 mg/tablet) Pyrilamine (10 mg/ml drops, or 12.5 mg/Juvelet and 25 mg/tablet) Phenylpropanolamine (20 mg/ml drops, or 25 mg/Juvelet and 50 mg/tablet	< 6 yr: 1 drop/2 lb body weight qid 6–12 yr: 1 Juvelet tid > 12 yr: 1 tablet or 2 Juvelets tid

tilted forward, and the patient is instructed to sniff during insufflation of the medicine.

2. *Cromolyn Sodium*

Cromolyn sodium, administered topically, has been shown to be clinically efficacious in the treatment of seasonal allergic rhinitis (see Chap. 4; 171). In experimental allergic rhinitis, both the early and late-phase clinical responses are diminished (172,173). The drug is most effective when used before the onset of symptoms and continued throughout the period of allergen exposure. Side effects have been minimal, consisting mostly of sneezing, nasal irritation, and stinging (174).

3. *Topical Corticosteroids*

The introduction of topical steroids for the treatment of allergic rhinitis in the United States during the 1960s greatly improved therapy (175–182). Systemic steroids have long been known to be efficacious in the treatment of allergic disease, but the risk of complications far outweighed their benefit for the prolonged management of allergic rhinitis. Topical steroids avoid these risk while achieving site-specific efficacy. A full description of the use of topical costicosteroids can be found in Chapter 4.

C. Immunotherapy

Because this topic is covered in Chapter 5, only a few comments will be made. Immunotherapy, the repeated injection of small amounts of known allergens, is beneficial in most patients with seasonal as well as perennial allergic rhinitis (183). This form of treatment is specific for the offending antigen and, therefore, all offending antigens responsible for symptoms must be defined before therapy. The decision to treat with immunotherapy commits the patient to an extended period of therapy and will surely be disappointing if a relevant antigen is omitted from the immunotherapy solution. The efficacy of immunotherapy, although clearly demonstrated for pollen allergens, house dust, and animal dander, is not as well proved for fungi. Allergens that are easily avoided, such as foods, should not be included in immunotherapy.

The decision to choose immunotherapy over pharmacologic therapy is best made by patient and physician preference, depending on the duration and severity of symptoms, as well as the degree of symptom control attained with other forms of therapy. Weekly injections are time-consuming, costly, and may be associated with adverse systemic allergic reactions. Daily medications themselves, however, may cause problems with compliance and adverse reactions. Both types of therapy are not mutually exclusive. A patient receiving immunotherapy with a symptomatic exacerbation during pollen season may benefit from the addition of antihistamines or topical nasal steroids.

D. Surgery

Surgery is not a treatment for allergic rhinitis, but it may play an important adjuvant role. Surgery can cure nasal airflow obstruction secondary to mechanical factors. Correcting a septal deviation can provide better access for topical therapy and may eliminate a predisposing factor for recurrent sinusitis. Other anatomical abnormalities (such as concha bullosa, medialized uncinate processes, and reversed middle turbinates) may predispose to chronic and recurrent acute sinusitis, compromising drainage from the paranasal sinuses (184). This area can be evaluated endoscopically and by coronal CT scans (185). The role of enlarged adenoids should also be considered. Consultation with a pediatric otolaryngologist can aid in the management of children with allergic rhinitis who are not responding to therapy, particularly those who have previously undergone surgical intervention.

In the past, dogma stated that children should not undergo septal surgery before the age of 16. This teaching was based on the assumption that surgical intervention would disrupt growth centers and that the child's nose would develop abnormally. Although there is some basis for this belief, it is best interpreted to mean that surgery should be limited to the difficult-to-manage patient and should be of limited scope. Submucous resection, therefore, does not have a place in the treatment of children. A child, however, should not be forced to suffer the consequence of an obstructing septal deviation until reaching age 16. Recent literature suggests that surgery in childhood is not necessarily followed by developmental sequelae (186).

VII. COMPLICATIONS

Orofacial and dental abnormalities, sinusitis, recurrent otitis media, and olfactory disturbances have been attributed to allergic rhinitis. The underlying factor in each of these processes is considered to be the development of nasal mucosal inflammation and edema, resulting in either total or partial nasal obstruction.

Orofacial and dental abnormalities have long been thought related to abnormalities in nasal respiratory function, both with nasal allergy (142,187–189) and with adenoidal hypertrophy (190). The classic long face syndrome, or adenoid facies, thought to be related to chronic mouth breathing, describes a child with a narrow maxillary arch and high palate, a vertical excess in lower third facial height, a steep mandibular plane angle, and an open bite. Principato, studying orthodontic patients and controls, found a correlation between elevated nasal airway resistance, orthodontic deformities, and increases in lower anterior vertical facial heights (191). Others, however, have found no evidence that nasal obstruction causes craniofacial abnormalities (192). Additional controlled studies should clarify this relationship.

Nasal allergy is thought to be a major cause of sinusitis in the pediatric population (193). Fifty-three percent of patients with perennial allergic rhinitis had abnormal sinus radiograms in one study, and treating these patients with antibiotics improved their symptoms (194). Inflammation and edema of the sinonasal mucosa results in poor drainage of the paranasal sinuses (195). A subsequent decrease in oxygen tension and pH within the sinus provides the perfect growth medium for anaerobic pathogens (196).

The role of allergic rhinitis in the pathogenesis of otitis media has not been resolved. That eustachian tube dysfunction caused by allergic rhinitis could predispose a patient to recurrent episodes of otitis media has been proposed (140,197,198). Bernstein (197) reported the presence of allergic rhinitis in 35 to 100 patients undergoing insertion of a second set of pressure equilization tubes for recurrent otitis media with effusion. Skoner and colleagues (198) challenged allergic and nonallergic patients intranasally with histamine. They noted subsequent eustachian tube dysfunction in the allergic rhinitis group but not in the control group, suggesting a hyperresponsiveness of the eustachian tube mucosa in those patients with allergic rhinitis. Local production of IgE has been noted in the middle ear space (197), indicating a possible direct role of the ear in hypersensitivity reactions. Antihistamines, on the other hand, have been clearly shown to be of no help in cases of otitis media uncomplicated by allergic rhinitis (199). The association between allergic rhinitis and recurrent otitis media, two very common problems of childhood, remains unclear.

Olfactory disturbances, especially anosmia, would be expected with any disease process resulting in airway obstruction that limits access to the superior part of the nasal cavity. Hyposmia has been reported in nasal allergic states (200–202), and Church (203) observed mucosal signs of allergy in 33 of 54 hyposmic patients. Treatment of nasal polyposis with systemic corticosteroids reversed the attendant anosmia in some patients (201,202). Furthermore, Goodspeed (202) associated this outcome with the reversal of attendant nasal or sinus disease.

VIII. SUMMARY

Allergic rhinitis and viral upper respiratory tract infection dominate the differential diagnosis of childhood rhinitis. A careful history, followed by a thorough physical examination, assists in distinguishing between these two entities and other diseases presenting with similar symptoms. Skin testing and RAST of antigens suggested by history confirm the diagnosis of allergic rhinitis. Therapy is then based on an understanding of the pathophysiology of allergic rhinitis. After avoidance, antihistamines and cromolyn sodium are first-line therapies; topical steroids and immunotherapy are reserved for more refractory cases. When therapy fails, reconsider the possibilities of sinusitis and adenoidal hypertrophy, which can be diagnosed endoscopically or by x-ray evaluation. Surgical consultation can assist in correcting confounding anatomical problems. The challenge of managing allergic rhinitis in childhood lies in understanding the role of development on the manifestations of illness.

ACKNOWLEDGMENTS

The authors wish to thank Alkis Togias, M.D., for his thoughtful review and Carol Dankelman for her secretarial assistance.

REFERENCES

1. Keith A. Human embryology and morphology. Baltimore: Williams & Wilkins, 1948:234–265.
2. Patten BM. Human embryology. New York: McGraw-Hill, 1968:317–320.
3. Stohl RS, Jurkiewicz JJ.Congenital posterior choanal atresia. Pediatrics 1985; 76:429–436.
4. Jaffe BF. Classification and management of anomalies of the nose. Otolaryngol Clin North Am. 1981; 14:989–1004.
5. Sessions RB. Nasal dermal sinuses—new concepts and explanations. Laryngoscope 1982; 92 (suppl 29):1–28.
6. Meyer CM, Cotton RT. Nasal obstruction in the pediatric patient. Pediatrics 1983; 72:766–777.
7. Dion MC, Jafek BW, Tobin CJ. The anatomy of the nose: external support. Arch Otolaryngol 1978; 104:145–150.
8. Mann DG, Sasaki CT, Suzuki M, Fukada H, Hernandez JR. Dilator naris muscle. Arch Otolaryngol 1977; 86:362–370.

9. Cauna N. Blood and nerve supply of the nasal lining. In: Proctor DF, Anderson IB, eds. The nose. Amsterdam: Elsevier Biomedical, 1982:45–70.
10. Bojsen-Moller F. Glandulae nasales anteriores in the human nose. Ann Otol Rhinol Laryngol 1965; 74:363–375.
11. Proctor DF, Adams GK. Physiology and pharmacology of nasal function and mucus secretion. Pharmacol Ther 1976; 2B:492–499.
12. Strohl KP, Hensely MJ, Hallet M, Saunders NA, Ingram RH Jr. Activation of the upper airway muscle before onset of inspiration in normal humans. J Appl Physiol 1980; 49:638–642.
13. Swift DL, Proctor DF. Access of air to the respiratory tract. In: Brain, DJ, Proctor, DF, Reid, LM, eds. Respiratory defense mechanisms. New York: Marcel Dekker, 1977, pp. 63–93.
14. Bridger GP, Proctor DF. Maximum nasal inspiratory flow and nasal resistance. Ann Otol Rhinol Laryngol 1970; 79:481–488.
15. Gray L. Deviated nasal septum. III. Its influence on the physiology and disease of the nose and ears. J Larnygol 1967; 81:953–986.
16. Mygind N, Pederson M, Nielsen M. Morphology of the upper airway epithelium. In: Proctor DF, Anderson, IB, (eds.) The nose. Amsterdam: Elsevier Biomedical, 1982:77–98.
17. Kayser R. Die exacte Messung der Luftdurchgangrgkeit der Nose. Arch Laryngol 1895; 3:101.
18. Hasegawa M, Kern EB. The human nasal cycle. Mayo Clin Proc 1977; 52:28–34.
19. Stoksted P. The physiologic cycle of the nose under normal and pathologic conditions. Acta Otolaryngol 1952; 42:175–179.
20. Jafek BW. Ultrastructure of the human nasal mucosa. Laryngoscope 1983; 93:1576–1599.
21. Rossmann CM, Lee R, Forrest JB, Newhouse MT. Nasal ciliary ultrastructure and function in patients with primary ciliary dyskinesia compared with that in normal subjects and in subjects with various respiratory diseases. Am Rev Respir Dis 1984; 129:161–167.
22. Tos M. Goblet cells and glands in the nose and paranasal sinuses. In: Proctor DF, Andersen IB, eds. The nose. Amsterdam: Elsevier Biomedical, 1982:99–144.
23. Leikauf GD, Veki IF, and Nadel JA. Bradykinin stimulates chloride secretion and prostaglandin E_2 release by canine tracheal epithelium. Am J Physiol 1985; 248:F48–F55.
24. Mostov KE, Blobel G. A transmembrane precursor of secretory component. The receptor for transcellular transport of polymeric immunoglobulins. J Biol Chem. 1982; 257:11816–11821.
25. Brandtzaeg P. Immune function of human nasal mucosa and tonsils in health and disease. In: Bienenstock J, ed. Immunology of the lung and upper respiratory tract. New York: McGraw-Hill, 1984.
26. Wilson WR, Allansmith MR. Rapid, atraumatic method for obtaining nasal mucus samples. Ann Otol Rhinol Laryngol 1976; 85:391–393.

27. Anderson I, Lundqvist G, Proctor DF. Human nasal mucosal function under four controlled humidities. Am Rev Respir Dis 1979; 119:619–627.
28. Brain DJ, Proctor DF, Reid LM, ed. Respiratory Defense Mechanisms, New York: Marcel Dekker, 1977.
29. Fry FA, Black A. Regional deposition of inhaled particles in the human nose. J Aerosol Sci 1973; 4:113–124.
30. Lippmann M. Deposition and clearance of inhaled particles in the nose. Ann Otol Rhinol Laryngol 1970; 779:519–528.
31. Ahronson EF, Menkes H, Gurtner G, Swift DL, Proctor DF. The effect of respiratory airflow rate on the removal of soluble vapors by the nose. J Appl Physiol 1974; 37:654–657.
32. Brain JD. The uptake of inhaled gases by the nose. Ann Otol Rhinol Laryngol 1970; 79:529–539.
33. Speizer FE, Frank, NR. The uptake and release of SO by the human nose. Arch Environ Health 1966; 12:725–728.
34. Taylor M. The origin and function of nasal mucus. Laryngoscope 1974; 84:612–636.
35. Boat TF, Cheng PW, Iyer RN, Carlson D, Polonoy I. Human respiratory tract secretions. Mucous glycoproteins of nonpurulent tracheobronchial secretions and sputum of patients with bronchitis and cystic fibrosis. Arch Biochem Biophys 1979; 177:95–104.
36. Roussel P, Degand, P, Lamblin G, Laine A, Lafitte JJ. Biochemical definition of human trachebronchial mucus. Lung 1978; 154:241–260.
37. Silberberg A. Basic rheological concepts. In: Elstein M, Parke DV, eds. Mucus in health and disease. New York: Plenum Press, 1976:181–190.
38. Rossen RD, Alford, RH, Butler, WI, Vannier WE. The separation and characterization of proteins intrinsic to nasal secretions. J Immunol 1966; 97:369–378.
39. Butler WT, Rossen RP, Waldmann TA. Mechanism of appearance of immunoglobulin A in nasal secretions in man. J Clin Invest 1967;46:1883–1893.
40. Rossen RD, Schade AL, Butler WT, Kasel JA. The proteins in nasal secretions: a longitudinal study of the IgA, IgG, albumin, siderophilin, and total protein concentrations in nasal washes from adult male volunteers. J Clin Invest 1966; 45:768–776.
41. Ishizaka K, Newcomb RM. Presence of IgE in nasal washes and sputum from asthmatic patients. J Allergy 1970; 46:197–204.
42. Naclerio RM, Meier HL, Kagey-Sobotka A, Adkinson NF Jr, Meyers DA, Norman PS, Lichtenstein LM. Mediator release after airway challenge with antigen. Am Rev Respir Dis 1983; 128:597–602.
43. Baumgarten CR, Togias AG. Naclerio RM, Lichtenstein LM, Norman PS, Proud D. Influx of kininogens into nasal secretions following antigen challenge of allergic individuals. J Clin Invest 1985; 76:191–197.
44. Watson ED, Hoffmann NJ, Simmens RW, Rosebury T. Aerobic and anaerobic

bacterial counts of nasal washings: presence of organisms resembling *Corynebacterium acnes*. J Bacteriol 1962; 83:144–148.
45. Fleming A. On a remarkable bacteriolytic element found in tissues and secretions. Proc R Soc (Biol) 1922; 93:306–317.
46. Lorin MI, Gaerlan PF, Mandel ID. Quantitative composition of nasal secretions in normal subjects. J Lab Clin Med 1972; 80:275–281.
47. Bascom R, Wachs M, Naclerio RM, Pipkorn U, Galli SJ, Lichtenstein LM. Basophil influx occurs after nasal antigen challenge: effects of topical corticosteroid pretreatment. J Allergy Clin Immunol 1988; 81:580–589.
48. Anderson I, Lundqvist G, Jensen PL, Proctor DF. Human response to controlled levels of sulfur dioxide. Arch Environ Health 1974; 28:31–39.
49. Hounam RF. The removal of particles from the nasopharyngeal (NP) compartment of the respiratory tract by nose blowing and swabbing. Health Physics 1975; 28:743–750.
50. Proetz AW. Applied physiology of the nose. St. Louis: Annals Publishing, 1941; 192–221.
51. Afzelius B. The immotile cilia syndrome and other ciliary diseases. Int Rev Exp Pathol 1979; 19:1–43.
52. Carson JL, Collier AM, Hu SS. Acquired ciliary defects in nasal epithelium of children with acute viral upper respiratory infections. N Engl J Med 1985. 312:463–468.
53. Homa B, Lindegren M, Anderson JM. pH effects on ciliomotility and morphology of respiratory mucosa. Arch Environ Health 1977; 32:216–226.
54. King M. Viscoelastic properties of airway mucus. Fed Proc 1980; 39:3080–3085.
55. Chodosh S. Objective sputum changes associated with glyceryl guaiacolate in chronic bronchial diseases. Bull Physiopathol Respir 1973; 9:452–456.
56. Boyd EM. Respiratory tract fluid and expectorants. Pharmacol Rev 19564; 6:521–542.
57. Dolovich J, Kennedy L, Vickerson F, Kazim F. Control of the hypersecretion of vasomotor rhinitis by topical ipratropium bromide. J Allergy Clin Immunol 1987; 80:274–278.
58. Anderson I, Lundqvist G, Jensen PL, Proctor DF. Human response after 78 hours' exposure to dry air. Arch Environ Health 1974; 29:319–324.
59. Maceri DR. Nasal trauma. In: Cummings, CW, Fredrickson JM, Harker, LA, Krause CJ, Schuller DE, eds. St. Louis: CV Mosby, 1986:611–624.
60. Dawes JDK and Pritchard M. Studies of the vascular arrangement of the nose. J Anat 1953; 87:311–322.
61. Cauna N. Hinderer KH. Fine structure of blood vessels of the human nasal respiratory mucosa. Ann Otol Rhinol Laryngol 1969; 78:865–879.
62. Rao SS, Potdar A. Nasal airflow with body in various positions. J Appl Physiol 1970; 28:162–165.
63. McCaffrey TV, Kern EB. Response of nasal airway resistance to hypercapnia and hypoxia in man. Ann Otol Rhinol Laryngol 1979; 88:247–252.
64. Drettner B. Vascular reactions of the human nasal mucosa on exposure to cold.

Acta Otolaryngol Supp 1961; 166:1–109.
65. Gsic B, Krajina Z, Lakic L, Konic V, Bobic I. Damage to the respiratory mucous membrane of rats exposed to cold. Acta Otolaryngol 1964; 57:342–351.
66. Hall LJ, Jackson RT. Effects of alpha and beta adrenergic agonists on nasal blood flow. Ann Otol Rhinol Laryngol 1968; 77:1120–1129.
67. McLaurin JW, Shipman WF, Rosedale R, Jr. Oral decongestants. Laryngoscope 1961; 71:54–67.
68. Eccles R, MacClean AG. Relaxation of smooth muscle following contraction elicited by sympathetic nerve stimulation in vivo. Br J Pharmacol 1977; 61:551–558.
69. Eccles R, Wilson H. The parasympathetic secretory nerves of the nose of the cat. J Physiol 1973; 230:213–223.
70. Borum P. Nasal methacholine challenge. A test for the measurement of nasal reactivity. J Allergy Clin Immunol 1979; 63:253–257.
71. Bentley AJ, Jackson RT. Changes in the patency of the upper nasal passage induced by histamine and antihistamine. Laryngoscope 1970; 80:1859–1870.
72. Secher C, Kirkegaard J, Borum P, Maansson A, Osterhammel P, Mygind N. Significance of H_1 and H_2 receptors in the human nose. Rationale for topical use of combined antihistamine preparations. J Allergy Clin Immunol 1982; 70:211–218.
73. Malcolmson KG. The vasomotor activities of the nasal mucous membrane. J Laryngol Otol 1959; 73:73–98.
74. Mohun M. Incidence of vasomotor rhinitis during pregnancy. Arch Otolaryngol 1943; 37:699–709.
75. Proetz AW. Further observations of effects of thyroid insufficiency on the nasal mucosa. Laryngoscope 1950; 60:627–633.
76. Holmes TH, Goddell H, Wolf S, Wolff HG. The nose; an experimental study of reactions within the nose in human subjects during varying life experiences. Springfield, IL: Charles C Thomas, 1950.
77. Cauna N., Hinderer KH, Wentges RT. Sensory receptor organs of the human nasal resiratory mucosa. Am J Anat 1969; 124:187–210.
78. Brubaker A. The physiology of sneezing. JAMA 1919; 73:585–587.
79. Gwaltney JM Jr. The common cold. In: Mandell GL, Douglas RG, Jr, Bennett JE, eds. New York: John Wiley & Sons, 1979: 429–434.
80. Angell-Jumes JE and Day M de B. Nasal reflexes. Proc R Soc Med 1969; 62:1287–1293.
81. Evertt HC. Sneezing in response to light. Neurology 1964; 14:483–490.
82. Barrow CS, Alarie Y, Stock MF. Sensory irritation and incapacitation evoked by thermal decomposition products of polymers and comparisons with known sensory irritants. Arch Environ Health 1978; 33:79–88.
83. Dixon WE, Brodie TG. Contributions to the physiology of the lungs. J Physiol 1903; 29:97–173.
84. Craig AB. Underwater swimming and loss of consciousness. JAMA 1961; 176:255–258.

85. Sercer A. Investigations dur l'influence relectorie de la cavitie nasale sur le pourmon der meme cote. Acta Otolaryngol 1930; 14:82–90.
86. Kaufman J, Wright GW. The effect of nasal and nasopharyngeal irritation on airway resistance in man. Am Rev Respir Dis 1969; 100:626–630.
87. Kaufman J, Chen JC, Wright GW. The effect of trigeminal resection on reflex bronchoconstriction after nasal and nasopharyngeal irritation in man. Am Rev Respir Dis 1970; 101:768–769.
88. Sedee GA. Relation between the functions of nose and lung on the same side of the body. Int Rhinol 1969; 7:7–14.
89. Silverstein EB, Lewis JT, Quenelle DJ. Study of the physiologic relationship of lower and upper airways with xenon-133. Ann Otol Rhinol Laryngol 1980; 89:62–64.
90. Eccles R. Neurological and pharmacological considerations. In: Proctor DF, Anderson IB, eds. The nose. Amsterdam: Elsevier Biomedical, 1982:191–214.
91. Boles R. Neuroanatomy for the otolaryngologist. In: Paparella M, Shumrick D, eds. Otolaryngology. Philadephia: WB Saunders, 1980: 148–151.
92. Boles R. Neuroanatomy for the otolaryngologist. In: Paparella M, Shumrick D, eds. Otolaryngology. Philadelphia: WB Saunders, 1980: 166–170.
93. Angaard A, Denset O. Adrenergic innervation of the nasal mucosa in the cat. Acta Otolaryngol 1974; 78:232–241.
94. Richerson HB, Seebohm PM. Nasal airway response to exercise. J Allergy 1968; 41:269–284.
95. Rooker DW, Jackson RT. The effects of certain drugs, cervical sympathetic stimulation and section on nasal patency. Ann Otol Rhinol Laryngol 1967; 78:403–414.
96. Barnes PJ. Neuropeptides in the lung: localization, function and pathophysiological implications. J Allergy Clin Immunol 1987; 79:285–295.
97. Uddman, R. Sundler F. Vasoactive intestinal peptide nerves in human upper respiratory tract. Otol Rhinol Laryngol 1979; 41:221–226.
98. Kurrian SS, Blank MA, Sheppard MN, Stanley PJ, Mackay IS, Cole PJ, Bloom SR, Polak JM. Vasoactive intestinal peptide (VIP) in vasomotor rhinitis. IRCS Med Sci 1983; 11:425–426.
99. Pevsner J, Trifiletti RR, Strittmatter SM, Snyder SH. Isolation and characterization of an olfactory receptor protein for odorant pyrazines. Proc Natl Acad Sci USA 1985; 82:3050–3054.
100. Pevsner J, Reed RR, Feinstein PG, Snyder SH. Molecular cloning of odorant binding protein: member of a ligand carrying family. Science 1988; 241:336–339.
101. Rouviere H. Anatomy of the human lymphatic system. A compendium. Ann Arbor: Edward Brothers, 1938.
102. Blackley CH. Experimental researches on the causes and nature of catarrhalis aestivus (hay-fever). London: Baliere, Tindall, and Cox, 1873.
103. Taylor G, Shivalker PR. Changes in nasal airway resistance on antigenic challenge in allergic rhinitis. Clin Allergy 1971; 1:63–73.

104. McLean J, Clarkowski A, Solomon W, Mathews K. An improved technique for nasal inhalation challenge tests. J Allergy Clin Immunol 1976; 57:153–163.
105. Connell J. Quantitative intransal pollen challenge. J Allergy 1968; 41:123–139.
106. Ishizaka K, Ishizaka T, Hornbrook MM. Physicochemical properties of a human reaginic antibody. IV. Presence of a unique immunoglobulin as a carrier of reaginic activity. J Immunol 1966; 97:75–80.
107. Ishizaka T, Foreman JC, Sterk AR, Ishizaka K. Induction of calcium flux across the rat mast cell membrane by bridging IgE receptors. Proc Natl Acad Sci USA 1979; 76:5858-5861.
108. Baumgarten CR, Nichols RC, Naclerio RM, Lichtenstein LM, Proud D. Plasma kallikrein during experimentally induced allergic rhinitis: role in kinin formation and contribution of TAME-esterase activity. J Immunol 1986; 137:977–982.
109. Baumgarten CR, Nichols R, Naclerio RM, Proud D. Concentration of glandular kallikrein in human nasal secretions increases during experimentally induced allergic rhinitis. J Immunol 1986; 137:1323–1328.
110. Castells M, Schwartz LB. Tryptase levels ion nasal lavage fluid as an indicator of the early allergic reaction. J Allergy Clin Immunol 1988; 82:348–355.
111. Creticos PS, Peters SP, Adkinson NF Jr, Naclerio RM, Hayes EC, Norman PS, Lichtenstein LM. Peptide leukotriene release after antigen challenge in patients sensitive to ragweed. N Engl J Med 1984; 310:1626–1630.
112. Shaw RJ, Fitzharris P, Cromwell O, Wardlaw AJ, Kay AB. Allergen-induced release of sulphidopeptide leukotrienes (SRS-A) and LTB_4 in allergic rhinitis. Allergy 1985; 40:1–8.
113. Freeland H, Pipkorn U, Schleimer RP, Bascom R, Lichtenstein LM, Naclerio RM, Peters SP. Leukotriene B_4 as a mediator of early and late reactions to antigen in humans. The effect of systemic glucocorticoid treatment in vivo. J Allergy Clin Immunol 1989; 83:634–642.
114. Bascom R, Pipkorn U, Gleich SJ, Lichtenstein LM, Naclerio RM. Effect of systemic steroids on eosinophils (EOS) and major basic protein (MBP) during nasal antigen challenge [Abstract]. J Allergy Clin Immunol 1986; 77:146.
115. Naclerio RM, Proud D, Togias AG, Adkinson NF Jr, Meyers DA, Kagey-Sobotka A, Plaut M, Norman PS, Lichtenstein LM. Inflammatory mediators in late antigen-induced rhinitis. N Engl J Med 1985; 313:65–70.
116. Dolovich J, Hargreave FE, Chalmers R, Shier KJ, Gauldie J, Bienenstock J. Late cutaneous allergic responses in isolated IgE-dependent reactions. J Allergy Clin Immunol 1973; 52:38–46.
117. Robertson DG, Kerigan AT, Hargreave FE, Chalmers R, Dolovich J. Late asthmatic responses induced by ragweed-pollen allergen. J Allergy Clin Immunol 1974; 54:244–254.
118. Booij-Nord H, de Vries K, Sluiter HJ, Orie NGM. Late bronchial obstructive reaction to experimental inhalation of house dust extract. Clin Allergy 1972; 2:43–46.
119. Allansmith MR, Baird RS, Greiner JV, Bloch KJ. Late-phase reaction in ocular anaphylaxis in the rat. J Allergy Clin Immunol 1984; 73:49–55.

120. Iliopoulos O, Proud D, Lichtenstein LM, Kagey-Sobotka A, Creticos P, Adkinson NF Jr, MacDonald SM, Norman PS, Naclerio RM. Relationships between the early, late, and rechallenge responses to nasal challenge [Abstract]. J Allergy Clin Immunol 1987; 79:253.
121. Pipkorn U, Proud D, Lichtenstein LM, Schleimer RP, Peters SP, Adkinson NF Jr, Kagey-Sobotka A, Naclerio RM. Effect of short-term systemic glucocorticoid treatment on human nasal mediator release after antigen challenge. J Clin Invest 1987; 80:957–961.
122. MacGlashan DW Jr, Schleimer RP, Peters SP, Schulman ES, Adams GK, Sobotka AK, Newball HH, Lichtenstein LM. Comparative studies of basophils and mast cells. Fed Proc 1983; 42:2504–2510.
123. Bryan WTK, Bryan MP. Significance of mast cells in nasal secretions. Trans Am Acad Ophthalmol Otolaryngol 1959; 63:613–627.
124. Okuda M, Ohtsuka M. Basophilic cells in allergic nasal secretions. Arch Otorhinolaryngol 1977; 214:283–289.
125. Okuda M, Kawabori S, Otsaka H. Electron microscope study of basophilic cells in allergic nasal secretions. Arch Otorhinolaryngol 1978; 221:215–220.
126. Hastie R, Heroy JH, Levy DA. Basophil leukocytes and mast cells in human nasal secretions and scrapings studied by light microscopy. Lab Invest 1979; 40:554–561.
127. Okuda M, Ohtsuka H, Kawabori S. Basophil leukocytes and mast cells in the nose. Eur J Respir Dis 1983; 64(suppl 128):7–14.
128. Ohtsuka H, Denburg J, Dolovich J, Hitch D, Lapp P, Rajan RS, Bienenstock J, Befus D. Heterogeneity of metachromatic cells in the human nose: significance of mucosal mast cells. J Allergy Clin Immunol 1985; 76: 695–702.
129. Enerback L, Pipkorn U, Granerus G. Intraepithelial migration of nasal mucosal mast cells in hay fever. Int Arch Allergy Appl Immunol 1986; 80:44–51.
130. Okuda M, Sakaguchi F, Suzuki F, Ohtsuka H, Kawabori S. Ultrastructural heterogeneity of the basophilic cells in the allergic nasal mucosa. Ann Allergy 1985; 154:152–157.
131. Dolovich J, Hargreave FE, Chalmers R, Shier KJ, Gauldie J, Bienenstock J. Late cutaneous allergic responses in isolated IgE-dependent reactions. J Allergy Clin Immunol 1973; 52:38–46.
132. deMonchy JGR, Kauffman HF, Venge P, Koeter GH, Jansen HM. Sluiter HJ, De Vries K. Bronchoalveolar eosinophilia during allergen-induced late asthmatic reactions. Am Rev Respir Dis 1985; 131:373–376.
133. Connell JT.The priming effect and its relationship to histopathologic changes in allergic rhinitis [Abstract]. J Allergy 1968; 41:101–102.
134. Bascom R, Pipkorn U, Proud D, Dunnette S, Gleich SJ, Lichtenstein LM, Naclerio RM. Major basic protein and eosinophil-derived neurotoxin concentrations in nasal lavage fluid after antigen challenge: effect of systemic corticosteroids and relationship to eosinophil influx. J Allergy Clin Immunol 1988; 84:197–205.
135. Frigas E, Loegering DA, Gleich GJ. Cytotoxic effects of the guinea pig eosinophil major basic protein on tracheal epithelium. Lab Invest 1980; 42:35–43.

136. Connell JT. Quantitative intranasal pollen challenge. III. The priming effect in allergic rhinitis. J Allergy 1969; 43:33–44.
137. Bacon JR, McLean JA, Mathews KP, Banas JM. Priming of the nasal mucosa by ragweed extract by an irritant (ammonia). J Allergy Clin Immunol 1981; 67:111–116.
138. Wachs M, Proud D, Lichtenstein LM, Kagey-Sobotka A, Norman PS, Naclerio RM. Observations on the pathogenesis of nasal priming. J Allergy Clin Immunol 1989; 84:492–501.
139. Khalife J, Capron M, Cesbron J-Y, Tai P-C, Taelman H, Prin L, Capron A. Role of specific IgE antibodies in peroxidase (EPO) release from human eosinophils. J Immunol 1986; 137:1659–1664.
140. Bluestone CD. Eustachian tube function and allergy in otitis media. Pediatrics 1978; 61:757–760.
141. Marks MB. Significance of discoloration in the lower orbitopalpebral grooves in allergic children (allergic shiners). Ann Allergy 1963; 21:26–32.
142. Marks MB. Allergy in relation to orofacial dental abnormalities in children: a review. J Allergy 1965; 36:293–302.
143. Meyers WA. A "nasal crease," a physical sign of allergy. JAMA 1960; 174:1204–1206.
144. Ownby D, Bailey J. Comparison of MAST with radioallergosorbent and skin tests for diagnosis of allergy in children. Am J Dis Child 1986; 140:45–48.
145. Bousquet J. In vivo methods for study of allergy: skin tests, techniques, and interpretation. In: Middleton E Jr, Reed CE, Ellis EF, Adkinson NF, Jr, Yunginger JW, eds. Allergy: principles and practice. St Louis: CV Mosby, 1986:419–436.
146. Zetterstrom O, Johansson SGO. IgE concentrations measured by PRIST in serum of healthy adults and in patients with respiratory allergy. Allergy 1981; 36:537–547.
147. Wide L, Bennich H, Johansson SGO. Diagnosis of allergy by an in-vitro test for allergen antibodies. Lancet 1967; 2:1105–1107.
148. Norman P. Correlations of RAST with in vivo and in vitro assays. In: Evans R, ed. Advances in diagnosis of allergy. RAST. Miami: Symposia Specialists 1975; 45–60.
149. Brostoff J, Pack S, Merritt T. A new multiple specific IgE assay-MAST. Lancet 1984; 2:748–749.
150. Gilles JGG, Mareschal JP, Saint-Remy JR. Latex allergosorbet test (LAST): a new immunoassay for specific IgE with latex particles. J Allergy Clin Immunol 1988; 82:35–39.
151. Seltzer JM, Halpern GM, Tsay Y. Correlation of allergy test results obtained by IgE FAST, RAST, and prick-puncture methods. Ann Allergy 1985; 54:25–30.
152. Juhn JP. Imaging of the paranasal sinuses. J Allergy Clin Immunol 1986; 77:6–8.
153. Schwachman H, Kulczycki LL, Mueller HL, Flake CG. Nasal polyposis in patients with cystic fibrosis. Pediatrics 1962;30:389–401.
154. Briant TD, Fitzpatrick PJ, Berman J. Nasopharyngeal angiofibroma: a 20 year study. Laryngoscope 1978; 88:1247–1251.

155. Snow JB. Neoplasms of the nasopharynx in children. Otolaryngol Clin N Am 1977; 10:11–24.
156. Black MJ, Remsen KA. Rhinitis medicamentosa. Can Med Assoc J 1980; 122:881–884.
157. Jacobs RL, Freedman PM, Boswell RN. Nonallergic rhinitis with eosinophilia (NARES syndrome). J Allergy Clin Immunol 1981; 67:253–262.
158. Stewart TW. Vasomotor rhinitis: neglected cause of nasal congestion. Postgrad Med 1980; 67(1):171–180.
159. Fowles EP. Unilateral vasomotor rhinitis due to interference with the cervical sympathetic system. Arch Otolaryngol 1943; 37:710–713.
160. Golding-Wood P. Vidian neurectomy and other transantral surgery. Laryngoscope 1970; 80:1179–1188.
161. Collins-Williams C, Hung F, Bremmer K. House dust mite and house dust allergy. Ann Allergy 1976; 37:12–17.
162. Nelson HS, Hirsch SR, Ohman JL Jr, Platts-Mills TAE, Reed CE, Solomon WR. Recommendations for the use of air cleaning devices in the treatment of allergic respiratory disease. J Allergy Clin Immunol 1988; 82:661–669.
163. Golden JA, Nadel JA, Boushey HA. Bronchial hyperirritability in healthy subjects after exposure to ozone. Am Rev Respir Dis 1978; 118:287–294.
164. Simons FER, Simons KJ. Pharmacologic treatment of rhinitis. Clin Rev Allergy 1984; 2:237–242.
165. Drovin MA. H_1 antihistamines: perspective on the use of conventional and new agents. Ann Allergy 1985; 55:797–801.
166. Backhouse CI, Brewster BS, Lockhart JDF, Mareksha S, Purvis CR, Valle-Jones J. Terfenadine in allergic rhinitis. A comparative trial of a new antihistamine versus chlorpheniramine and placebo. Practitioner 1982; 226:347–351.
167. Richards DM, Brogden RM, Heel RL. Astemizole. A review of its pharmacodynamic properties and therapeutic efficacy. Drugs 1985; 29:34–56.
168. Schuller DE, Turkewitz D. Adverse effects of antihistamines. Postgrad Med 1986; 79(2):75–86.
169. Weiner N. Norepinephrine, epinephrine, and the sympathomimetic amines. In: Gilman AG, Goodman LS, Rall TW, Murad F, eds. The pharmacological basis of therapeutics. New York: Macmillan Publishing 1985:172–174.
170. Petruson B. Treatment with xylometazoline (Otrivin) nosedrops over a six week period. Rhinology 1981; 19:167–172.
171. Welsh PW, Stricker WE, Chu C, Naessens JM, Reese ME, Reed CE, Marcoux JP. Efficacy of beclomethasone nasal solution, flunisolide, and cromolyn in relieving symptoms of ragweed allergy. Mayo Clin Proc 1987; 62(2):125–134.
172. Pelikan Z, Pelikan-Filipek M. The effects of disodium cromoglycate and beclomethasone dipropionate on the immediate response of the nasal mucosa to allergen challenge. Ann Allergy 1982; 49:283–292.
173. Pelikan Z. The effects of disodium cromoglycate and beclomethasone dipropionate on the late nasal mucosa response to allergen challenge. Ann Allergy

1982; 49:200–212.
174. Taylor G, Shivalker PR. Disodium cromoglycate: laboratory studies and clinical trials in allergic rhinitis. Clin Allergy 1971; 1:189–192.
175. Norman PS, Winkenwerder WL. Suppression of hay fever symptoms with intranasal dexamethasone aerosol. J Allergy 1965; 36:284–292.
176. Smith RE. Dexamethasone nasal aerosol in nasal polyps and hypertrophic allergic rhinitis. Ann Allergy 1965; 23:273–276.
177. Norman PS, Winkenwerder WL, Agbayani AF, Migeon CJ. Adrenal function during the use of dexamethasone aerosols in the treatment of ragweed hay fever. J Allergy 1967; 40:57–61.
178. Kobayashi R, Tinkelman P, Reese M, Sykes S. Effectiveness of Beconase AQ in treating seasonal rhinitis in children ages 5 to 12 years [Abstract]. J Allergy Clin Immunol 1987; 79:152.
179. Mygind N. Topical steroid treatment for allergic rhinitis and allied conditions. Clin Otolaryngol 1982; 7:343–347.
180. Dickson DJ, Cruikshank JM. Comparison of flunisolide nasal spray and terfenadine tablets in hayfever. Br J Clin Pract 1984; 38:416–421.
181. Physician's Desk Reference, 43rd ed. Oradell, NJ. Medical Economics, 1988:2103.
182. Physician's Desk Reference, 43rd ed. Oradell, NJ: Medical Economics, 1988; 1004–1005.
183. Norman PS. An overview of immunotherapy: implications for the future. J Allergy Clin Immunol 1980; 65:87–96.
184. Stammberger H. Endoscopic endonasal surgery—concepts in treatment of recurring rhinosinusitis. Part I. Anatomic and pathophysiologic considerations. Otolaryngol Head Neck Surg. 1986; 94:143–147.
185. Kennedy DW, Zinreich SJ, Rosenbaum AE, Johns ME. Functional endoscopic sinus surgery. Theory and diagnostic evaluation. Arch Otolaryngol 1985; 111:576–582.
186. Healy GB. An approach to the nasal septum in children. Laryngoscope 1986; 96:1239–1242.
187. Balyeat RM, Bowen R. Facial and dental deformities due to perennial nasal allergy in childhood. Int J Orthodont 1934; 20:445.
188. Duke WW. Deformity of the face caused by nasal allergy in childhood. Arch Otolaryngol Head Neck Surg 1930; 12:493–498.
189. Todd TW, Cohen MB, Broadbent BH. The role of allergy in the etiology of orthodontic deformity. J Allergy 1938; 10:246–248.
190. Linder-Aronson S. Nasorespiratory function and craniofacial growth. In: McNamara JA Jr, ed. Nasorespiratory function and craniofacial growth series. Ann Arbor: University of Michigan, 1979, pp. 121–147.
191. Principato JJ, Kerrigan JP, Wolf P. Pediatric nasal resistance and lower anterior vertical face height. Otolaryngol Head Neck Surg 1986; 95:226–229.
192. Klein JC. Nasal respiratory function and craniofacial growth. Arch Otolaryngol

1986; 112:843–849.

193. Shurin P. Inflammatory diseases of the nose and paranasal sinuses. In: Bluestone CD, Stool SE, eds. Pediatric otolaryngology. Philadelphia: WB Saunders, pp. 781–790.

194. Rachelefsky GS, Goldberg M, Katz RM, Boris G, Byepes MT, Shapiro MJ, Mickey MR, Finegold S, Siegel SC. Sinus disease in children with respiratory allergy. J Allergy Clin Immunol 1978; 61:310–344.

195. Carenfelt C, Lundberg C. The role of local gas composition in the production of maxillary sinus empyema. Acta Otolaryngol 1978; 85:116–121.

196. Carenfelt C, Lundberg C. Purulent and nonpurulent maxillary sinus secretions with respect to pO_2, pCO_2, and pH. Acta Otolaryngol 1978; 84:138–144.

197. Bernstein JM, Lee J, Conboy K, Ellis E, Li P. Role of IgE mediated hypersensitivity in recurrent otitis media with effusion. Am J Otolaryngol 1983; 5:66–70.

198. Skoner DP, Doyle WJ, Fireman P. Eustachian tube obstruction (ETO) after histamine nasal provocation—a double-blind dose-response study. J Allergy Clin Immunol 1987; 79:27–31.

199. Canteken EI, Mandel EM, Bluestone CD. Lack of efficacy of a decongestant–antihistamine combination for otitis media with effusion ("secretory" otitis media) in children. N Engl J Med 1983; 308:297–301.

200. Proetz AW. Applied physiology of the nose. St. Louis: Annals Publishing, 1941:106.

201. Hotchkiss WT. Influence of prednisone on nasal polyposis with anosmia. Arch Otolaryngol 1956; 64:478–451.

202. Goodspeed RB, Gent JF, Catelanotto FA. Clinical trial of systemic corticosteroid therapy in anosmia. 5th Annual Meeting for the Association for Chemoreception Sciences, 1983, Abstract 51.

203. Church JA, Bauer H, Bellanti JA, Satterly RA, Henkin RI. Hyposmia associated with atopy. Ann Allergy 1978; 40:105–109.

7

Sinusitis

Gilbert A. Friday, Jr., and Philip Fireman
University of Pittsburgh School of Medicine and Children's Hospital of Pittsburgh
Piitsburgh, Pennsylvania

Aurapin Sukanich and Michael L. Steinberg
Children's Hospital of Pittsburgh
Pittsburgh, Pennsylvania

I. INTRODUCTION

Sinusitis is a common problem in children (1). It is a disease associated with infection of the paranasal sinuses, occlusion of the sinus ostia, and inflammation of the sinus and nasal mucosa. Symptoms, such as purulent rhinorrhea and nasal congestion, overlap with those of various forms of rhinitis or occur in conjunction with rhinitis. The headache of sinusitis (uncommon complaint in children) is primarily related to infection of the nasal passages about the sinus ostia (2). Sinus radiographs are required to make the diagnosis, but in some instances, they are less than reliable. Sinusitis is considered acute when present for fewer than 3 weeks and chronic when present for more than 6 weeks. The true prevalence of sinusitis is unknown, but closely parallels the incidence of acute infections of the upper respiratory tract. Therefore, most episodes of sinusitis are presumed to be infectious in etiology and more common during the late fall, winter, and early spring when upper respiratory infections are more common. However, sinusitis has also been described in association with allergic rhinitis as well as asthma, and a seasonal incidence coincident with an increase of atmospheric pollen has been suggested, but not definately documented. The possibility of a recurrent or persistent sinusitis associated with perennial allergic rhinitis related to an allergy to dust mites, animal danders, or molds has also been reported.

II. ANATOMY AND DEVELOPMENT OF THE PARANASAL SINUSES

The paranasal sinuses are a grouping of paired air-containing cranial cavities that develop as outpouchings of the nasal mucosa (Figs. 1 and 2) (1). The origins of the maxillary and ethmoidal sinuses are apparent by the third to fourth months of fetal life. The maxillary sinus, the first one to develop, starts as an evagination from the middle meatus. The anterior ethmoidal labyrinth is also derived from the middle meatus, whereas the posterior ethmoid cells derive from the superior meatus and are considered, by some authors, to be associated with sphenoid sinus growth. The ethmoid sinus is the only multicompartmentalized (honeycomb) sinus. The frontal sinuses become recognizable by 6–12 months after birth. The frontal sinuses, similar to the anterior ethmoidal cells and maxillary sinuses, are also derived from the middle meatus.

The ethmoid and maxillary sinuses first appear radiologically as air-filled spaces between the 3rd and 12th months of life. The frontal bone is not pneumatized until the first or second year of life, assuming its definitive shape by the third year and become radiologically visible between years 3 and 6.

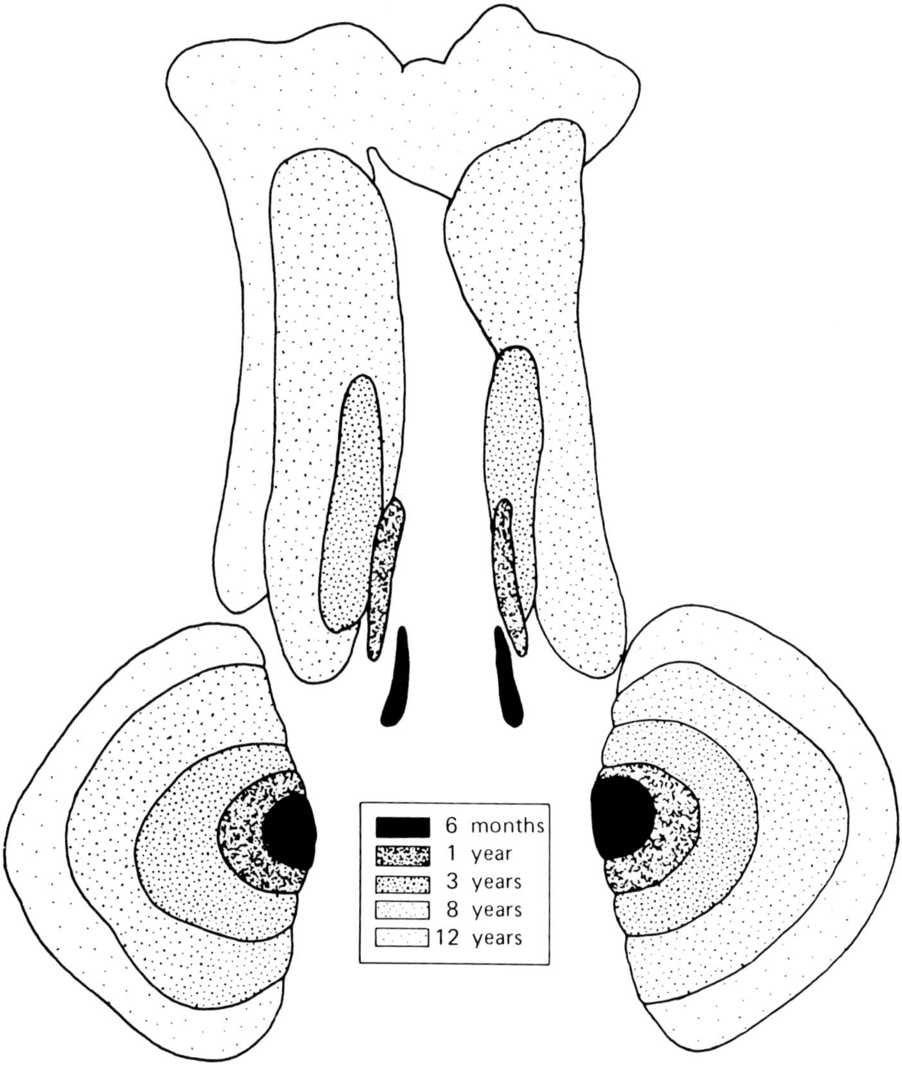

Figure 1 Development of the maxillary and frontal sinuses at various ages. (After Caffey.)

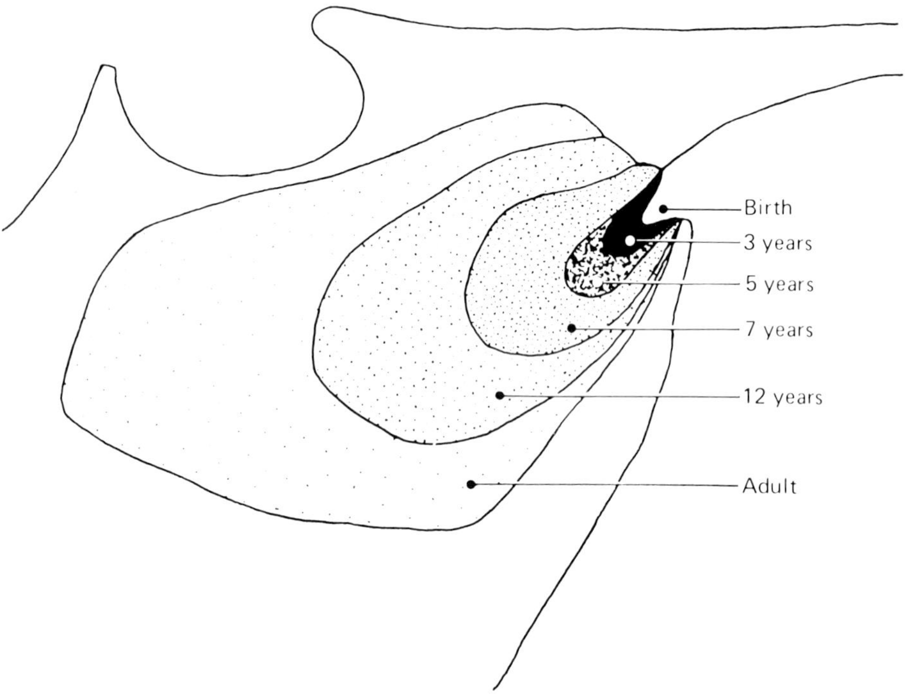

Figure 2 Development of the sphenoid sinus at various ages. (After Caffey.)

Occasionally, the frontal sinus develops as an expansion of one of the air cells on the ethmoidal infundibulum. The sphenoids, which form by about the third year of life, do not appear radiographically until the ninth year. The sphenoid sinus begins as an evagination from the posterior part of the nasal capsule. It is important to note that there is much variation in shape and size of the sinuses at all ages.

The mucous membranes lining the sinuses are made up of ciliated pseudostratified columnar epithelium, with interspersed goblet cells, or non-cilated columnar epithelium. As in other parts of the respiratory tract, the submucosa contains mast cells and can be infiltrated with neutrophils, lymphocytes, and plasma cells during inflammation.

The normal physiology of the sinuses resembles that of the adjacent nasal respiratory structures (1). The mucous membranes lining the sinuses function in a similar manner. Secretions are a mixture of viscid mucus from the seromucous glands and watery secretions from the anterior serous glands. Mucus, biologically mucin, is synthesized by mucous glands and goblet cells. There appears to be two layers of mucus in the airways; the gel layer (superficial viscid fluid) and the sol layer (underlying serous fluid). The tips of the cilia just touch the gel layer during forward movement. The cilia are always surrounded by and move the sol layer.

The adhesive properties of mucus and the strength and constant beating of the cilia are such that bacteria usually cannot penetrate to the epithelium. However, the protective mucous layer is less effective against viruses, which seem to possess a special affinity to receptors on the cilia. Mucous secretions contain activities derived from lysozymes and the lactoperoxidase–thiocyanate system, which decrease bacterial attachment, inhibit bacterial or viral replication, and destroy specific bacteria. Lactoferrin, originating from serous glands and from neutrophils, has a bacteriostatic activity that is potentiated by antibodies. Its antibacterial effect probably stems from its affinity for iron, which is necessary for bacteria to grow. When present in secretions, interferon, the synthesis of which is stimulated by viral infection, decreases viral multiplication.

Secretory IgA, consisting of polymetric IgA, its J chain, and a secretory piece, is also present in the mucosal secretions. Native secretory IgA does not fix complement. There is controversy over whether or not IgA can opsonize bacteria or other particles for phagocytosis. It appears that secretory IgA functions by aggregating particulate matter and soluble antigens. Thus, bacterial toxins may be neutralized. Viruses and bacteria are prevented from attaching to cells and tissues and, thereby, IgA may inhibit microbial replication. Secretory IgA appears to play an important role in protecting the upper respiratory tract from infection, and IgA deficiency is frequently associated with recurrent sinusitis. A few persons who lack secretory IgA do not have an increased number or more severe respiratory or sinus infections. These IgA deficient persons may be protected by increased quantities of IgG and, especially, by the compensatory appearance of IgM in their secretions. The IgG present in respiratory secretions is mainly from passive transfer from the serum (3).

III. PATHOPHYSIOLOGY

The three key elements in the understanding of the pathophysiology of sinusitis include the patency of the ostia, the appropriate function of the ciliary apparatus, and the quantity of secretions. One or more abnormalities in these factors will lead to retention of secretions in the paranasal sinuses, followed by secondary infection and subsequent sinusitis.

The pathogenesis of sinusitis usually involves blockage of the ostia. This can be initiated by infection, allergy, structural abnormalities, or any edema of the nasal mucosa, which will impede ventilation and appropriate drainage of the sinuses. Viral and bacterial infections and, in certain instances, fungi will also impair the ciliary activity of the epithelial cells lining the sinuses. The result is accumulation of mucous secretions, followed by bacterial multiplication and an influx in inflammatory cells that convert mucus to mucopus. Death of mucosal cells may result from viral multiplication, and some degree of sloughing of respiratory epithelium is part of the natural course of the disease. Ordinarily, regeneration of the mucosa is prompt, and the outcome is benign. However, when acute sinusitis is not resolved, but becomes chronic, the epithelial lining may be irreversibly damaged. This may lead to thickening of the mucosa and the development of mucoceles or polyps.

The most commonly found pathogens of sinusitis in children are similar to those found in adults (Table 1; 4–8). The predominant organisms in two-thirds of acute sinusitis infections include *Streptococcus pneumoniae*, nontypable *Haemophilus influenzae*, and *Branhamella catarrhalis*. Other aerobic organisms less frequently found are *S. veridans*, *S. pyogenes*, and *Staphylococcus aureus*. Anerobic bacteria may be found in chronic infections and include bacteroides and streptococci (7). Viruses are occasionally isolated and include rhinovirus, adenovirus, influenza type A, and parainfluenza virus (4,6). There are occasional reports of fungal sinusitis caused by *Aspergillus*, *Mucor*, *Candida*, or other species (8).

Table 1 Principle Bacteria, Viruses, and Fungi Isolated from Sinuses

Aerobic Bacteria	Viruses
S. pneumoniae	Rhinovirus
H. influenzae	Adenovirus
B. catarrhalis	Influenza virus type A
	Parainfluenza
Anaerobic Bacteria	Fungi
Streptococci	*Aspergillus*
Bacteroides	*Candida*

Table 2 Signs and Symptoms of Sinusitis

Cough
Purulent nasal discharge
Headache, facial pain, and tenderness
Fever
Fetor oris

Pathogenic bacteria, fungi, and viruses have been cultured from sinus secretions obtained by direct needle aspiration of the maxillary antra or by direct antral swabbing under local anesthesia (4,9). There is a poor correlation between the predominant species of bacteria cultured from the sinus aspirate and those found in nasopharynx or throat cultures (4,7,9).

Signs and symptoms of sinusitis are noted in Table 2. These symptoms include rhinorrhea, which may be purulent, occasional fever, headache and facial pain, sore throat, and postnasal drainage, along with fetor oris. Coughing that persists during the day, and especially at night, is frequent. Children with sinusitis have fewer complaints of facial pain and headache than adults and adolescents.

IV. DISEASES ASSOCIATED WITH SINUSITIS (Table 3)

A. Upper Respiratory Infections

Sinusitis most commonly follows a viral upper respiratory infection (URI), which is common in childhood. It is very difficult to determine when this URI has progressed to sinusitis. Estimates of the frequency with which acute sinusitis complicates upper respiratory infections may vary from 0.5 to 5.0%. The mechanism of sinusitis after an URI appears to be the following: the acute rhinitis results in an edematous obstruction of the sinus ostia and a decrease in paranasal sinus ciliary action. Subsequently, there is accumulation of mucus in the sinuses, followed by a superimposed secondary bacterial infection, and a conversion of mucus to mucopus. Mucopus further impairs ciliary function and increases the swelling around the ostia (10).

During the course of an apparent viral URI there are two common circumstances in which bacterial infection of the paranasal sinuses should be suspected. The more common is when the symptoms of a URI persist beyond 10 days without appreciable improvement. The nasal discharge and cough

Table 3 Conditions Predisposing to Sinusitis

Sinus osteal obstruction:
Mucosal swelling: URI, allergy, trauma, swimming, and topical decongestants
Mechanical obstruction: choanal atresia, adenoid hypertrophy, deviated septum, polyps, foreign body, and neoplasms
Ciliary dysfunction
Viral URI
Immotile cilia syndrome (Kartagener's)
Medication
Secretion alteration
Viral URI
Cystic fibrosis
Immune deficiency

remain persistent, although the patient may not appear particularly ill. The second, less common presentation, is a URI that seems more severe than usual. High temperature, purulent nasal discharge, and periorbital swelling and facial pain may be present.

B. Allergic Rhinitis

Sinusitis in children can also be associated with allergic rhinitis. This IgE-mediated hypersensitivity disorder of the nasal mucous membranes causes edema and increased production of seromucous secretions. Studies suggest that a child with allergic rhinitis who has persistent cough, chronic rhinorrhea, fatigue, and irritability, and who does not benefit from adequate antihistamines and decongestant therapy, should be evaluated for sinusitis (11).

C. Asthma

Frequent association of asthma and sinusitis has been appreciated in the past and, recently, has been reexamined (12–15). Asthma is a respiratory disease characterized by an increased responsiveness of the bronchi to various stimuli and manifested by a widespread narrowing of the airways that is reversible in severity, either spontaneously or as a result of therapy. The possibility that sinusitis might be a causal mechanism in developing asthma, in addition to being a frequently associated finding, has been postulated. Three potential hypotheses on the contribution of sinusitis to the pathogenesis of asthma are

(1) bacteria-laden mucopurulent material from the infected sinuses could drip into the pharynx, and by infectious extension, involve the mucous membranes of the lower respiratory tract, causing inflammation of the bronchial mucosa, and increasing bronchial airway hyperreactivity. (2) Infections of the respiratory tract are known to enhance β-adrenergic blockade (16). Because a partial blockade is present in patients with asthma, infected sinuses, being part of the respiratory tract would enhance the blockage, resulting in an increase in hyperreactivity of the bronchial tree. (3) Existence of a nasaobronchial reflex, mediated through the parasympathetic nervous system, has also been proposed over the past several years (12–15, 17). This theory suggests that stimulation of neural receptors in the nose and sinuses can activate the afferent fibers that form part of the trigeminal nerve. Collaterals from the trigeminal nerve fibers enter the reticular formation at which connection is made with the dorsal vagal nucleus. Parasympathetic fibers then proceed to the bronchial musculature, causing bronchospasm.

D. Immunodeficiency Disorders

Acute recurrent, as well as chronic sinus infections, may frequently develop in immunocompromised children. Deficiency in humoral or cell-mediated immunity, abnormal neutrophil or macrophage function, or a combination of these immunological defects, may predispose to sinus infections. Signs and symptoms vary in these children, who may appear similar to those patients who are immunocompetent, or whose symptoms may be more exaggerated or even more subtle initially (18).

Patients with altered humoral immunity, such as infantile X-linked agammaglobulinemia, common variable immunodeficiency, IgG and IgG subclass deficiencies, IgA deficiency, and immunodeficiency with ataxia–telangiectasia, have inadequate serum, as well as secretory, antibody response to infections. Such patients are more likely to have infections with pyogenic bacteria, particularly those with polysaccharide capsules such as *S. pneumoniae*, *H. influenzae*, *Pseudomonas*, or *Neisseria meningitidis*.

Patients with primary abnormal cell-mediated immunities, as well as secondary immunodeficiency, such as those who are receiving corticosteroid therapy, cytotoxic drugs, and patients with malignancies including leukemia, lymphoma, and Hodgkin's disease, are more susceptible to various fungal, viral, and parasitic pathogens such as *Pneumocystis carinii*.

The pathogens that are more likely to cause infection in the patient with poor neutrophil or marcrophage function, such as chronic granulomatous disease and Chediak-Higashai syndrome, as well as therapy with corticosteroids and cytotoxic drugs, are *S. aureus* and gram-negative bacterial species, such as *Klebsiella*, *Pseudomonas*, and *Serratia*. These patients are also at risk for infection with fungi, such as *Aspergillus* and *Nocardia*.

E. Cystic Fibrosis

Chronic pansinusitis occurs commonly in cystic fibrosis as a result of increased viscosity of secretions and obstruction of sinus ostia by the frequently associated nasal polyps. In a review of radiographic examinations of the paransal sinuses of 187 patients followed in the cystic fibrosis clinic of Children's Hospital of Pittsburgh from 1959 to 1971, 185 patients consistently had homogeneously opaque maxillary and ethmoid sinuses (19). The sinuses contained thick tenacious and purulent secretions. The organisms commonly recovered from sinus aspirates in cultures of surgical specimens include *P. aeruginosa, S. aureus, H. influenzae*, and anaerobes (20).

V. DIAGNOSTIC PROCEDURES

Diagnostic procedures that have been used for sinusitis include radiography, ultrasound, transillumination, rhinoscopy, and antral puncture (Table 4). Anteroposterior occipital (Water's view) and lateral radiographs of the paranasal sinuses can establish a diagnosis of paransal sinusitis most practically and effectively. Diffuse opacification, except possibly in infants (21), and an air–fluid level are considered diagnostic (Figs. 3 and 4). Mucosal thickening may be due to infection (22) or possibly to allergy (Fig. 5).

The diagnosis of sinusitis by A-mode ultrasound studies have been useful only if the sinuses are completely opaque on radiographic examinations (4). The frontal sinuses may possibly be screened by this method. The ethmoid and spenoid sinuses are not accessible to ultrasound examination. In general, A-mode ultrasound is used primarily for the detection of retained secretions

Table 4 Diagnostic Methods

Radiography
Computed tomography
Magnetic resonance imaging
Fiberoptic rhinoscopy
Maxillary aspiration (antral puncture)
A-Mode ultrasound
Transillumination

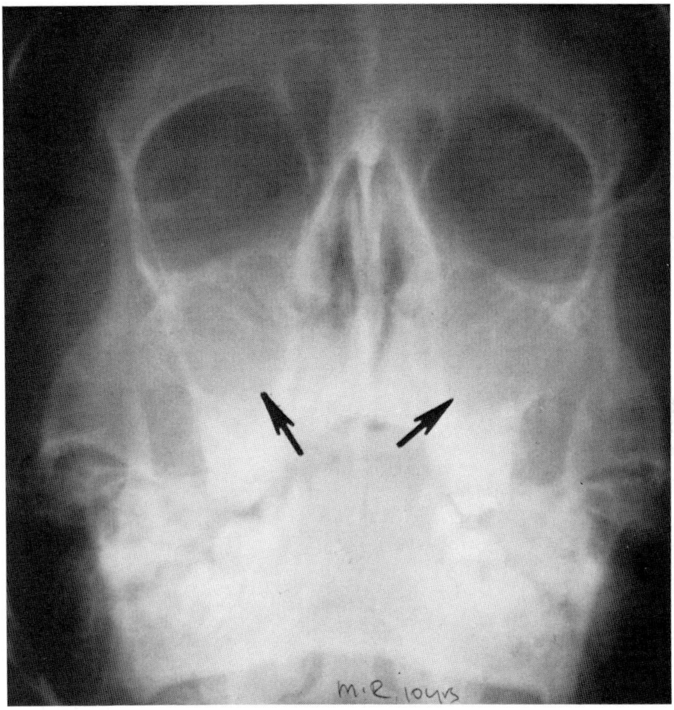

Figure 3 Maxillary antra are opaque (arrows).

within the sinus and not for mucosal thickening. Its clinical usefulness has yet to be completely defined (23).

Transillumination may be useful in screening adults, but it is not useful in detecting sinusitis in children (Fig. 6). Fiberoptic rhinoscopy can be particularly helpful in direct visualization of purulent secretions emanating directly from the sinus ostia.

Antral puncture is a most useful procedure in correlating radiographic evidence of sinusitis with bacteriology (4,7). It is not to be used clinically in the initial evaluation of sinusitis under most circumstances. Yet, for persistent infection or suspicion of an unusual organism in a compromised host, documenting the specific pathogen by aspiration and culture with microbial sensitivity tests will help in choosing the appropriate antibiotic.

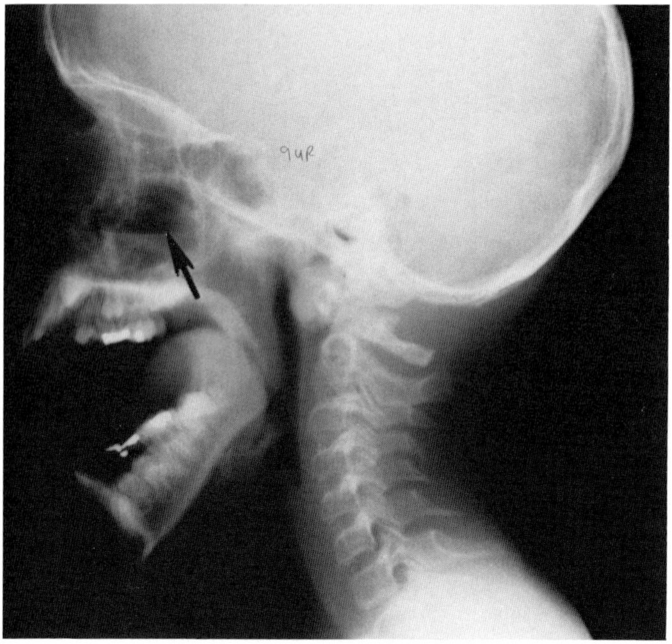

Figure 4 Maxillary sinusitis with air-fluid level (arrow).

Computed tomography (CT) scanning (Fig. 7) and magnetic resonance imaging (MRI) studies (Fig. 8) are quite definitive for such complications as orbital cellulitis and extension of sinusitis into the central nervous system. These studies are not currently practical for most patients with uncomplicated sinusitis because of the expense and inconvenience.

In an uncomplicated sinusitis in children, the diagnosis can usually be made from the history and physical examination. Sinus radiographs may be helpful and CT scans in selected patients with potential complication are necessary. Sinus aspiration may be indicated if there is clinical unresponsiveness to conventional therapy, sinusitis in an immunosuppressed patient, severe symptoms such as headache or facial pain, or life-threatening disease at the time of clinical presentation.

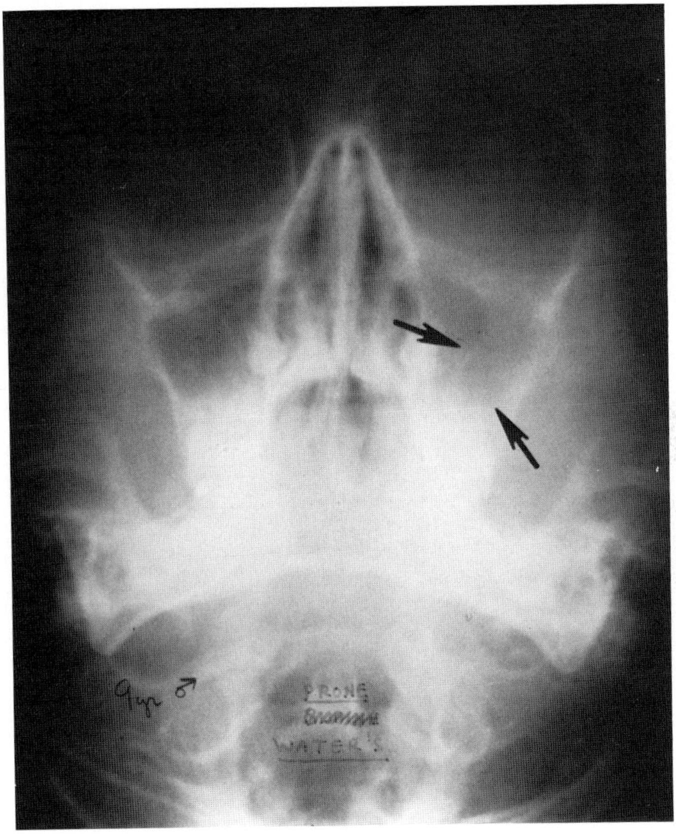

Figure 5 Increased mucosal thickening of maxillary sinuses (arrows).

VI. MEDICAL AND SURGICAL TREATMENT OF SINUSITIS

A. Medical Management (Table 5)

Acute sinusitis is usually associated with bacterial infection, and the primary focus of the management of acute and chronic sinusitis is proper antibiotic treatment. Amoxicillin is the first drug of choice in the treatment of acute sinusitis. If β-lactamase-producing bacteria are suspected, then amoxicillin–potassium clavulanate, trimethoprim–sulfamethoxazole, erythromycin-sulfisoxazole or cefaclor may be used. Treatment for 10–21 days is usually

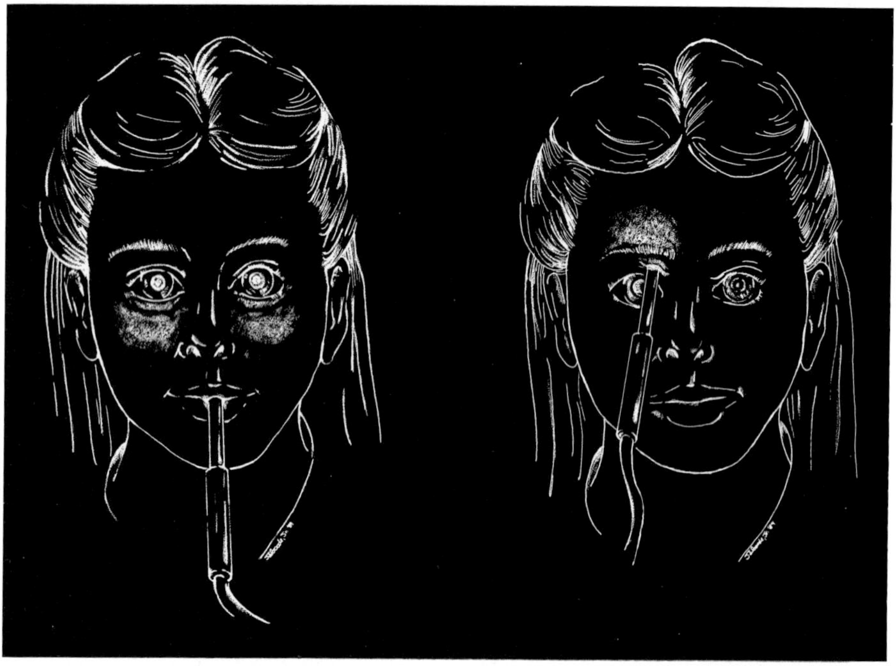

Figure 6 Transillumination.

adequate for most patients with acute sinusitis. The relief of sinus pain can usually be accomplished by the use of analgesics such as aspirin, acetaminophen, or a nonsteroidal anti-inflammatory drug, such as ibuprofen. The application of moist heat over the affected sinuses may also ease the discomfort. A vasoconstrictor in the form of an α-adrenergic nose drop or nasal spray, such as phenylephrine or oxymetazoline, may be useful in promoting sinus drainage. The use of topical or oral decongestants has not been evaluated adequately for efficacy in the management of acute sinusitis. The inhalation of warm air saturated with water is also quite useful for symptomatic relief.

In instances of recurrent sinusitis associated with allergy, the use of antihistamines, topical cromolyn, and topical nasal steroids can also be prescribed to decrease nasal mucosal edema and promote drainage of secretions. At times, a short course of prednisone, 3–4 days, may be useful to further promote decrease in nasal mucosal edema and encourage sinus drainage.

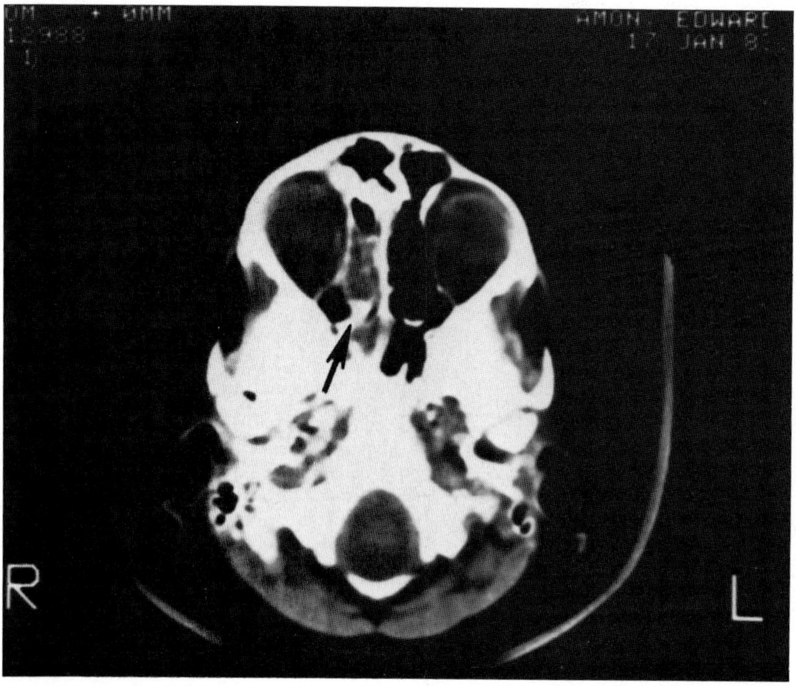

Figure 7 Computerized tomography scan showing ethmoidal sinusitis (arrows).

a short course of prednisone, 3–4 days, may be useful to further promote decrease in nasal mucosal edema and encourage sinus drainage.

If medical management is not effective after a second course of antibiotics, antral lavage may be entertained, both diagnostically (culture and sensitivity results) and therapeutically, for drainage of a closed-spaced infection (9). In the allergic rhinitis patient, immunotherapy with appropriate allergens should be helpful in management of allergic rhinitis and, potentially, decrease the frequency of sinusitis.

B. Surgical Management

Failure of medical therapy in a persistent or chronic sinusitis is an indication for consideration of surgical intervention to eliminate mechanical obstructions,

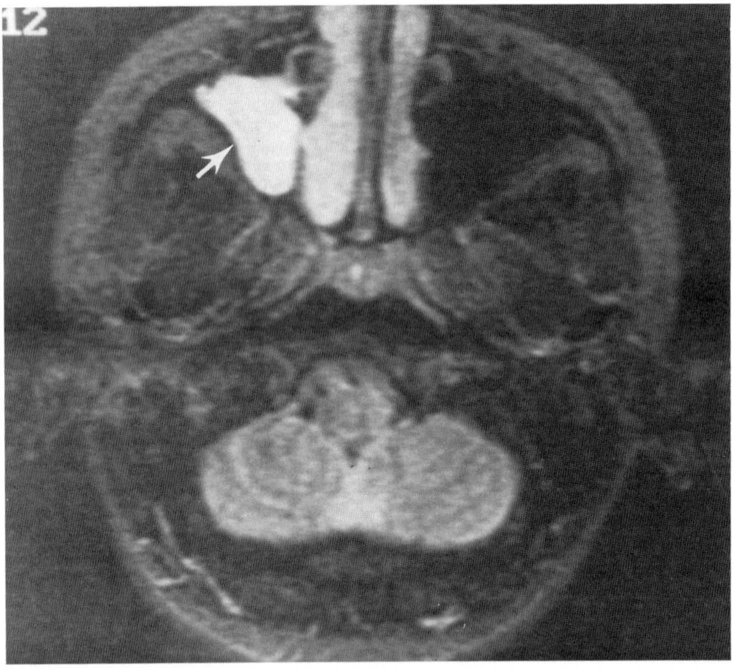

Figure 8 Acute sinusitis. Axial MRI image shows marked mucosal thickening and fluid within the right maxillary antrum. Slight mucosal thickening is also seen on the left.

drain infected sinuses, and establish new or better drainage systems for the sinuses (Table 6). An important distinction between adult and pediatric sinus drainage procedures is that surgery is rarely used for removal of diseased tissue in children, as is commonly performed in adults (24,25).

Table 5 Medical Management

Antibiotics
Analgesics
Decongestants
Antihistamines
Cromolyn
Steroids
Humidity and heat

A procedure commonly employed in young children is intranasal antrostomy or the creation of a nasoantral window between the nasal cavity and the maxillary sinus (Fig. 9; 25). This surgically created ostium is a routine part of the Caldwell–Luc procedure (refers to an anterior approach to the maxillary sinus through the canine fossa of the maxilla and formation of an antrostomy into the inferior meatus). The Caldwell–Luc procedure is generally avoided in children because of the increased likelihood of damage to unerupted teeth.

Recently, intranasal endoscopic surgical procedures—such as polypectomy, middle meatus antrostomy, intranasal ethmoidectomy, and sphenoidotomy—have been developed to facilitate treatment.

Other less commonly employed surgical procedures are ethmoidectomy and trephination of the frontal sinuses in patients who are not responding to medical therapy or in whom complications are threatening or present. Procedures for removal of diseased tissue, such as the Caldwell–Luc procedure, ethmoidectomy, and frontal sinus obliterative procedures, should be restricted to complicated cases or to patients with underlying systemic conditions such as cystic fibrosis, immotile cilia syndrome (cilia dyskinesia), or immune deficiencies.

Antibiotic treatment of sinusitis in cystic fibrosis patients is often accomplished during treatment of pulmonary exacerbations. It usually consists of a semisynthetic penicillin, such as ticarcillin, and an aminoglycoside, such as tobramycin. These are the antibiotics usually given both prophylactically and therapeutically in the perioperative period in which nasal and paranasal sinus surgery is performed (26).

C. Nasal Polyps

Even though nasal polyps are rare in children, they are the most common nasal masses, aside from intranasal foreign bodies. They are seen as gelatinous, semitranslucent, round or pear-shaped, and pale entities found most commonly in the middle meatus, extending to the nasal cavity or projecting posteriorly

Table 6 Surgical Management

Sinus aspiration
Nasoantral window
Polypectomy
Caldwell–Luc
Ethmoidectomy

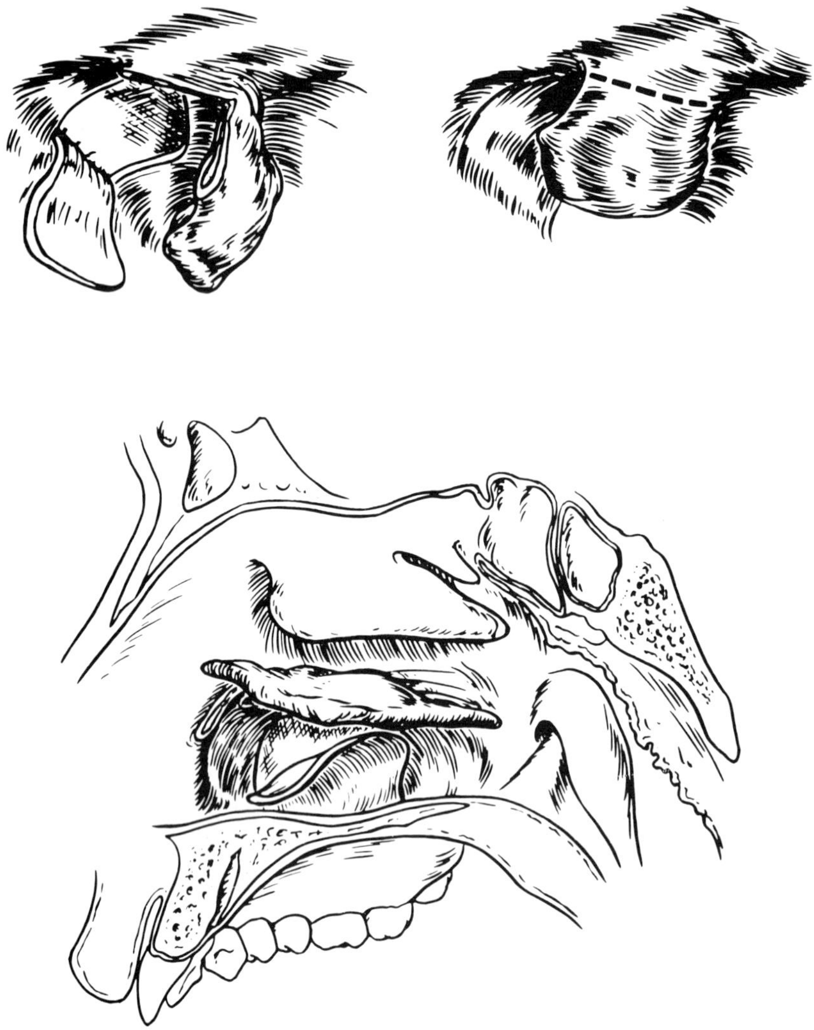

Figure 9 Intranasal antrostomy Fracture of the inferior turbinate and creation of a 1 × 2-cm mucoperiostal flap in the inferior meatus preceded by the formation of a bony window.

into the nasopharynx (choanal polyp; Fig. 10). Nasal polyps in children requiring surgical intervention are infrequent. For example, a study at the Children's Hospital of Pittsburgh from 1964 to 1978 showed only 0.3% (120 patients) of the total otolaryngological surgical admissions were for removal of nasal polyps (27).

The mass of a nasal polyp is made up chiefly of edema fluid, with sparse fiber cells and a few mucous glands. Nasal polyps appear to be derived from, and contain most of the cellular and chemical elements found in the respiratory mucosa (28). They seem to be void of sensory vasomotor and secretomotor enervation. The histology of polyps varies in different diseases. The polyps from atopic patients have thickening of the epithelial basement membranes, numerous eosinophils, and a neutral mucin. In contrast, polyps from cystic

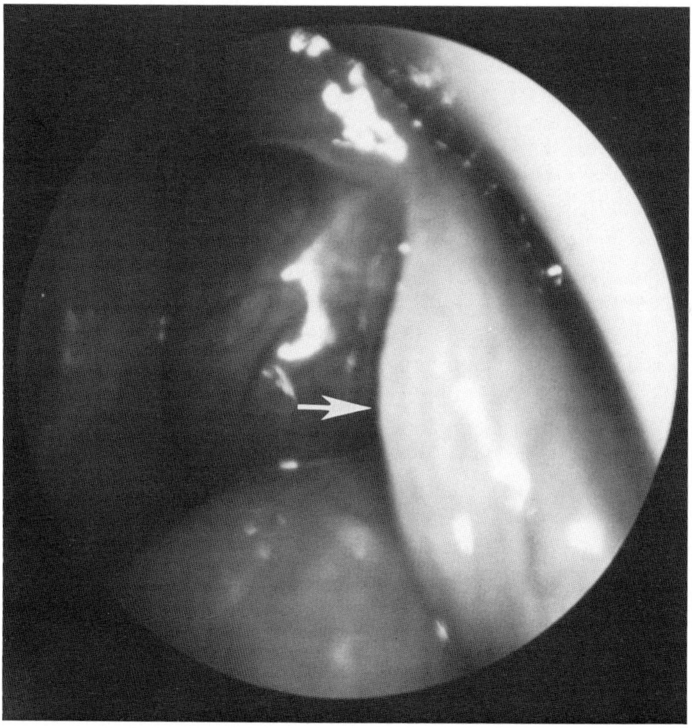

Figure 10 Nasal polyp (arrow).

fibrosis patients have a barely visible basement membrane, a lack of eosinophils, and a preponderance of acid mucin. The pathogenesis of nasal polyps is not known. Concomitant mucosal injury, interference with sinus drainage, and hinderance of ciliary action will create a static environment that is susceptible to bacterial invasion, resulting in sinusitis. Sinusitis causes more venous stasis and mucosal edema, which leads to further enlargment of polyps.

Nasal polyps in children are occasionally associated with allergy. One study found that 3% of patients with single polyps, and 59% of patients with multiple polyps, without concomitant cystic fibrosis, had a history of allergy (27). Pediatric patients with nasal polyps, after exclusion of cystic fibrosis, deserve an allergic evaluation. If clinically relevant IgE-mediated disease is found, allergy management would be indicated.

Asthma is not commonly associated with nasal polyps in children (29). Polyposis, rhinitis, and asthma, in association with aspirin or other nonsteroidal inflammatory drug intolerance, is a well-known clinical triad in older patients, but it is seen rarely in children.

D. Complications of Sinusitis

Complications of sinusitis occur, but are less common since the introduction of antibiotics (Table 7). Serious complications include orbital cellulitis, abscess formation, cavernous sinus thrombosis, meningitis, subdural empyema, and osteomyelitis. Osteomyelitis usually occurs in the frontal sinus area because of venus drainage into the diploic veins of the skull. Because the frontal sinuses are not well developed in children, this is not a problem until later years.

Sinus infections have been associated with lower respiratory tract infections and asthma. The relationship between asthma and sinusitis has been frequently reported. However, the definitive controlled study has never been reported and, at this point, we must conclude that there are no data to support a

Table 7 Complication of Sinusitis

Orbital cellulitis and abscess
Cavernous sinus thrombosis
Meningitis, brain abscess, subdural empyema
Osteomyelitis
Polyps, mucoceles
Asthma

nasobronchial reflex as a factor in chronic asthma (30,31). However, treatment of sinusitis or sinobronchitis will, in most instances, improve the asthmatic symptom (9,11,13,14,24).

E. Immunodeficiency

Recognition of an immunodeficiency state in the patient with sinusitis warrants the same treatment as seen with other patients with sinusitis, with the addition of measures to replace or reconstitute the immune deficiency, depending upon the type of immunodeficiency. Organisms of low-grade virulence are more common pathogens in the immunodeficient patient. Early irrigation or aspiration of the sinuses to establish bacteriological diagnosis may be essential in these compromised patients so that appropriate antibiotic therapy can be promptly instituted. Patients with specific immune defects will also benefit from immunological replacement, such as gamma globulin therapy and bone marrow transplantation (18). Various measures have been recommended for preventing infection in immunocompromised hosts, such as immunization with pneumococcal vaccine, and prophylactic antibiotic therapy in children 3 years of age and older.

VII. SUMMARY

Sinusitis is frequently associated with allergic rhinitis. Signs and symptoms of persistent cough, purulent nasal discharge, headache, sore throat with postnasal draining, and bad breath, suggests sinusitis clinically and associated wheezing suggests concomitant asthma. Diagnostic procedures most clinically useful are roentgenograms of the paranasal sinuses, which should help establish the diagnosis. A CT scan or MRI is needed in selected patients. Treatment is primarily with broad-spectrum antibiotics that cover the spectrum of bacteria such *Streptococcus pneumonae*, *Haemophilus influenzae*, and *Branhamella catarrhalis* for a period of 10–21 days. Surgical treatment for sinusitis is rarely needed in children unless complicated by immunodeficiencies, cystic fibrosis, and other predisposing abnormalities and complications. When allergic rhinitis is present, skin testing will help define the etiologic allergens. Appropriate management of the allergic rhinitis with enviromental control measures, mediations, and immunotherapy should alleviate the symptoms and may help prevent sinusitis in individual allergic children.

REFERENCES

1. Rohr PS, Spector SL. Sinusitis: pathophysiology, diagnosis and management. Immunol Allergy Clin N Am 1987; 7:383–391.
2. Dalessio DJ. Headache and other head pain, 3rd ed. New York: Oxford University Press, 1972:477–505.
3. Rachelefsky GS, Katz RM, Siegal SC. Disease of paranasal sinuses in children. Curr Probl Pediatr 1982; 12:1–57.
4. Wald ER, Milmoe W, Bowen AD, Ledesma-Medina J, Salamon BS, Bluestone CL. Acute maxillary sinusitis in children. N Engl J Med 1981; 304:749–754.
5. Brook I. Bacteriologic features of chronic sinusitis in children. JAMA 1981; 246:967–969.
6. Evans FO, Jr, Sydnor JB, Moore WEC, Moore CR, Manwaring JL, Brill AL, Jackson RT, Hanna S, Skaar BS, Holdeman LV, Fitz-Hugh GS, Sande MA, Gwaltney JM Jr. Sinusitis of the maxillary antrum. N Engl J Med 1975; 293:735–739.
7. Frederick J, Braude AI. Anaerobic infection of the paranasal sinuses. N Engl J Med 1974; 290:135.
8. Goldstein MF, Atkins PC, Cogan FC, Kornstein MJ, Levine RS, Zweiman B. Allergic aspergillus sinusitis. J Allergy Clin Immunol 1985; 76:515–524.
9. Friedman R, Ackerman M, Wald E, Casselbrant M, Friday G, Fireman P. Asthma and bacterial sinusitis in children. J Allergy Clin Immunol 1984; 74:185–189.
10. Slavin RG. Nasal polyps and sinusitis. In: Middleton E Jr, Reed CE, Ellis EF, Adkinson, NF Jr, Younginger JW, eds. Allergy principles and practice. Clinical Science, vol 2. St Louis: CV Mosby, 1988:1291–1303.
11. Rachelefsky GS, Goldberg M, Katz RM, Boris G, Gyepes MT, Shapiro MJ, MIckey MA, Finegold SM, Siegal SG. Sinus disease in children with respiratory allergy. J Allergy Clin Immunol 1978; 61:310–314.
12. Sluder G. Asthma as a nasal reflex. JAMA 1919; 73:589–591.
13. Slavin RG. Relationship of nasal disease and sinusitis to bronchial asthma. Ann Allergy 1982; 49:76–80.
14. Slavin RG, Cannon RE, Friedman WH, Palstange E, Sundaram M. Sinusitis and bronchial asthma. J Allergy Clin Immunol. 1980; 66:250–259.
15. Rachelefsky GS, Katz RM, Siegal SC Chronic sinus disease with associated reactive airway disease in children. Pediatrics 1984; 73:526–529.
16. Szentivanyi A. The beta adrenergic theory of the atopic abnormality in bronchial asthma. J Allergy 1968; 42:203–232.
17. Gottlieb MJ. Relation of intranasal disease in the production of bronchial asthma. JAMA 1925; 85:105–108.
18. Page R, Friday G, Stillwagon P, Skone D. Caliguiri L, Fireman P. Asthma and selective immunoglobulin subclass deficiency: improvement of asthma after immunoglobulin replacement therapy. J Pediatr 1988; 112:127–131.
19. Ledesma-Medina J, Osman MZ, Girdany BR. Abnormal paranasal sinuses in

patients with cystic fibrosis of the pancreas: radiological findings. Pediatr Radiol 1980; 9:61-64.
20. Shapiro ED, Milmoe GJ, Wald ER, Rodman JB, Bowen A. Bacteriology of the maxillary sinuses in patients with cystic fibrosis. J. Infect Dis 1982; 146:589-593.
21. Glasier CM, Mallory GB, Steele RW. Significance of opacification of the maxillary and ethmoid sinuses in infants. J Pediatr 1989; 114:45-50.
22. Axelsson A, Greiselius N, Childerez N, Jensen C. The correlation between the radiological examination and the irrigation findings in maxillary sinusitis. Acta Otoaryngol 1970; 69:302-306.
23. Healy GB. Methods of examination. In: Bluestone CD, Stool SE, eds. Pediatric otolaryngology, vol 1. Philadelphia: WB Saunders, 1983; 689-704.
24. Friedman WH, Katsaneonis GP, Slavin RG, Kannel P, Lindord P. Sphenoethmoidectomy: its role in the asthmatic patient. Otolaryngol Head Neck Surg 1982; 90:171-177.
25. Fisher SR, Newman CE. Surgical perspectives on allergic airway disease. J Allergy Clin Immunol 1988; 81: 361-375.
26. Crockett DM, McGill TJ, Friedman EM, Healy GB, Salkeld LJ. Nasal and paranasal sinus surgery in children with cystic fibrosis. Ann Otol Rhinol Laryngol 1987; 96:367-372.
27. Schramm VL, Effron MZ. Nasal polyps in children. Laryngoscope 1980; 90:1488-1495.
28. Taylor M. Histochemical studies of nasal polypi. J Laryngol Otol. 1973; 77:326.
29. Settipane GA, Chafee FH. Nasal polyps in asthma and rhinitis. J Allergy Clin Immunol 1977; 59:17-21.
30. McFadden EF, Jr. Nasal-sinus-pulmonary reflexes and bronchial asthma. J Allergy Clin Immunol 1986; 78:1-3.
31. Friday GA, Fireman P. Sinusitis and asthma: clinical and pathogenetic relationships. Clin Chest Med. 1988; 9:557-565.

8

Nasal Obstruction and Facial Development

Gina M. Trask and Peter A. Shapiro
University of Washington School of Dentistry, Seattle, Washington

I. INTRODUCTION

Nasal obstruction in children can be caused by a variety of factors such as allergic rhinitis, adenoid hypertrophy, polyps, congenital nasal deformities, neoplasms, and recurrent upper respiratory infections. The relationship between nasal obstruction and facial development is not completely understood. Furthermore, the extent to which the clinician can influence facial development therapeutically is controversial. This chapter will review the scientific literature concerning these controversies and provide the clinician with guidelines to address the problem of nasal obstruction in children.

II. HISTORICAL PERSPECTIVE

There has been long-standing disagreement between two groups: those who support the functional matrix theory, that is, that function dictates facial form; and others who believe that facial structure is governed strictly by heredity. This controversy is evident for the effects of altered respiration on facial development.

Morrison (1), in a historical review of the literature, cited a number of authors who reported a relationship between nasal obstruction and palatal form. Others, including Duke (2), Bowen (3), Cohen (4), and Straub (5), stated that chronic allergy influenced dentofacial development. They felt that an altered mode of breathing could result in a high and narrow palate, protruded maxillary incisors, a retrusive mandible, and a long, narrow face. Figure 1 diagrams some common anatomical relationships.

Some authors believed that genetic factors were responsible for facial type. Ballard (6) and Gwynne-Evans (7) conducted a 15-year longitudinal study on the relationship between dentofacial morphology and upper respiratory conditions. They concluded that orofacial structure remained constant during growth, and variations were determined by inheritance. Gwynne-Evans (7) stated that "the facial mask is innate to the individual and resists change by any means." Ranley (8) proposed a composite view, stating that the chondrocranium is influenced by both intrinsic genetic and local environmental factors.

III. CLINICAL HUMAN STUDIES

In 1960, Linder-Aronson and Backstorm (9) evaluated 115 children about 10 years of age. They compared dental occlusion in mouth and nose breathers and evaluated the influence of adenoid size and nasal resistance on facial

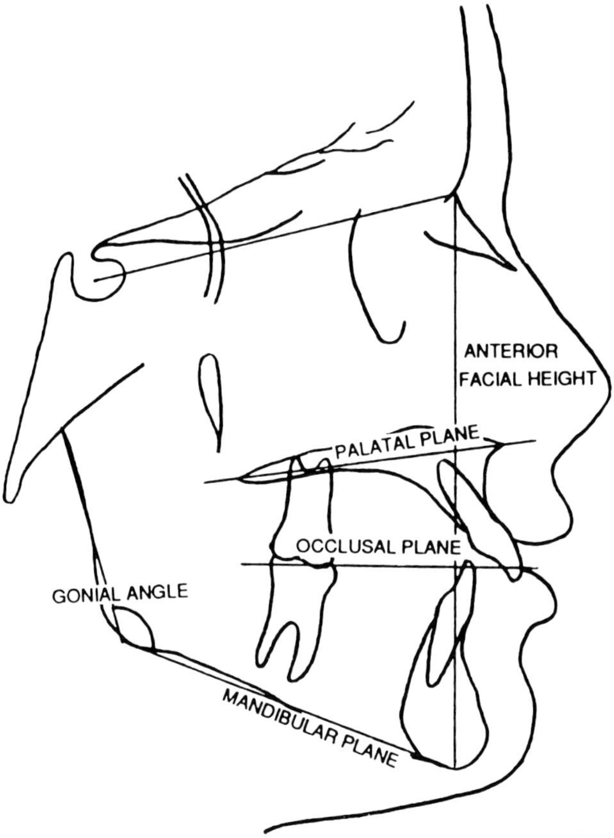

Figure 1 Common anatomical relationships: anterior facial height, gonial angle, mandibular plane, palatal plane, and occlusal plane.

dimensions. Subjects were categorized as mouth or nose breathers by observation, with the aid of moisture condensation on mirrors, and by movement of cotton held before the nose. The investigators concluded that children with long, narrow jaws had greater nasal resistance. Although the height of the palate was greater in habitual mouth breathers, no direct correlation could be shown between mouth breathing and malocclusion.

Linder-Aronson (10) then performed a more complex cross-sectional evaluation of children to identify any correlation between airway obstruction from adenoid hypertrophy and dentofacial characteristics. Eighty-one children scheduled for adenoidectomy were studied before and after the procedure and were compared with 81 age and sex-matched controls. The children with obstructed noses had longer faces, retrognathic maxilla and mandible, decreased sagittal depth of the bony nasopharynx, and a tendency to hold the tongue in a lower position. When facial photographs were analyzed, only 25% of the children scheduled for adenoidectomy and 4% of the controls were judged to display the characteristic "adenoid facies." Therefore, although differences existed between the two groups, the author discouraged using the facial pattern as a diagnostic characteristic of nasal airway obstruction.

Other studies also found a relationship between airway obstruction and facial characteristics. Dunn (11) tried to limit the amount of genetic variability in the subjects by evaluating frontal and lateral cephalometric radiographs from 33 pairs of 7- to 12-year-old monozygotic twins. The pairs were characterized as being similar or different for adenoid size. In the group with significant adenoidal size difference, the gonial angle increased as the nasopharyngeal size decreased. The gonial angles were similar in the group of pairs with similar adenoidal size.

Woodside and Linder-Aronson (12) evaluated lateral radiographs taken serially on 127 males from 6 to 20 years of age. They demonstrated a relationship between airway obstruction in the nose or nasopharynx and increased lower anterior face height. Quick and Gundlach (13), in a study of pretreatment lateral cephalographs of 155 patients, also found that the size of the nasopharynx was smaller in the long-faced group.

Another form of restricted nasal respiration, unilateral choanal atresia, was studied by Freng (14). Eleven males with choanal atresia were matched with normal controls on the basis of age, sex, and ethnic background. The length of both the maxilla and mandible were significantly shorter in the choanal atresia group.

Nasal obstruction resulting from atopic disease has been studied extensively. Marks (15) hypothesized that malocclusions seen in allergic rhinitis patients were a result of venous stasis. Eastman (16) felt that airway maintenance would take precedence over other factors in determining the postural position of structures that form the airway. He theorized that, in allergic patients, the mouth breathing that frequently occurs alters the environmental matrix of the dentition.

Only recently has more controlled research been undertaken. Hannuksela (17) evaluated the effect of moderate and severe atopy on the facial skeleton of 100 11-year-old children. Groups were determined by the degree of allergy and size of the adenoids. Overall, with increasing severity of allergy and increasing adenoidal size, dorsal rotation of the mandible and an anterior lowering of the nasal floor occurred. The author concluded that atopy may lead to disturbances in growth of the facial skeleton.

In Sassouni's (18) study comparing perennial allergic rhinitis children and controls, he reported that the 37 children with allergic disease had a significantly larger palatomandibular angle and a longer upper and lower facial height. Evaluation of the posterioanterior radiographs showed that the bilateral orbital breadth and the bizygomatic dimensions were narrowed in the allergic group. His observation of long and narrow faces in the atopic children is in agreement with several previously mentioned studies of mouth breathers.

Bresolin and coauthors (19) also evaluated the effects of mouth breathing and allergic rhinitis on dental and skeletal relationships. Thirty allergic children were compared with 15 age-matched controls. The allergic subjects had positive histories for allergic rhinitis, positive immediate skin tests and were judged by parent and physician to have been chronic mouth breathers. The controls were nonallergic and apparent nose breathers. Both skeletal and dental differences were found. The allergic group had longer faces, more divergent mandibular angles, more retrusive profiles, increased palatal heights, and narrower maxillary intermolar widths (Fig. 2).

In a study that used similar methods, Trask (20) and associates analyzed the effects of perennial allergic rhinitis on dental and facial skeletal characteristics. Twenty-five allergic children, who were apparent mouth breathers, their 25 siblings who were not atopic and were apparent nose breathers, and 14 nasal-breathing control subjects were examined medically, dentally, and cephalometrically. The allergic subjects, compared with controls, had longer faces and more retrusive profiles. However, the retrusive characteristic was also present in the nonallergic siblings and, therefore, could not be ascribed to the apparent mode of breathing.

Although most of the current research demonstrates a relationship between impaired nasal respiration and dentofacial characteristics, there is still no consensus on this issue. Koski and Lahdemaki (21), in a study of lateral head radiographs of 15 children from 7 to 16 years of age with obstructing adenoids, found these children had smaller gonial angles than a control group of 40 girls from 6 to 9 years of age. However, in a longitudinal study of cephalometric radiographs of 12 subjects from 9 months to 18 years, Handelman and Osborne (22) did not demonstrate a relationship between nasopharyngeal airway obstruction and the mandibular plane angle.

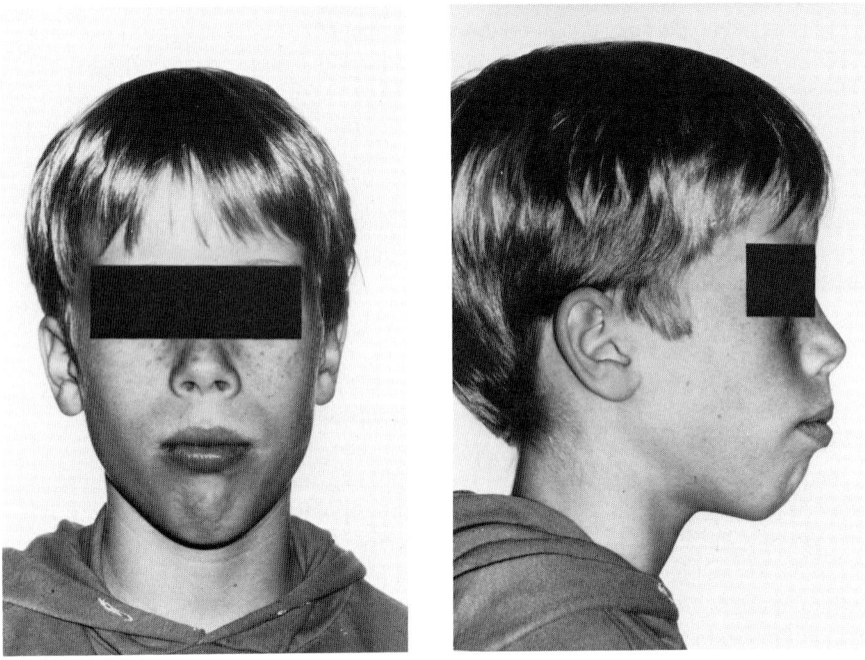

(a)

Figure 2 Frontal and profile views of two boys with allergic rhinitis. The boy in (a) has the typical facies attributed to children with allergic rhinitis, while the boy in (b) has a more normal facial pattern.

IV. INDUCED NASAL OBSTRUCTION IN ANIMALS

To eliminate some variables present in human studies, Harvold (23) investigated the effects of induced nasal obstruction on rhesus monkeys. Nine pairs of monkeys were studied. In one of each pair the nasal apertures were occluded with silicone nose plugs, forcing the animals to breathe exclusively through their mouths. The other animal of the pair served as a control. After 15 months, the following changes were observed in the experimental animals, but not in the controls: notching of the upper lip, an alteration in tongue morphology,

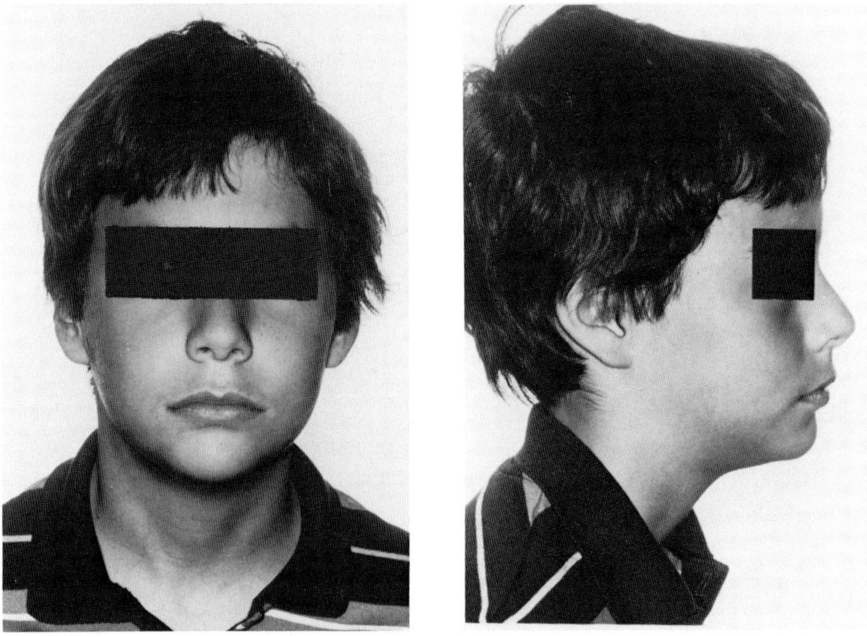

(b)

increased total face height and gonial angles, and decreased maxillary and mandibular intercanine width.

In studying 42 additional rhesus monkeys (21 experimental and 21 age- and sex-matched controls), Harvold (24) found similar facial changes in the experimental animals. He also studied the animals electromyographically and found that individual animals recruited different muscle combinations to aid in oral breathing. This led to variable changes in dental, skeletal, and facial characteristics.

Miller and co-workers (25) also examined the muscular changes resulting from changes in mode of breathing. Experimental rhesus monkeys had their nasal cavity obstructed, whereas age-matched controls did not. Rhythmic muscle activity increased in a variety of facial muscle groups in the first months following nasal obstruction. After approximately 5 months, tonic discharge became important. The authors concluded that long-term changes in craniofacial function correlate with soft-tissue changes and precede morphological adaptation of the cranioskeleton.

Tomer (26) studied the effects of nasal obstruction on mandibular growth in eight pairs of rhesus monkeys. The nose of one member of each pair was obstructed with silicone plugs. After 3 years of observation, the experimental monkeys displayed an increased facial height and gonial angle, an increased mandibular plane angle, and an increase in the angle between the posterior border of the ramus and a line drawn between the condyles.

Ramadan (27) investigated the relationship between nasal obstruction and facial form in growing albino rabbits. Four-week-old rabbits underwent nasal electrocauterization; in 20 animals no nasal obstruction was found, in 20 animals unilateral obstruction was created, and in the remaining 20 bilateral nasal obstruction was produced. At maturity (6 months of age), the animals with bilateral nasal obstruction displayed narrower and shorter alveolar arches.

Animal studies clearly show a relationship between mode of breathing, muscular activity, and craniofacial morphology. However, in most of the studies, the effects of nasal obstruction in individual animals was highly variable. As many of the authors have indicated, we cannot directly extrapolate these findings to human beings.

V. METHODS OF DETERMINING MODE OF BREATHING

Some of the confusion in the literature concerning the effects of respiration on facial deveopment may be due to the difficulty in determining the subject's actual mode of breathing. The methods for this determination have ranged from simple observation, holding an object in front of the airway, measuring the nasopharyngeal space cephalometrically, measuring the nasal resistance, to any combination of the above. Each technique has limitations. Some of the methods do not quantify respiration. Those that do, use equipment that tends to be bulky, cumbersome, and unnatural feeling. Consequently, the subject may alter his/her mode of breathing subconsciously. Also, young children have difficulty performing the procedures necessary to get accurate readings. One limitation common to all methods is that subjects may undergo cyclic respiration, switching from nasal to oral respiration at different times of the day.

The techniques used to measure airflow and nasal resistance have varied, partially explaining why the results of the studies using these devices have also varied. Vig (28) studied 28 subjects divided into three categories: normals, lip incompetent without long faces, and lip incompetent with long faces. Neither long-faced morphology nor lip incompetence was a reliable indicator of mouth breathing. Linder-Aronson (10) and Sassouni (18) found a correlation between nasal airflow and craniofacial morphology; Watson (29) found no relationship.

VI. RESULTS OF INTERVENTION

Although most current literature demonstrates a relationship between nasal obstruction and craniofacial development, there is little information about the value of intervention. Miller, et al. (30) studied neuromuscular changes in eight rhesus monkeys during 2 years of nasal obstruction (caused by silicone plugs) and 18 months after plug removal. During the nasal obstruction period various muscles exhibited rhythmic or tonic responses. Within 1 week after removal of the nasal obstruction, this rhythmic activity stopped. However, tonic discharge still occurred in the genioglossus, geniohyoid, inferior obicularis oris, and lip-elevator fibers during the postobstruction period. The authors reported that experimentally induced nasal obstruction appeared to establish an altered drive of certain craniofacial muscles, which then became the normal mode. The original stimulus was supplanted by a learned central synaptic control of the specific muscles.

The effect of reversing nasal obstruction in human subjects is uncertain. Sassouni and co-workers (18) conducted a pilot study of 12 children with perennial allergic rhinitis. After 2½ years of treatment for allergy, no significant dentofacial changes were found. Linder-Aronson (31) analyzed the effect of adenoidectomy on the dentition and nasopharynx. He followed 37 children who had adenoidectomies and who seemed to change from mouth breathing to nose breathing, and 37 matched controls. After 1 year the children who underwent adenoidectomy had a significantly greater increase in the following areas: upper and lower incisors to the sellanasion and mandibular planes, width of the upper dental arch between the first molars, and sagittal depth of the nasopharynx. These children were evaluated 5 years postsurgery (32). An association between adenoidectomy and the establishment of a more horizontal growth pattern of the mandible was found in girls, but not in boys. Coversely, Hannuksela (33) showed no significant differences between variables studied in children with enlarged adenoids and those children who had undergone adenoidectomy.

VII. CLINICAL IMPLICATIONS

Although most current research demonstrates some relationship between mode of breathing and facial development, there are many unanswered questions concerning the actual cause and effect relationships. At what proportion of oral versus nasal respiration does facial development become adversely affected? Is the effect on facial development progressive with longer periods of nasal impairment? Are the results of these changes reversible with interception? The answers to these and other questions will be found only with controlled longitudinal evaluations of subjects, treated and untreated, who are defined by objective measures of facial growth and respiratory patterns. Until these studies have been undertaken, the clinician should be cautious in recommending aggressive treatment to specifically affect facial development. However, there is justification for trying to correct problems of medical importance to the patient, especially if they are undesirable influences on facial development. A good example of such a problem is symptomatic nasal obstruction. Correction of that problem may have beneficial effects on chronic rhinorrhea, hyponasal speech, recurrent middle ear problems, and recurrent sinusitis, as well as on facial development.

As noted previously, some patients who appear to be mouth breathers have patent nasal airways, and others who appear to have nasal obstruction breathe normally. If a patient appears to have some upper airway impairment, a thorough history and examination should be performed. A complete history should include familial patterns, onset, duration, exacerbating and ameliorating factors, and chronic versus intermittent nature. Physical examination should include visualization of nasal mucosa: color, edema, presence of polyps, and the nature of secretions. A history of chronic airway obstruction with a patent nose may be indicative of enlarged adenoids. A lateral head radiograph can be used to evaluate adenoidal size. However, because any radiograph is only two-dimensional, one must be cautious in drawing conclusions about adenoidal size and airway patency.

A positive history of chronic rhinitis and its associated symptoms may indicate allergy. Allergic rhinitis is known to be the most common cause of chronic nasal obstruction in children. Treatment, such as avoidance of allergens, pharmacologic intervention, and appropriately used immunotherapy, are likely to decrease the symptoms of chronic nasal disease.

Surgical intervention to alter obstructing turbinates has been advocated by some practitioners. However, there is no long-term data that demonstrates this procedure reduces nasal obstruction for any substantial period postsurgery. The effect of turbinate surgery on the growth and function of the nasal structure in children also is unknown.

There are three major issues of importance to orthodontists related to nasal obstruction. The first is that children who grow with a divergent facial pattern present orthodontic problems that are difficult to treat. Second, nasal obstruction may be related to abnormal tongue function and muscle balance, both factors that may negatively affect the stability of orthodontic treatment. Third, orthodontists are sometimes asked to widen narrow palates to decrease nasal resistance. This procedure, commonly called palatal expansion, can be used only if the posterior teeth are in crossbite, otherwise an iatrogenic malocclusion could be created. Also there is no information on the long-term effects of mechanical enlargement of the nasal airway. For example, if the patient is allergic, will the tissues enlarge to fill the space?

Orthodontic treatment procedures used to affect dentofacial development are used most effectively while the child is still growing. Therefore, the physician who notes malocclusion features, such as palatal constriction, mandibular retrognathism, or anterior open bite should consider referring the patient to an orthodontist as soon as the problem is discovered. Similarly, the orthodontist should consider medical referral of patients who present with apparent nasal obstruction.

Most research indicates a relationship between nasal obstruction and altered facial growth. Nevertheless, the data are not conclusive. Our ability as clinicians to alter some aspects of facial growth is variable. Therefore, specific and aggressive treatment to affect mode of respiration or facial growth should be undertaken with caution, and patients should be made aware of the present limitations.

REFERENCES

1. Morrison WW. The interrelationship between nasal obstruction and oral deformities. The action of obstructed nasal breathing upon the mouth and the facial structures, an historical review. Int J Orthod 1931; 17:453–458.
2. Duke WW. Asthma, hay fever, urticaria, and allied manifestations of allergy. St Louis: CV Mosby, 1926.
3. Bowen R. Dental and palate deformities due to perennial nasal allergy in childhood. Balyeat-Bowen, Hay Fever Asthma Clin 1939; 8:2.
4. Cohen MB. Orthodontic problems associated with allergy. Angle Orthod 1937; 7:150–154.
5. Straub WJ. Frequency of allergy in orthodontic patients. J Am Dent Assoc 1947: 31:334–342.
6. Editorial. The mouth breather. Br Med J 1957; X:1109.
7. Gwynne-Evans E. Discussion on the mouthbreather. Proc R Soc Med 1958; 51:279–282.
8. Ranley DM. Theories of craniofacial growth. In: Ranley DM, ed. A synopsis of craniofacial growth. New York: Appleton-Century-Crofts, 1980.
9. Linder-Aronson S, Backstrom A. A comparison between mouth and nose breathers with respect to occlusal and facial dimensions. Odont Rev 1960; 2:343–376.
10. Linder-Aronson S. Adenoids—their effect on mode of breathing and nasal airflow and their relationship to characteristics of the facial skeleton and the dentition.

Acta Otolaryngol Suppl 1970; 265:1–132.
11. Dunn GF, Green LJ, Cunat JJ. Relationship between variation of mandibular morphology and variation of nasopharyngeal airway site in monozygotic twins. Angle Orthod 1973; 43:129–135.
12. Woodside DG, Linder-Aronson S. The channelization of upper and lower anterior face heights compared to population standards in males between ages 6 to 20 years. Eur J Orthod 1979; 1:25–40.
13. Quick CA, Gundlach KH. Adenoid facies. Laryngoscope 1978;88:327–333.
14. Freng A. Dentofacial development in long lasting nasal stenosis. Scand J Dent Res 1979; 87:260–267.
15. Marks MB. Allergy in relation to orofacial dental deformities in children: a review. J Allergy 1965; 36:293–302.
16. Eastman GA. Oropharyngeal muscular interrelationships in chronic nasorespiratory allergy—a cephalometric study [Dissertation]. Ann Arbor: University of Michigan, 1963.
17. Hannuksela A. The effect of moderate and severe atopy on the facial skeleton. Eur J Orthod 1981; 3: 187–193.
18. Sassouni V, Friday G, Shnorhokian H, Beery Q, Fullo T, Miller D, Murphy S, Landay R. The influence of perennial allergic rhinitis on facial type and a pilot study of the effect of allergy management on facial growth patterns. Ann Allergy 1985;54:493–497.
19. Bresolin D, Shapiro GG, Shapiro PA, Chapko MK, Dassel S. Mouthbreathing in allegic children: its relationship to dentofacial development. Am J Orthod 1983; 83:334–340.
20. Trask GM, Shapiro GG, Shapiro PA. The effects of perennial allergic rhinitis on dental and skeletal development: a comparison of sibling pairs. Am J Orthod Dentofacial Orthop 1987; 92:286–293.
21. Koski K, Lahdemaki P. Adaptation of the mandible in children with adenoids. Am J Orthod 1975; 68:660–665.
22. Handelman CS, Osborne G. Growth of the nasopharynx and adenoid development from one to eighteen years. Angle Orthod 1976; 46:243–259.
23. Harvold EP, Vargervik K, Chierici G. Primate experiments on oral sensation and dental malocclusions. Am J Orthod 1973; 63:494–508.
24. Harvold EP, Tomer BS, Vargervik K, Chierici G. Primate experiments on oral respiration. Am J Orthod 1981; 79:359–373.
25. Miller AJ, Vargervik K. Neuromuscular adaptation in experimentally induced oral respiration in the rhesus monkey (*Macaca mulatta*). Arch Oral Biol 1980; 25:579–589.
26. Tomer BS, Harvold EP. Primate experiments on mandibular growth direction. Am J Orthod 1982; 82:114–119.
27. Ramadan MF. Effect of experimental nasal obstruction on growth of alveolar arch. Acta Otolaryngol 1984; 110:566–570.
28. Vig PS, Sarver DM, Hall DJ, Warren DW. Quantitative evaluation of nasal airflow

in relation to facial morphology. Am J Orthod 1981; 79:263–272.

29. Watson RM, Warren DW, Fischer ND. Nasal resistance, skeletal classification, and mouth breathing in orthodontic patients. Am J Orthod 1968; 54:367–379.
30. Miller AJ, Vargervik K. Neuromuscular changes during long-term adaptation of the rhesus monkey to oral respiration. In: McNamara JA Jr, ed. Naso-respiratory function and craniofacial growth, Monograph no 9, Ann Arbor: University of Michigan, 1979.
31. Linder-Aronson S. Effects of adenoidectomy on dentition and nasopharynx. Am J Orthod 1974; 65:1–15.
32. Linder-Aronson S, Woodside DG, Lundstrom A. Mandibular growth direction following adenoidectomy. Am J Orthod 1986; 89:273–284.
33. Hannuksela A. The effect of moderate and severe atopy on the facial skeleton. Eur J Orthod 1981; 3:187–193.

9

Nonallergic Rhinitis in Children: The Diagnosis and Management Options

John W. Georgitis
Bowman Gray School of Medicine of Wake Forest University, Winston-Salem, North Carolina

I. INTRODUCTION

When evaluating children with chronic nasal complaints, the most common diagnosis, by far, is allergic rhinitis. Nonallergic rhinitis of childhood, on the other hand, comprises a lesser but still significant percentage of rhinitis (1,2). The true prevalence of nonallergic rhinitis is unknown, but, in our studies, 33–45% of adults and children fit the diagnostic category of nonallergic rhinitis. Nonallergic rhinitis embraces a variety of acute and chronic rhinitic disorders and, therefore, is a frustrating entity to treat. Nonallergic rhinitis is best defined by the negative features or, rather, that it is *not* allergic rhinitis.

II. DEFINITION

Nonallergic rhinitis is a constellation of chronic rhinitis complaints that cannot be directly attributed to an allergen (1). A better diagnostic definition is the chronic rhinitis patient with negative skin tests to appropriate allergens for the geographic area (Table 1).

III. CLASSIFICATIONS

Nonallergic rhinitis may be grouped into specific classifications based upon the nasal cell influxes and other laboratory findings (3). Some laboratory studies are quite simple and easy to perform, whereas others are expensive and labor-intensive. The selection of effective therapy can be based upon the rhinitis classification. Specific pharmacologic agents work better for certain classifications than for others.

For rhinitis classification, the important factor is the presence or absence of cellular components in the nasal secretions. This can be done simply by counting the different cell types present. When the percentage of eosinophils is > 30%, the patient is defined as having eosinophilic nonallergic rhinitis (4,5). However, several nasal samples or smears may be needed before this percentage of eosinophils is seen. Therefore, it is recommended that a sample or smear be done several times, even after the patient has begun therapy.

If the cellular influx is predominantly neutrophilic, one should examine for obvious infectious causes of rhinitis or the common infectious complications associated with rhinitis, such as sinusitis, nasopharyngitis, or otitis media. If these infectious causes are absent and the nasal sample repeatedly shows high percentages of neutrophils, the patient has neutrophilic nonallergic rhinitis. However, there should be a constant surveillance for infectious causes while treating patients with neutrophilic nonallergic rhinitis.

Table 1 Categories of Nonallergic Rhinitis

Eosinophilic nonallergic rhinitis
With eosinophilia only
With nasal polyp present
With coexisting aspirin sensitivity
With coexisting asthma
Neutrophilic nonallergic rhinitis
Basophilic nonallergic rhinitis
Acellular nonallergic rhinitis
Vasomotor rhinitis
Endocrine-induced rhinitis
Pregnancy, menstrual cycles
Metabolic rhinitis
Hypothyroidism
Rhinitis medicamentosa
Chronic decongestant use
β-antagonist therapy
Reserpine therapy
Anatomic obstructive rhinitis
Deviated nasal septum or spurs
Adenoidal hypertrophy
Nasal polyps

When the cellular influx is basophilic, the patient may be classified as basophilic nonallergic rhinitis or nasal mastocytosis (6,7). To differentiate these cells requires electron microscopy of a nasal biopsy sample or special mast cell stains of the nasal samples.

Lymphocytes may be present on the nasal sample but this has been rarely described in chronic rhinitis. A lymphocyte influx probably reflects the presence of common viral infections, such as the common cold. However, it is possible that lymphocytes will appear in response to chronic fungal infections or mycobacterial causes of rhinitis. Table 2 lists infectious causes of chronic rhinitis (2).

If there is an absence of cells on the nasal sample or smear, the classification of nonallergic rhinitis are quite varied and can be difficult to treat. As seen from Table 1, there are important systemic causes for chronic rhinitis that need to be excluded (8,9). A detailed history and physical examination will help lead to the cause or to the pharmacologic therapy that causes the rhinitis. For example, excessive use of local decongestants results in rhinitis

Table 2 Infectious Causes of Rhinitis

Bacteria	Viruses	Fungi	Protozoa
Streptococcus pneumoniae	Herpex simplex	*Blastomyces dermatitidis*	*Leishmania* spp.
Haemophilus influenzae	Varicella–zoster	*Paracoccidioides*	
Streptococcus pyogenes	Rhinovirus	*brasiliensis*	
Staphylococcus aureus	Coronavirus	*Cryptococcus*	
Neisseria meningitidis	Parainfluenza	*neoformans*	
Cornyebacterium diphtheriae	Adenovirus	*Rhinosporidium seeberi*	
Klebsiella rhinoscleromatis	Influenza	Mucorales	
Calymmatobacterium	Respiratory syncytial virus	*Aspergillus* spp.	
Myobacterium leprae			
Treponema pallidum			

medicamentosa. Alternatively, a metabolic disorder, such as hypothyroidism, normal fluctuations of female sex hormones, or persistant elevations of estrogens during pregnancy, may cause chronic nasal congestion. With effective thyroid replacement or completion of the pregnancy, this nasal congestion will resolve. In terms of anatomical causes for rhinitis listed in Table 1, nasopharyngeal tumors, nasal polyps, deviated septum, and adenoidal hypertrophy can cause the nasal symptoms through obstruction of the nasal airway. With effective removal of the nasal polyps or adenoidal tissues, there is more effective airflow and mucociliary clearance, thereby leading to resolution of the rhinitis.

IV. ETIOLOGY

For nonallergic rhinitis, the etiology is as varied as the list of classifications. With eosinophilic nonallergic rhinitis and neutrophilic nonallergic rhinitis, the history and physical examinations often suggests an allergic cause, especially with the presence of eosinophils on nasal smear. However, after extensive allergy skin testing, there is no obvious IgE-mediated sensitivity. To identify an antibody-mediated cause for the chronic rhinitis, some authors have proposed that IgG4 acts similarly to IgE and is elevated in atopic families (10–14). Routine skin tests in this situation fail to identify allergen specific IgE or IgG4. There are immunoassays available that measure allergen-specific IgG4. However, many experts have found that IgG4 is produced by allergen immunotherapy and, therefore, is a protective antibody (15–18). Until future studies resolve this controversy surrounding IgG4, there is no need to measure allergen-specific IgG4 in patients. Another theory proposes that there is a second IgE antibody, IgE2 not detected by standard skin testing or radioimmunoassays for IgE. Additional immunological studies are needed to prove that such an antibody exists and, more importantly, is the cause for nonallergic rhinitis. Finally, there may be local histamine-releasing factors in the nasal mucosa and secretions that result in nonspecific mast cell degranulation (19–27). These factors are an active area of research for several centers.

With noninflammatory nonallergic rhinitis, the etiology is often a systemic disorder. The one exception is vasomotor rhinitis in which symptoms are intense, yet appear and resolve within minutes. In vasomotor rhinitis, there is no underlying systemic disorder (28). The rhinorrhea of vasomotor rhinitis has no specific cellular influx. Many authors have proposed that vasomotor rhinitis is a condition of autonomic imbalance that causes rhinitis symptoms. Unfortunately, there has been no extensive investigation into the pathophysiology of vasomotor rhinitis.

Finally, with the pervasion of illicit drug use, these causes should be considered in children with chronic unclassified rhinitis. The exposure to these drugs may be active patient use or passive exposure through inhaling the smoke or gases. It is a sad commentary on our society that this type of rhinitis classification even needs to be included for children, but the good diagnostician will consider all possible causes, even though it is a pediatric patient.

V. PATHOPHYSIOLOGY

The mechanisms causing allergic rhinitis are well studied, but not those for nonallergic rhinitis (29–37). Therefore, assumptions are made concerning nonallergic rhinitis because its clinical presentation is similar to allergic rhinitis. The nasal mast cell is thought to be the major focal point for nonallergic rhinitis. In allergic rhinitis, there is cross-linkage of allergen-specific surface-bound IgE, resulting in mediator release from the mast cell. The mast cell also can release mediators after exposure to hyperosmolar solutions, cold dry air, and the calcium ionophore, A23817 (38). With release of mediators (Table 3), other inflammatory cells migrate to the site (39–41). In the nose, these cells may be neutrophils, eosinophils, basophils, and other unidentifiable lymphoid-type mononuclear cells (42). The classification of nonallergic rhinitis is based upon the major cells present in the nasal secretions (i.e., neutrophils, eosinophils, or basophils). With appearance of these inflammatory cells, there is further perpetuation of the inflammatory response in nasal tissues. For nonallergic rhinitis, only cold, dry air nasal challenges have been used to study mast cell mediator release into nasal lavages samples (43,44). In these experiments, some of the cold air-challenged subjects are atopic individuals. Togias and co-workers (43) have demonstrated that prostaglandin D_2 (PGD_2), histamine, leukotriene C4 (LTC_4), tosyl argenine methyl ester (TAME) esterase, and kinins are released into the nasal lavage samples, thereby indicating that mast cells can respond to cold air. In another series, which included nonallergic and allergic rhinitis patients, Wilson and associates found no difference between the two patient groups in histamine and heparin concentrations in nasal turbinate tissues (45). However, the nonallergic subjects had more mast cells present on staining than the allergic rhinitis patients. This may reflect that the mast cells in the allergic group had degranulated and could not be stained easily. Further nasal challenge studies involving nonallergic subjects have, unfortunately, the distinct problem of which stimulus to use to provoke rhinitis.

In addition to the mast cells, lipid mediators, and inflammatory cells present in chronic rhinitis, neuropeptides are released from peripheral nerve endings and are potent mediators of edema and inflammation (46–48). There are a

Table 3 Inflammatory Mediators

Preformed, rapidly released
Histamine
High-molecular-weight neutrophil chemotactic factor
Eosinophil chemotactic factors of anaphylaxis
Kinogenases
Prekallikrein activator
Hageman factor "activator"
Arylsulfatase A
Serotonin
Exoglycosidases (β-hexoseaminidase, β-glucoronidase, β-galactosidase)
Lymphocyte chemotactic factors
Eosinophil chemotactic factor oligopeptides
Granule matrix-associated
Heparin
Tryptase
Arylsulfatase B
Superoxide dismutase
Proteoglycans
Chymoptryptic proteases
Peroxidase
Newly generated or secondary
Arachidonic acid derivatives
LTC_4, LTD_4, LTE_4
Hydroperoxyeicosatetraenoic acids
Hydroxyeicosatetraenoic acids
Prostaglandins
Thromboxanes
Platelet-activating factor
Superoxide, H_2O_2
Adenosine
Bradykinin
Prostaglandin-generating factor of anaphylaxis

limited number of studies involving neuropeptides for either allergic or nonallergic rhinitis.These sensory neuropeptides include substance P (sP), somatostatin (SOM), vasointestinal peptide (VIP), and calcitonin gene-related peptide (CGRP). These sensory neuropeptides are potent mediators of vasodilation; of secretion by exocrine glands, smooth-muscule contractions, and relaxation, and affect leukocyte function. Substance P, SOM, and CGRP are elevated locally in tissues during immediate hypersensitivity and inflammation. In the nose, evaluation of neuropeptide release and action has not been well studied.

In the skin, substance P can produce a classic wheal-and-flare reaction similar to allergen (49). Substance P has also been found in afferent nerve endings in the nasal mucosa (46). Substance P can directly cause vasodilation, extravasation of plasma proteins, and contraction of airway smooth muscle, and increased mucous production. Substance P can also modulate acetylcholine release from parasympathetic nerve endings or may activate central reflex pathways. It directly provokes mast cell degranulation and is present in nasal secretions of allergic subjects after allergen and methacholine challenge (50,51). In one study, Walker and associates found small increases in SOM and GCRP in nasal secretions of allergic subjects undergoing rye grass challenge (52). There was no change in sP concentration of allergic subjects. In a different study, Devillier and co-workers examined the effect of topical sP on nasal resistance in allergic rhinitis subjects and normal subjects (53). Substance P evoked cutaneous flushing in all subjects and, in allergic subjects, sP caused greater increase in nasal resistance, when compared with normal subjects. Pretreatment with an anticholinergic, oxytropium bromide, had no effect on the sP increase in nasal resistance. Substance P appears to be cell-selective because only mast cells released leukotrienes and histamine upon exposure of sP, whereas basophils do not react to sP (48). On the other hand, SOM inhibits IgE-mediated histamine release from basophils, but not A23187 ionophore-induced release (54). Somatostatin has little inhibitory effect on mast cells. Similarly to sP, CGRP can directly increase microvascular permeability and stimulate epithelial cell secretion (48).

More importantly, neuropeptides can modulate inflammation and tissue repair (48). Substance P stimulates chemotaxis of monocytes and polymorphonuclear leukocytes. It also induces generation of thromboxane A_2, O_3^-, and H_2O_2 by activated macrophages. Substance P also stimulates synthesis and release of lysosomal enzymes, LTC_4, PGE_2, and thromboxane B_2. Substance P and CGRP enhance smooth-muscle and fibroblast proliferation. Therefore, further investigations of the neuropeptides may prove valuable for nonallergic rhinitis.

Another explanation for nonallergic rhinitis includes basic anatomy, especially nasal vascular structures (55,56). The nasal turbinates are highly vascular tissues with rapid fluctuations in turbinate size, resulting in the nasal cycle. The physiological purpose of the nasal cycle is not adequately explained, but this cycle leads to alternating nasal airflow from one nasal passage to the opposite passage about every 3–4 hr. This cycling clearly is affected by circulating hormones because exercise and elevated epinephrine concentrations leads to nasal decongestion. Alternatively, menstruation and pregnancy results in increased turbinate engorgement and complaints about severe nasal congestion. With partuition, the women report the nasal congestion and rhinitis resolve quickly.

In summary, the pathophysiology of nonallergic rhinitis may be due nonspecific stimulation of mast cells, local sensory neuropeptide release, exaggerated vascular responses, or combinations of these. It is well known that young children are prone to recurrent respiratory tract infections. Petruson and Hansson (56) examined the nasal mucosal changes in 12 children thought to be representative of over 100 cases with recurrent infections. Histopathological findings showed that goblet cells varied widely from being absent to being the major cell type of epithelium. Ciliated cell numbers were frequently decreased or were abnormal in appearance. An absence of ciliary dynein arms was found in one child, and four children had abnormal cilia. The epithelial cell surface was normal in only two children, with varying obstruction, and the remainder of the children showed a range from disruptive epithelial surface to reactive cells. More importantly, microabscesses were present in five patients with increased mucosal vascularity in the subepithelial area. The basement membrane was thicker than normal in all but one case. Fibrosis was present in the older children. In 9 of 12 patients, the predominant types of inflammatory cells seen in biopsy specimens were lymphocytes and plasma cells in the lamina propria. This shows that repeated infections can lead to nasal dysfunction, with findings consistent with chronic inflammation.

VI. CLINICAL FEATURES

Children may not directly complain about symptoms; therefore, the history is often based upon the parental observations. Patients and parents often will report a wide variety of symptoms, and this reporting may be fragmented and disjointed. Similarly to those with allergic rhinitis, nonallegic rhinitis patients will complain about nasal itching, rhinorrhea, congestion, postnasal drip, and cough (2,4,5). The nasal symptoms of itching may be located in the nose or extend to the ears and eyes and can be episodic or continuous. The rhinorrhea can be clear or mucoid. The patients may not actually complain about itching, but may just constantly rub their nose or do the "allergic salute." More commonly, patients complain about postnasal drip or "drainage in their throats." In some patients, the complaint may be frequent sore throats, dry throats, or constant clearing of their throats. In the toddler and young child, parents may report a "rattly" type of breathing, a "wheezing that they hear." Some parents may report that they can feel the wheezing on their child's back. In addition to these prominant symptoms of rhinitis, there are other or indirect symptoms of rhinitis. For example, children or parents may report the child is a chronic mouth breather, has chronic snoring, or complaints about frequent headaches. Patients may report about "being stopped-up" or a "popping" in the ears. There also may be a history of chronic hoarseness. These are associated symptoms that are indirectly connected to the chronic rhinitis. Other associative symptoms include chronic fatigue, malaise, irritable behavior, and behavioral problems (1,2). Furthermore, there may be a history of poor school performance, upset stomach, chronic stomatitis, decreased appetite, and restless sleep. These symptoms may occur in any combination and severity but certain patterns do emerge and help in categorizing the rhinitis.

With eosinophilic nonallergic rhinitis, the patient reports symptoms classically associated with allergic rhinitis. They will describe nasal, eye, or ear itching; complain about a clear rhinorrhea; and comment on repetitive sneezing. These symptoms may seem to have a seasonal pattern or correlate with environmental exposures. With further investigation, one finds the nonallergic triggers such as tobacco smoke, gas fumes and irritants, rapid climatologic changes (high- and low-pressure trends), or irritant dust exposure.

With noneosinophilic nonallergic rhinitis, the patients report more about severe nasal congestion and comment less about nasal itching, repetitive sneezing, or rhinorrhea. There is no obvious seasonal or environmental variation to the symptoms. Patients may report that symptoms intensify with recumbancy, which is due to the normal increase in nasal turbinate size and nasal resistance with lying down.

Vasomotor rhinitis is the other nonallergic rhinitis with a distinct history. These patients will complain bitterly about nasal congestion, sneezing, and a profuse watery rhinorrhea. These symptoms will appear rapidly and resolve quickly within minutes. There may or may not be obvious precipitants or provocateurs. For example, a vasomotor rhinitis patient will have symptoms after exposure to bright lights or cooking odors.

VII. PHYSICAL FINDINGS

It must be noted that use of a topical vasoconstrictor may be needed in cases in whom there is extensive tissue edema. Basically, this should be done to examine for anatomical causes of rhinitis such as polyps, septal deviations and spurs, or foreign bodies. Before using topical vasoconstrictors, the examiner may want to obtain the nasal secretion sample because the topical sympathomimetics may alter the nasal specimen.

Externally, one may see obvious allergic shiners, the characteristic bluish discoloration below the lower eyelid. This area may also be mildly edematous. With the constant rubbing of the nose, one may see a nasal crease present.

In eosinophilic nonallergic rhinitis, the examiner may see pale or blue, edematous turbinates with variable degrees of obstruction. There may be a clear sheen to the mucosal surface or extensively profuse secretions on the nasal floor. The secretions may be clear or contain flecks of thick white mucus. Examination of the pharyngeal area may reveal tonsillar hypertrophy with dilated surface vessels, but more commonly, the tonsils are unimpressive in size or appearance. On the other hand, the posterior pharyngeal wall has a follicular hyperplasia, giving it the appearance of a "cobblestone road." Mucus can occasionally be seen along the lateral walls. Often, there is nontender cervical adenopathy present just below the angle of the jaw.

In nonallergic noninfectious rhinitis with neutrophils, the nasal cavity has an appearance similar to eosinophilic rhinitis. The major difference is not in the mucosal surface, but rather, the secretions. The rhinorrhea frequently is mucoid or purulent in gross appearance. Secretions may be thick and rather tenacious. With the extensive drainage, the posterior pharyngeal wall will develop the follicular appearance.

Very little has been written about basophilic rhinitis and the physical findings, yet one must assume that nasal mucosa will have an appearance similar to that of eosinophilic rhinitis.

In vasomotor rhinitis, the physical examination can be quite unimpressive. If there is an absence of active symptoms, the physical examination confirms this. The nasal mucosa will appear normal in color, have little edema of the nasal turbinates, and exhibit normal appearance of the nasal secretions. Alternatively, with active symptoms, the mucosa may become edematous and have a profuse watery rhinorrhea present.

In rhinitis medicamentosa, the nasal mucosa will have a beefy red appearance, with varying degrees and odors of secretions (58). The edema may vary from minimal to extensive obstruction of the nasal cavity. Bascially this is an inflammed mucosa from excess topical decongestant use.

The last major çategory of rhinitis involves infections. The history may be the same as for other nonallergic rhinitis categories. However, the rhinitis can be caused by a variety of infectious agents and may be associated with a subtle immunodeficiency such as IgG subclass deficiency. The nasal tissues will appear red and inflamed. The nasal secretions will be mucoid to purulent in gross appearance, therefore, similar to neutrophilic rhinitis. The color of secretion may range from light yellow to thick gray-green.

VIII. LABORATORY STUDIES AND DIFFERENTIAL DIAGNOSIS

Laboratory studies are used to classify chronic rhinitis, since the patients have nondiagnostic findings on allergy skin testing. Studies may need to be repeated several times or throughout the course of treatment. Most studies can be done in the office, whereas other studies are performed in a research laboratory setting.

A. Nasal Smear and Nasal Cytology

Foremost in the evaluation of chronic rhinitis is the nasal smear or cytology (59–61). To obtain a smear, the patient blows into wax paper and the secretions are transferred to a glass slide and air-dried before staining. In the younger child, unable to blow on demand, simple squeezing the external nares together and movement downward to the nasal tip can produce sufficient secretions. Hansel's stain is used to identify the number of eosinophils present, or a simple Wright's stain may be done for leukocyte identification (Fig. 1). A minimum of 100 stained cells should be counted to identify the preponderant cell type. Alternatively, a simple graduation may be used by the number of cells seen in oil immersion: $<$ 1 cell/field = $<$ 50 cells total ($<+$); 1 cell/field = 50–100 cells total ($+/-$); 2–5 cells/field = 100–300 cells total ($+$); 6–15 cells/field = 400–1000 cells total ($++$); 16–30 cells/field = 1000–2000 cells total ($+++$), and $>$30 cells/field = $>$ 2000 cells total ($++++$). From the cells noted, a percentage of cells present (eosinophils, neutrophils, and others) can be reported.

The nasal cytological examination is of value in cases in whom there is minimal or no secretions noted on examination (59,60). There are several methods used to obtain cytological specimens (Table 4). The method used should be based upon the desired information needed. Scraping methods are uncomfortable, yet yield samples of the epithelial surface, such as goblet cells, ciliated cells, and inflammatory cells. The submucosa is not obtained with the scraping method and cell–cell architecture is not maintained. If one needs an evaluation of the submucosa or the intact cell–cell architecture, then a mucosal biopsy is needed. Biopsy methods require local anesthesia, and there is extensive bleeding and discomfort associated with the biopsy.

Fortunately, in children, the nose-blowing and nasal-scraping methods are usually all that are needed to characterize the cells. Biopsy specimens are taken infrequently in children with chronic rhinitis.

From the nasal smear and cytological studies, the patient may be placed into a major rhinitis category by using the predominant cell present on the specimen.

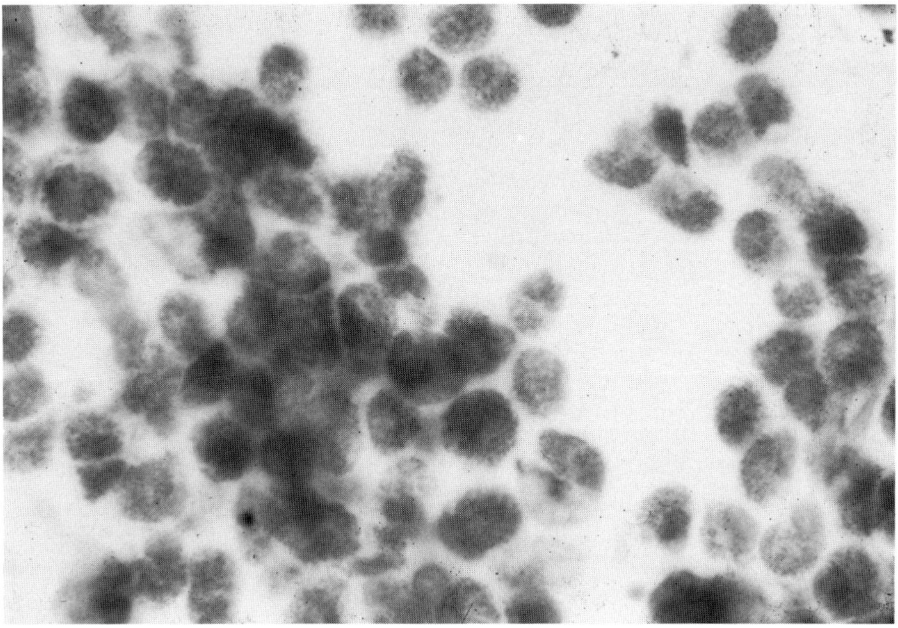

Figure 1 Hansel's stain of nasal secretions demonstrating eosinophils.

It must be stressed that multiple specimens may be necessary at separate office visits. It eosinophils are the major cell present, the subject is classified as having eosinophilic rhinitis. Similarly, if the cell predominance is neutrophils or basophils, then the rhinitis is neutrophilic or basophilic. On the other hand, in specimens with numerous bacteria present, one must explore for infectious causes of the rhinitis.

B. Rhinolaryngopharyngoscopy

With the advent of flexible fiberoptic scopes, the office or outpatient evaluation of chronic rhinitis has become more extensive and informative (62). Rhinolaryngopharyngoscopy is considered a laboratory procedure because the subject will need local anesthesia before examination. More importantly, this evaluation is not needed for every chronic rhinitis subject, especially if the history, examination skin testing, and nasal smear cytology is classic for the

Table 4 Nasal Cytological Specimen Sources

Nasal secretions
Nasal scrapings
Cotton tips
Calcium alginate
Cerumen spoon
Flexible plastic scoop (rhinoprobe)
Nasal biopsy

rhinitis category. It is recommended that rhinopharyngoscopy be used for complicated cases or for cases unresponsive to standard medical therapy.

Rhinopharyngoscopy allows the examiner to visualize the middle and posterior portions of the nasal passage that are not readily visible with the standard nasal speculum or during indirect laryngoscopy. Specifically the patency of the sinus ostia and the presence of purulent secretions can be directly visualized with rhinopharyngoscopy. Deviations in the nasal septum or septal spurs can be easily seen in middle to posterior portions. Finally, and especially importantly in pediatric practice, the adenoidal tissues can be directly visualized for size, appearance, and the degree of obstruction of the posterior choanae.

With the introduction of rigid nasopharyngoscopes, nasopharyngeal and sinus surgery is now being done routinely in adult outpatients. Procedures such as ostial enlargement, sinus lavage for culture and sensitivity, septal repair, and turbinate biopsy or turbinectomy can be done through a rigid nasopharyngoscope. Its use in children is yet to be determined.

C. Quantitative Antibodies and Allergen-Specific Antibodies

Allergy skin testing is a common practice, yet it has distinct limitations, especially in the evaluation of nonallergic rhinitis. The skin test demonstrates specific IgE antibody on dermal mast cells (63). The assumption is that similar IgE antibodies are present on the nasal mucosal and submucosal mast cells. In essence, the skin test is an indirect bioassay for the presence of IgE on nasal mast cells. A positive skin test result consists of a classic wheal-and-flare reaction 15–20 min after application of the allergen. However, in young children ($<$ 2 years of age), histamine and inhaled allergen skin tests will result in smaller wheal-and-flare reactions, compared with those of adults (64).

The nonallergic subject, however, has the skin findings that are negative or equivocal (reactions that are the same size or slightly larger than the saline control). There are clinical conditions that can result in negative skin tests when true allergen sensitivity exists. The liberal use of antihistamines, common in pediatric practice, can result in negative skin tests. Furthermore, the widespread presence of antihistamines in cough and cold preparations, especially the nonprescription preparations, afford the parents ample opportunity to give an antihistamine to their child. Parents often forget that they gave an antihistamine the day before the skin test. The remedy is to repeat the skin test at a later visit when the antihistamines have been withheld for at least 3 days.

Another consideration is the selection of allergens tested. In children, because of their small size, extensive series of allergic skin tests cannot be done as readily as in an adult. The evaluation must then be selective for the allergen tested. It is possible that the child does have a specific allergen sensitivity, but was not tested for that allergen.

The method of skin testing may also result in a negative skin test. In this situation, either the technique failed to deliver enough allergens to bind the IgE, or the potency of the specific allergen was not sufficient to stimulate mast cell mediator release.

Finally, there are reports of subjects with local nasal production of specific IgE, but whose skin tests are negative (65,66). One may continue to explore for the sensitivity by doing a total serum IgE. In general, atopic subjects will have higher total IgE than nonatopic subjects. Yet up to 20–30% of skin test-positive subjects will have low levels of total serum IgE. For general screening, a quantitative serum IgE measurement can be done first. If total serum IgE is elevated, further skin testing with other allergens may then be appropriate.

The other commonly used method of antibody determination is the solid-phase allergen-specific IgE immunoassays (67). These assays have been developed and refined for over two decades and are now readily available. They have the advantage of using serum and having no interference by antihistamines. The assays are dependent upon the stability of reagents and upon the reliability of the equipment used to measure the absorbance or radioactivity. In the patient with negative skin tests, a few selected serum allergen-specific IgE measurements could be done, but extensive testing with multiple allergens is fruitless. It must be noted that comparisons of skin testing, total serum IgE, and serum allergen-specific IgE tests have shown varying degrees of correlation with clinical history and with each other (68–71). However, the relatively high frequency of positive skin reactions favors this test over the serum allergen-specific IgE determinations.

Quantitative determinations of IgM, IgG, IgA, and IgG subclasses should be considered in selected cases of nonallergic rhinitis and chronic sinusitis. In the nonallergic patient with numerous bacteria or neutrophils present, the rhinitis and chronic infections may be due to selective immunodeficiency. There are reports of IgG subclass deficiencies present in children with recurrent respiratory complaints (72–77). In our experience, 20–30% of our referred patient population with documentable recurrent infections involving the upper airway (nose, ears, throat) have low IgG subclasses with normal total serum IgG.

Immunoglobulin A deficiency is the most common immunodeficiency known (78). Secretory IgA functions to prevent bacterial adherence to mucosal surfaces and, therefore, is the most prevalent antibody in nasal secretions. Selective IgA deficiency historically presents with recurrent respiratory infections, or it may be found in asymptomatic subjects.

Determination of allergen-specific IgG or allergen-specific IgG4 is another immunoassay often proposed for the chronic rhinitis patient (79). This last category of antibody analysis remains controversial and needs further investigation before being an acceptable diagnostic tool. These assays are readily available; however, the question remains unanswered about the physiological function of IgG4. Specifically, it is whether or not IgG4 has cytotoxic properties similar to IgE. Therefore, some people believe that IgG4 is capable of inducing mast cell mediator release (10–14). Others have shown that IgG4 is the predominant antibody produced by standard parenteral immunotherapy and, therefore, functions as a blocking antibody (15–18). Until further studies clarify how IgG4 functions, these IgG immunoassays are best used as research studies, not as diagnostic studies.

D. Radiological Studies

In nonallergic rhinitis, radiological studies are frequently used to identify other causes for chronic rhinitis. The sinus series remains the most valuable radiological evaluation. Specifically, the paranasal sinus cavities are evaluated for air–fluid levels, for opacification, or for mucosal thickening (Figs. 2–4). In children, most sinusitis involves maxillary and ethmoid sinusitis (80). A simple Water's view of the sinuses often gives an acceptable evaluation of the maxillary and ethmoid sinuses. If during the course of the evaluation, rhinopharyngoscopy can not be done on the child, a lateral neck film will help evaluate the posterior airway. The adenoid tissues may cause narrowing of the air column on lateral neck film. The laternal neck also involves study of the oropharyngeal area and tracheal column.

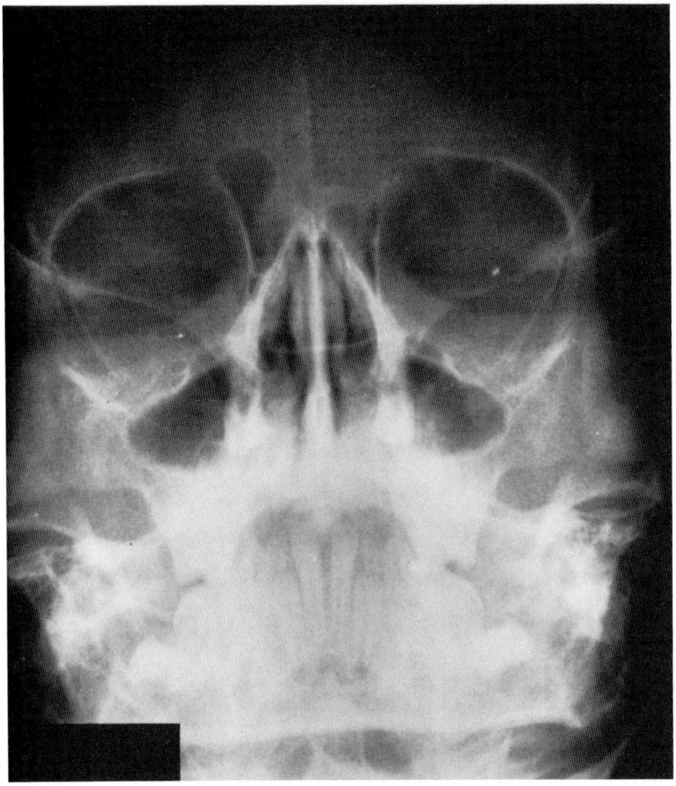

Figure 2 Water's view of paranasal sinuses demonstrating normal maxillary and ethmoid sinuses.

IX. EXPERIMENTAL STUDIES

Experimental studies are not readily available, but are utilized for investigations on the pathophysiology of allergic rhinitis. In selected cases, these studies may be useful in uncovering a true allergen sensitivity that is suspected clinically, but could not be documented by routine techniques, such as skin tests. Their use in children has yet to be defined.

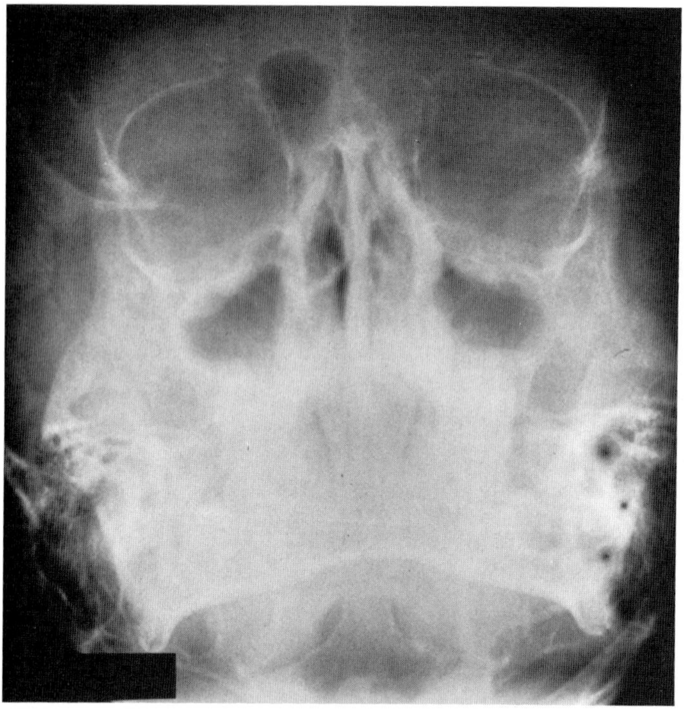

Figure 3 Water's view demonstrating mucosal thickening to the maxillary sinuses.

A. Nasal Provocation

There are several different types of nasal provocation (81). The ultimate purpose is to document the nasal tissues' response to the stimulus, albeit changes in airflow, mediator release, cell influx, or induction of late-phase reactions. Delivery of the stimulus to nasal tissue can done by multiple methods: (1) inhalation of pollen grains, (2) topical placement of fluid extracts, or (3) aerosolization of allergen extracts. Each method of delivery has its own advantages and disadvantages.

Selection of the stimulus is important when doing nasal provocation. The following have been used as nasal stimulants: histamine, methacholine, cold air, specific allergens, and specific inflammatory mediators (82,83). Methacholine evaluates the cholinergic reactivity of the nasal tissues. Specifically,

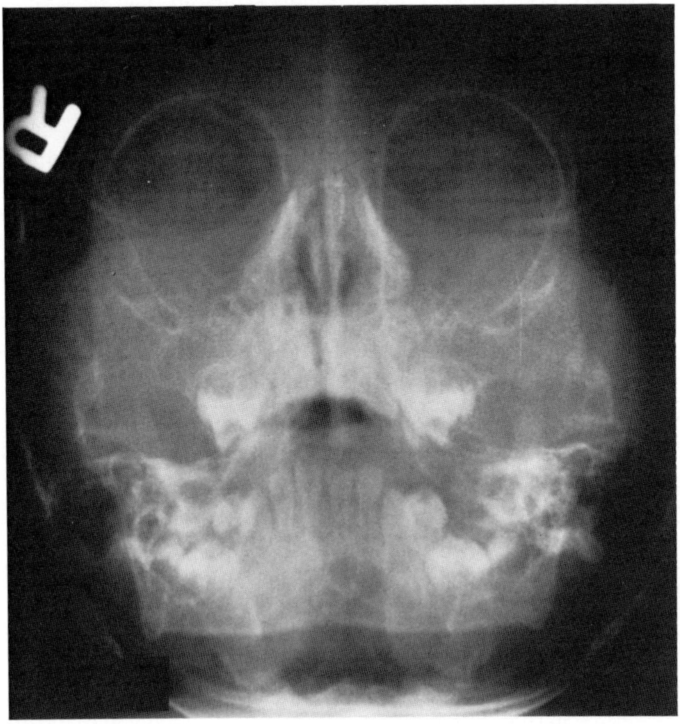

Figure 4 Water's view demonstrating opacification to the maxillary sinuses.

varying concentrations of methacholine (10–50 mg/ml) can sprayed or placed inside the nasal cavity. Clinical responses consist of profuse rhinorrhea and nasal congestion. From this type of nasal challenge, the volume of secretions may directly measured. The degree of obstruction may be quantitated by rhinomanometry. Topical treatment with ipratropium bromide, a parasympatholytic, can inhibit the secretory response to methacholine.

Histamine nasal provocation is done using a nasal spray or saturated paper disks (0.1–2.5 mg/ml) placed into the nasal passages (84). Histamine has a local vascular effect and directly stimulates sensory nerve endings. Histamine also causes local vasodilation, extravasation of serum protein into nasal secretions, and increase in the volume of nasal secretions Histamine stimulates sensory nerve endings, resulting in reflex sneezing. The histamine nasal provocation results in reproduction of major rhinitis symptoms that are similar to those seen with allergen challenge. Histamine, therefore, assesses nasal reactivity, but does not evaluate for any specific allegen sensitivity.

The allergic nasal challenge is basically the skin test evaluation of the nasal cavity (85,86). Varying dilutions of allergen may be sprayed, inhaled, or placed directly in the nasal cavity. The response is evaluated by measuring the volume of secretions produced, recording the number of sneezes, or assessing the degree of obstruction using rhinomanometry. The main purpose of allergic challenge is to measure local mediator production. Naclerio and others have convincingly shown that ragweed nasal challenge results in mast cell mediators released into secretions (29–37). Specifically, histamine, PGD_2, LTC_4 (D_4 and E_4), kinins, and TAME esterase can be found in secretions of allergic individuals.

The cold-air challenge utilizes nasal inhalation of cold, dry air to assess mediator release and the late-phase reaction. Naclerio and co-workers have shown that mast cell mediators (histamine, PGD2, TAME) are released into secretions during cold, dry air challenge (43,44,87). Extensive nasal challenge testing, however, has not been done exclusively in nonallergic subjects or subjects with only eosinophilic or neutrophilic nonallergic rhinitis.

B. Rhinomanometry

The measurement of inspiratory and expiratory nasal airflow is accomplished by using anterior or posterior rhinomanometry (88,89). Rhinomanometry involves the continuous measurement of nasal airflow (V) and differential pressure (ΔP) (Figs. 5–9). Airflow (V) is both laminar and turbulent during normal nasal breathing and can be directly measured with a pneumotachograph. Differential nasal pressure (ΔP) is the difference in pressure between the external air outside the nose and the retronasal space. Anterior rhinomanometry measures airflow through one nostril with a modified adaptor placed upon the external nares. The other nostril is occluded and indirectly measures retronasal pressure. With posterior rhinomanometry, a face mask is placed on the subject to measure total nasal airflow through both nostrils. Retronasal pressure is measured by use of a tube placed inside the mouth. A different method of posterior rhinomanometry involves use of body plethysomgraphy. With this technique, nasal airflow is calculated by subtracting the lower airway resistance from the total airway resistance.

From the rhinomanometry curves, nasal airway resistance is calculated assessing the degree of nasal patency, thereby, nasal resistance correlates well with the degree of nasal obstruction reported by the patient. Rhinomanometry

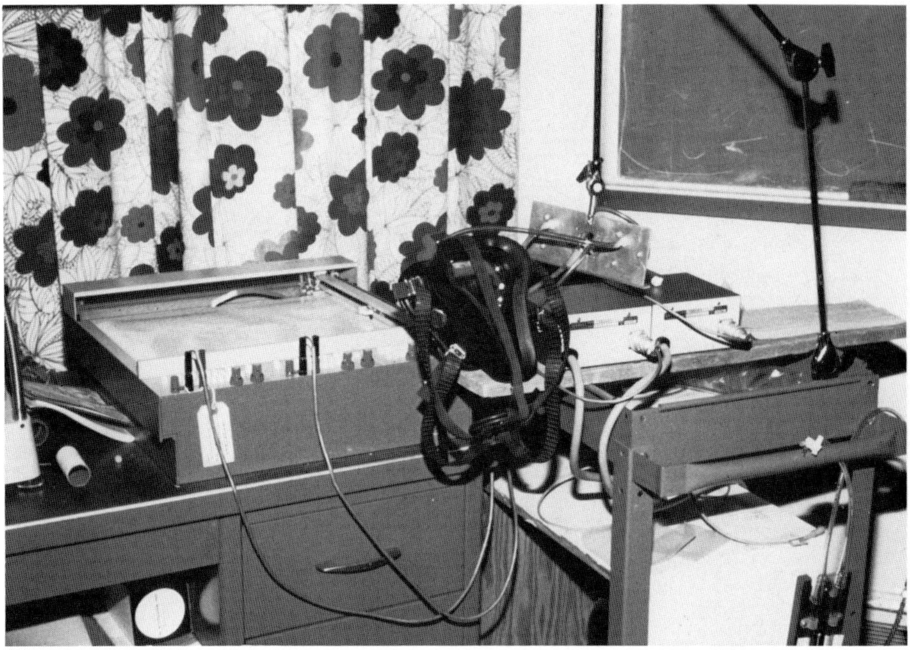

Figure 5 Rhinomanometry equipment showing pressure and flow transducers connected to an X/Y plotter.

can be done in children, but nasal resistance values are higher than those of adult subjects (89). The value of rhinomanometry is in the measurement of nasal obstruction and turbinate edema during nasal provocation. Rhinomanometry can also help identify an anatomical cause for nasal obstruction. For the latter, measurements of nasal resistance can be done before and after administering a topical decongestant. If the obstruction is anatomical, such as a deviated septum, there will be minimal change in the nasal resistance. Rhinomanometry may also be helpful in determining the effectiveness of medical or surgical treatment for nasal obstruction by determining nasal resistance before and after the therapy.

C. Nasal Antibodies and Mediators

Measurements of nasal antibodies or mediators remain purely experimental studies. In numerous publications, allergen-specific nasal IgE, IgA, and IgG

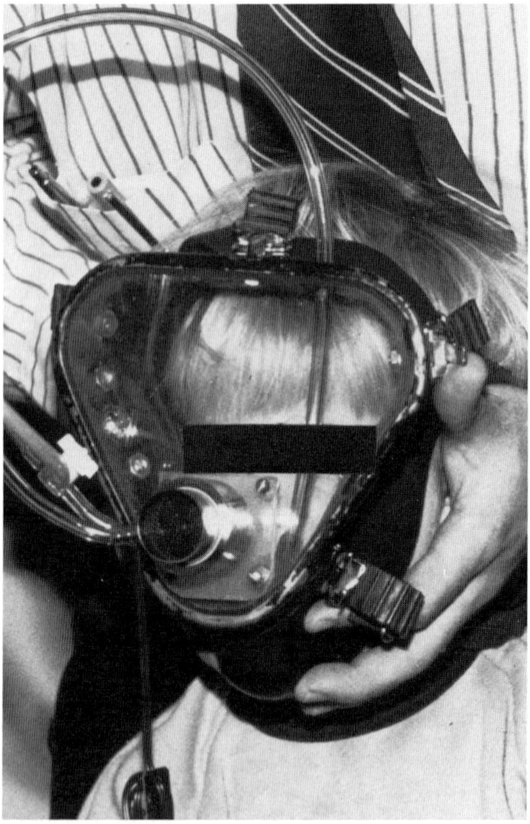

Figure 6 A 3-year-old child doing posterior rhinomanometry with a face mask and pneumotachometer in the mask. An oral tube is placed inside the mouth to measure differential pressure. The face pneumotachometer measures nasal airflow.

have been determined in allergic subjects (90–95). Nasal allergen-specific IgE is negative in subjects without active symptoms, but is present during active symptoms and, therefore, is more sensitive than serum allergen-specific IgE. The allergen-specific IgE in nasal secretions has fair to good correlations with the nasal provocation for pollens, dust mites, cat and dog dander, and molds (3). On the other hand, the appearance of allergen-specific IgA and IgG do not correlate with clinical response or correlate with the degree of clinical improvement of allergic subjects.

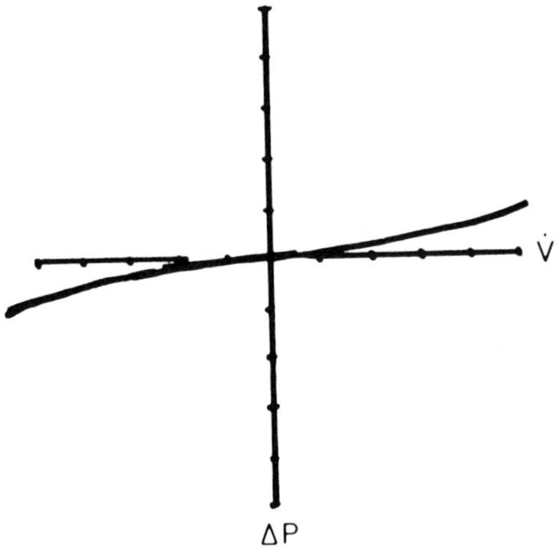

Figure 7 The nasal airflow curve generated by posterior rhinomanometry. Airflow in liters per second (L/sec) is on the horizontal axis and differential nasal pressure is on the vertical axis.

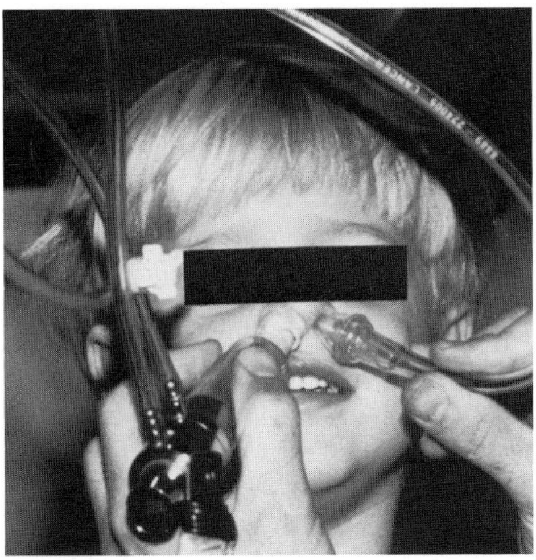

Figure 8 A 3-year-old child doing anterior rhinomanometry. One nasal tube with a pneumotachometer is placed inside one nostril; the other nasal tube blocks airflow and, thereby, measures nasal differential pressure.

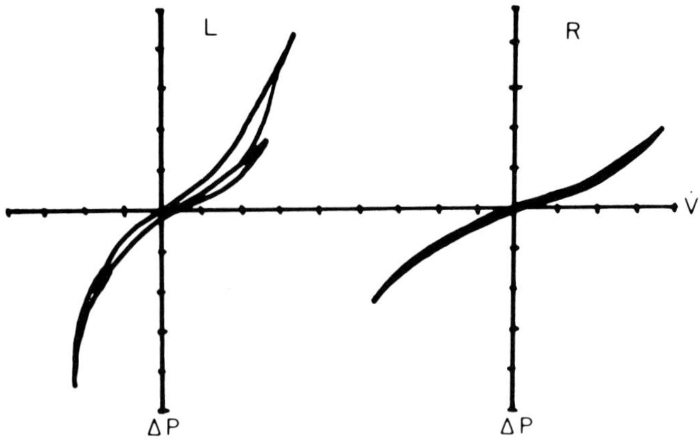

Figure 9 The nasal airflow curves for the left and right sides obtained with anterior rhinomanometry. Airflow in liters per second (L/sec) is on the horizontal axis and differential nasal pressure is on the vertical axis

Measurement of nasal mediators is used to study IgE-mediated allergic rhinitis. As previously mentioned, these studies examine for specific mast cell mediators and also other inflammatory mediators.

X. TREATMENT

Immunotherapy is not indicated for nonallergic rhinitis, therefore, pharmacotherapy remains the only acceptable therapeutic modality. However, infectious etiologies should be aggressively identified and treated in patients with nonallergic rhinitis. Anatomical causes for rhinitis also should be identified and corrected.

For eosinophilic nonallergic rhinitis, regular antihistamines and decongestants provide reasonable symptom control (4,5). However, intranasal corticosteroids are often needed and highly effective. Intranasal cromolyn, with or without corticosteroids, may be used for patients not controlled by corticosteroids alone. In recalcitant cases, secondary infections, such as sinusitis, should be considered and treated. Oral corticosteroids may be considered for difficult cases, but usually they are not needed in children with eosinophilic nonallergic rhinitis.

For neutrophilic nonallergic rhinitis, oral antihistamines and decongestants are frequently tried. Saline lavage or anticholinergic agents may provide effective symptomatic control. Antibiotics often are given, with variable response rates. Nasal corticosteroids or cromolyn, or both, may also be used to reduce the inflammation.

For basophilic rhinitis, antihistamines and decongestants are frequently prescribed, but corticosteroids are often required to control symptoms. Alternatively, intranasal cromolyn may be used as an alternative therapy for basophilic rhinitis. Antibiotics are rarely effective unless there is an underlying infection.

Vasomotor rhinitis is a difficult disorder to treat. Saline lavages have been helpful in some patients with congestion and postnasal drip symptoms. Oral antihistamines and decongestants may be effective in a few cases. For patients with profuse watery rhinorrhea, intranasal ipratropium bromide, once it is available, will be the treatment of choice for vasomotor rhinitis (96–99). In the meantime, intranasal atropine may be used as the anticholinergic agent.

For rhinitis medicamentosa, short-term systemic corticosteroids or long-term intranasal corticosteroids are often needed to allow the patient to stop their topical decongestant use. More importantly, the discontinuation of the decongestant medication is required to resolve the symptoms.

In systemic causes of rhinitis, treatment of the underlying disorder is foremost. If not successful, antihistamines may be effective for the rhinorrhea. Use of decongestants will help the congestion, but there should be careful monitoring of blood pressure. Intranasal corticosteroids may be added if symptom control is inadequate.

XI. COURSE AND COMPLICATIONS

The overall course for nonallergic rhinitis is unknown, but is is assumed that this is a life-long malady. Symptoms probably wax and wane over years. In terms of complaints, patients with nonallergic rhinitis are probably prone to recurrent sinusitis and otitis, similar to allergic rhinitis patients. Recurrent antibiotic use is commonplace for nonallergic rhinitis. With severe nasal congestion and obstruction, facial growth disturbances can occur. If there is recurrent otitis, a hearing defect may develop, depending upon the degree of scarring of the tympanic membrane. As the female child enters into adolescence and puberty, the cyclic changes in sex hormones will affect nasal function, resulting in worsening of rhinitis symptoms before menses. In addition, pregnant adolescents can experience the classic symptoms of rhinitis encountered during pregnancy. Rhinitis of pregnancy often presents in the first or second trimester and intensifies as the pregnancy progresses. The woman frequent reports symptoms of cyclic nasal congestion, profuse rhinorrhea, and repetitive sneezing. The symptoms resolve after completion of the pregnancy.

In summary, nonallergic rhinitis can be classified into different subgroups based upon the cells present in nasal smears or cytological samples. Future investigations need to concentrate on the natural causes and provocateurs, as well as to document the normal and abnormal nasal responses to these stimuli. For treatment, intranasal corticosteroids and intranasal cromolyn are highly effective for most forms of nonallergic rhinitis. The overall prognosis and course on nonallergic rhinitis is currently unknown.

ACKNOWLEDGMENT

This work is supported in part by NIH Grant No. 5 R29 AI24598.

REFERENCES

1. Pearlman DS. Chronic rhinitis children. J Allergy Clin Immunol 1988; 81:962–966.
2. Georgitis JW. Allergic rhinitis and non-allergic rhinitis: current concepts and treatment. Immunol Allergy Clin North Am 1987; 7:221–234.
3. Meltzer EO, Schatz M, Zeiger RS. Allergic and nonallergic rhinitis. In: Middleton E Jr, Reed CE, Ellis EF, Adkinson NF Jr, Yunginger JW, eds. Allergy: principles and practice. St. Louis: CV Mosby, 1988:1253–1289.
4. Jacobs RL, Freedman PM, Boswell RN. Non-allergic rhinitis with eosinophilia (NARES syndrome). J Allergy Clin Immunol 1981; 67:252–262.
5. Mullarkey MF. Eosinophilic nonallergic rhinitis. J Allergy Clin Immunol 1988; 82:941–949.
6. Connell JT. Nasal mastocytosis. J Allergy 1969; 43:182.
7. McKenna EL. Nasal mastocytosis. Laryngoscope 1974; 84:112–125.
8. Eccles R. Neurological and pharmacologic considerations. In: Procter DF, Andersen IB, eds. The nose: upper airway physiology and the atmospheric environment. Amsterdam: Elsevier Biomedical, 1982: 205–206.
9. Stevenson DD, Pleskow WW, Simon RA, et al. Aspirin-sensitive rhinosinusitis and asthma: a double-blind crossover study of treatment with aspirin. J Allergy Clin Immunol 1984; 73:500–507.
10. Fagan DL, Slaughter CA, Capra JD, Sullivan TJ. Monoclonal antibodies to immunoglobulin G_4 induces histamine release from human basophils in vitro. J Allergy Clin Immunol 1982; 70:399–404.
11. Gwynn CM, Morrison-Smith J, Leon Leon G, Stanworth DR. IgE and IgG_4 subclass in atopic families. Clin Allergy 1986; 19:227–240.
12. Stanworth DR. Immunochemical aspects of human IgG_4. Clin Rev Allergy 1983; 1:183–195.
13. Hindocha P, Wood CBS. Histamine release from human leukocytes by IgG_4 subclass in the sera of allergic children. Allergy 1985; 40:523–528.

14. Djurup R, Malling H-J. High IgG_4 antibody level is associated with failure of immunotherapy with inhalant allergens. Clin Allergy 1987; 17:459–468.
15. Vijay HM, Perlmutter L. Inhibition of reagin-mediated PCA reactions in monkeys and histamine release from human leukocytes by human IgG_4 subclass. Int Arch Allergy Appl Immunol 1977; 58:78–87.
16. Halpern GM. Recent application of IgG_4 in diagnosis and management of allergic disease. Immunol Allergy Pract 1986; 8:386–396.
17. Aalberse RC, van der Gaag XX, van Leeuwen J. Serologic aspects of IgG_4 antibodies. I. Prolonged immunization results in an IgG_4-restricted response. J Immunol 1983; 130:722–726.
18. Nakagawa T, de Weck AL. Membrane receptors for the IgG_4 subclass on human basophils and mast cells. Clin Rev Allergy 1983; I:197–206.
19. Kaplan AP, Haak-Frendscho M, Fauci A, Dinarello C, Halbert E. A histamine-release factor from activated human mononuclear cells. J Immunol 1985; 135:2027–2032.
20. Theuson DO, Speck LS, Lett-Brown MA, Grant JA. Histamine-releasing activity (HRA) I. Production by mitogen or antigen-stimulated human mononuclear cells. J Immunol 1979; 123:626–632.
21. Ezeumuzie IC, Assem ESK. A study of histamine release from human basophils and lung mast cells by products of lymphocyte stimulation. Agents Actions 1983; 13:222–230.
22. Schulman ES, Liu MC, Proud D, MacGlashan DW Jr, Lichtenstein LM, Plaut M. Human lung macrophages induce histamine release from basophils and mast cells. Am Rev Respir Dis 1985; 131:230–235.
23. Liu MC, Proud D, Lichtenstein LM, et al. Human lung macrophage-derived histamine-releasing activity is due to IgE-dependent factors. J Immunol 1986; 136:2588–2595.
24. Zheutlin LM, Ackerman SJ, Gleich GJ, Thomas LL. Stimulation of basophil and rat mast cell histamine release by eosinophil granule-derived cationic proteins. J Immunol 1984; 133:2180–2185.
25. Orchard MA, Kagey-Sobotka A, Proud D, Lichtenstein LM. Basophil histamine release induced by a substance from stimulated human platelets. J Immunol 1986; 136:2240–2244.
26. Warner JA, Pienkowski MM, Plaut M, Norman PS, Lichtenstein LM. Identification of histamine releasing factor(s) in the late phase of cutaneous IgE-mediated reactions. J Immunol 1986; 136:2583–2587.
27. White M, Kaliner MA. Neutrophils and mast cells I. neutrophil-derived histamine-releasing activity. J Immunol 1987; 139:1624–1630.
28. Bickmore JT. Vasomotor rhinitis: an update. Laryngoscope 1981; 91:1600–1605.
29. Naclerio RM, Proud D, Togias AG, et al. Inflammatory mediators in late antigen-induced rhinitis. N Engl J Med 1985; 313:65–70.
30. Pellikan Z. Late and delayed responses of the nasal mucosa to allergen challenge. Ann Allergy 1978; 41:37–47.

31. Schumacher MJ, Pain MCF. Nasal challenge testing in grass pollen hay fever. J Allergy Clin Immunol 1979; 64:202–208.
32. Dvoracek JE, Yunginger JW, Kern EB, Hyatt RE, Gleich GJ. Induction of nasal late-phase reactions by insufflation of ragweed-pollen extract. J Allergy Clin Immunol 1984; 73:363–368.
33. Naclerio RM, Meier HL, Kagey-Sobotka A, et al. Mediator release after nasal airway challenge with allergen. Am Rev Respir Dis 1983; 128:597–602.
34. Naclerio RM, Meier HL, Kagey-Sobotka A, Norman PS, Lichtenstein LM. In vivo model for the evaluation of topical antiallergic medications. Arch Otolaryngol 1984; 110:25–27.
35. Proud D, Togias A, Naclerio RM, Crush SA, Norman PS, Lichtenstein LM. Kinins are generated in vivo following nasal airway challenge of allergic individuals with allergen. J Clin Invest 1983; 72:1678–1685.
36. Pipkorn U, Proud D, Lichtenstein LM, Kagey-Sobotka A, Norman PS, Naclerio RM. Inhibition of mediator release in allergic rhinitis by pretreatment with topical glucocorticosteroids. N Engl J Med 1987; 316:1506–1510.
37. Pipkorn U, Proud D, Lichtenstein LM, et al. Effect of short-term systemic glucocorticoid treatment in human nasal mediator release after antigen challenge. J Clin Invest 1987; 80:957–961.
38. Galli SJ, Lichtenstein LM. Biology of mast cells and basophils. In: Middleton EM Jr, Reed CE, Ellis EF, Adkinson NF Jr, Yunginger JW, eds. Allergy: principles and practice. St Louis: CV Mosby, 1988:106–134.
39. Holgate ST, Robinson C, Church MK. Mediators of immediate hypersensitivity. In: Middleton EM Jr, Reed CE, Ellis EF, Adkinson NF Jr, Yunginer JW, eds. Allergy: principles and practice. St Louis: CV Mosby, 1988:135–163.
40. Mathews KP. Mediators of anaphylaxis, anaphylactoid reactions and rhinitis. J Rhinol 1987; 1:17–26.
41. Burrall BA, Payan DG, Goetzl EJ. Arachidonic acid-derived mediators of hypersensitivity and inflammation. In: Middleton EM Jr. Reed CE, Ellis EF, Adkinson NF Jr, Yunginger, JW eds. Allergy: principles and practice. St Louis: CV Mosby 1988:164–178.
42. Bascom R, Pipkorn U, Lichtenstein LM, Naclerio RM. The influx of inflammatory cells into nasal washings during late response to antigen challenge. Am Rev Respir Dis 1988; 138:406–412.
43. Togias AG, Naclerio RM, Proud D, et al. Nasal challenge with cold, dry air results in release of inflammatory mediators: possible mast cell involvement. J Clin Invest 1985; 76:1375–1381.
44. Iliopoulos O, Proud D, Norman PS, Lichtenstein LM, Kagey-Sobotka A, Naclerio RM. Nasal challenge with cold, dry air induces a late-phase reaction. Am Rev Respir Dis 1988; 138:400–450.
45. Wilson J, Reilly K, Salter D, et al. Nasal histamine and heparin in chronic rhinitis. Ann Otol Rhinol Laryngol 1988; 97:389–392.
46. Uddman R, Malm L, Sundler F. Substance-P-containing nerve fibers in the nasal mucosa. Arch Otorhinolaryngol 1983; 238:9–16.

47. Lundblad L, Lundberg JM, Brodin E, Anggard A. Origin and distribution of capsaicin-sensitive trigeminal neurons. Acta Otolaryngol 1983; 96:485–493.
48. Payan DG, McGillis JP, Renold FK, Mitsuhashi M, Goetzl EJ. Neuropeptide modulation of leukocyte function. In: Jankovic BD, Markovic BM, Spector NH, eds. Neuroimmune interactions: proceedings of the second international workshop on neuroimmunomodulation. Ann NY Acad Sci 1987; 496:182–191.
49. Devillier P, Regoli D, Asseraf A, Descours B, Marsac J, Renoux M. Histamine release and local response of rat and human skin to substance P and other mammalian tachykinins. Pharmacology 1986; 32:340–347.
50. Shanahan F, Denburg JA, Fox J, Bienenstock J, Befus D. Mast cell heterogeneity: effects of neuroenteric peptides on histamine release. J Immunol 1985; 135:1331–1337.
51. Tonneson P, Hindberg I, de Muckadell OBS, Mygind N. Effect of nasal allergen challenge on serotonin, substance P and vasoactive intestinal peptide in plasma and nasal secretions. Allergy 1988; 43:310–317.
52. Walker KB, Serwonska MH, Valone FH, et al. Distinctive patterns of release of neuroendocrine peptides after nasal challenge of allergic subjects with ryegrass. J Clin Immunol 1988; 8:108–113.
53. Devillier P, Dessanges JF, Rakotosihanaka F, et al. Nasal response to substance P and methacholine in subjects with and without allergic rhinitis. Eur Respir J 1988; 1:356–361.
54. Goetzl EJ, Payan DG. Inhibition by somatostatin of the release of mediators from human basophils and rat leukemic basophils. J Immunol 1984; 133:3255–3259.
55. Naclerio RM, Proctor DF. The anatomy and physiology of the upper airway. In: Middleton EM Jr, Reed CE, Ellis EF, Adkinson NF Jr, Yunginger JW, eds. Allergy: principles and practice, St Louis: CV Mosby, 1988:579–591.
56. Petruson B, Hansson H-A. Nasal mucosal changes in children with frequent infections. Arch Otolaryngol 1987; 113:1294–1300.
57. Ricketti AJ. Allergic rhinitis: In: Patterson R, ed. Allergic diseases diagnosis and management. Philadelphia; JB Lippincott, 1985:218.
58. Meltzer EO. Evaluation rhinitis: clinical, rhinomanometric and cytologic assessments. J Allergy Clin Immunol 1988; 82:900–908.
59. Meltzer EO, Jalowayski AA. Nasal cytology in clinical practice. Am J Rhinol 1988; 2:47–54.
60. Fair B, Hackett SF, Winther B, Hendley JO. A method of measuring polymorphonuclear leukocyte concentrations in nasal mucus. Acta Otolaryngol Suppl 1984; 413:15–18.
61. Selner JC. Visualization techniques in the nasal airway: their role in the diagnosis of upper airway disease and measurement of therapeutic response. J Allergy Clin Immunol 1988; 82:909–916.
62. Bousquet J. In vivo methods for study of allergy. In: Middleton EM Jr, Reed CE, Ellis EF, Adkinson NF Jr, Yunginger JW, eds. Allergy: principles and practice. St. Louis: CV Mosby 1988:419–436.

63. Van Asperen PP, Kemp AS, Mellis CM. Skin test reactivity and clinical allergen sensitivity in infancy. J Allergy Clin Immunol 1984; 73:381–386.
64. Mygind N, Dirksen A, Johnsen NJ, Weeke B. Perennial rhinitis: an analysis of skin testing, serum IgE and blood and smear eosinophilia in 201 patients. Clin Otolaryngol 1978; 3:189–196.
65. Stevens WJ, Vermeire PA. Serum IgE determinations in patients suffering from asthma, rhinitis, cough and various combinations of these disorders. Prog Respir Res 1980; 14:51.
66. Homburger HA, Katzmann JA. Methods of laboratory immunology. In: Middleton EM Jr, Reed CE, Ellis EF, Adkinson NF Jr, Yunginger JW, eds. Allergy: principles and practice. St Louis: CVV Mosby, 1988:409–411.
67. Pepys J, Roth A, Carroll KB. RAST, skin and nasal test and the history in grass pollen allergy. Clin Allergy 1975; 5:431–442.
68. Pascual HC, Reddy PM, Nagaya H, et al. Agreement between radioallergosorbent test and skin test. Ann Allergy 1977; 39:325–327.
69. Bousquet J, Lebel B, Dhivert H, Bataille Y, Martinot B, Michel FB. Nasal challenge with pollen grains, skin-prick tests and specific IgE in patients with grass pollen allergy. Clin Allergy 1987; 17:529–536.
70. Negrini AL, Troise C, Voltolini S. ELISA in diagnosis of respiratory allergy. Allergy 1985; 40:238–241.
71. Oxelius VA. Chronic infections in a family with hereditary deficiency of IgG_2 and IgG_4. Clin Exp Immunol 1974; 17:19–27.
72. Schur PH, Borel H, Gelfand EW, Alper CA, Rosen FS. Selective gamma-G globulin deficiencies in patients with recurrent pyogenic infections. N Engl J Med 1970; 283:631–634.
73. Smith TF, Morris EC, Bain RP. IgG subclasses in nonallergic children with chornic chest symptoms. J Pediatr 1984; 105:896–900.
74. Umetsu DT, Ambrosino DM, Quinti I, Siber GR, Geha RS. Recurrent sinopulmonary infections and impaired antibody response to bacterial capsular polysaccharide antigen in children with selective IgG-subclass deficiency. N Engl J Med 1985; 313:1247–1251.
75. Frijd A, Oxelius V-A, Rynnel-Dagoo B. A prospective study demonstrating an association between IgG_2 concentrations and susceptibility to otitis media in children. Scan J Infect Dis 1985; 17:115–120.
76. Madassery JV, Kwon OH, Lee SY, Nahm MH. IgG_2 subclass deficiency: IgG subclass assays and IgG_2 concentrations among 8015 blood donors. Clin Chem 1988; 34:1407–1413.
77. Buckley RH, Immunodeficiency. J Allergy Clin Immunol 1983; 72:627–641.
78. Homburger HA, Klatzmann JA. Methods in laboratory immunology. In: Middleton EM Jr, Reed CE, Ellis EF, Adkinson NF Jr, Yunginger JW, eds. Allergy principles and practice, St Louis: CV Mosby, 1988:411–412.
79. Conner BL, Roach ES, Laster W, Georgitis JW. Magnetic resonance imaging of the paranasal sinuses: frequency and type of abnormalities. Ann Allergy (in press).

80. McLean JA. Nasal rhinomanometry and experimental nasal challenges. N Engl Soc Allergy Proc 1982; 3:397–404.
81. Druce HM, Wright RH, Kossoff D, Kaliner MA. Cholinergic nasal hyperreactivity in atopic subjects. J Allergy Clin Immunol 1985; 76:445–452.
82. Raphael GD, Druce HM, Baraniuk JN, Kaliner MA. Pathophysiology of rhinitis I. assessment of the sources of protein in methacholine-induced nasal secretions. Am Rev Respir Dis 1988; 138:413–420.
83. Georgitis JW. Nasal provocation testing (NPT) with histamine: comparison of disk vs spray. J Allergy Clin Immunol 1986; 77:139.
84. Georgitis JW. Nasal hyperreactivity in allergic rhinitis: correlation with end point titrations (EPT). J Allergy Clin Immunol 1986; 77:181.
85. Georgitis JW. Changes in effective nasal airway diameter during grass allergen challenges. J Allergy Clin Immunol 1987; 79:254.
86. Togias AG, Proud D, Lichtenstein LM, et al. The osmolarity of nasal secretions increases when inflammatory mediators are released in response to inhalation of cold, dry air. Am Rev Respir Dis 1988; 37:625–629.
87. Clement PAR, Hirsch C. Rhinomanometry—a review. ORL J Otorhinolaryngol Relat Spec 1984; 46:173–191.
88. Georgitis JW. The applicability of rhinomanometry in non-atopic children: comparison of three techniques. J Allergy Clin Immunol 1985; 75:614–620.
89. Schumacher MJ, Pain MCF. Intranasal immunotherapy with polymerized grass pollen allergens. Allergy 1982; 37:241–248.
90. Nickelsen JA, Goldstein S, Mueller U, Wypych J, Reisman RE, Arbesman CE. Local intranasal immunotherapy for ragweed allergic rhinitis I. Clinical response. J Allergy Clin Immunol 1981; 68:33–40.
91. Nickelsen JA, Goldstein S, Mueller U, Wypych J, Reisman RE, Arbesman CE. Local intranasal immunotherapy for ragweed allergic rhinitis II. Immunological response. J Allergy Clin Imunol 1981; 68:41–45.
92. Nickelsen JA, Georgitis JW, Mueller UR, et al. Local intranasal immunotherapy for ragweed-allergic rhinitis III. A second year of treatment. Clin Allergy 1983; 13:509–519.
93. Welsh PW, Zimmermann EM, Yunginger JW, Kern EB, Gleich GJ. Preseasonal intranasal immunotherapy with nebulized short ragweed extract. J Allergy Clin Immunol 1981; 67:237–242.
94. Georgitis JW, Nickelsen JA, Wypych JI, Kane JH, Reisman RE. Local nasal immunotherapy: efficacy of low-dose aqueous ragweed extract. J Allergy Clin Immunol 1985; 75:496–500.
95. Borum P, Mygind N, Larsen S. Ipratropium treatment of rhinorrhea in patients with perennial rhinitis. Clin Otolaryngol 1983; 8:267–272.
96. Borum P. Intranasal ipratropium: inhibition of methacholine induced hypersecretion. Rhinology 1978; 16:225–233.
97. Sanwikarja S, Schmitz PIM, Dieges PH. The effect of locally applied ipratropium aerosol on the nasal methacholine challenge in patients with allergic and nonallergic rhinitis. Ann Allergy 1986; 56:162–166.

98. Jokinen K, Sipila P. Intranasal ipratropium in the treatment of vasomotor rhinitis. Rhinology 1983; 21:341–345.
99. Knight A. Intranasal Atrovent vs placebo in vasomotor rhinitis. Ann Allergy 1985; 55:305.

10

Relationship Between Rhinitis and Sinusitis and Asthma

Gail G. Shapiro
School of Medicine, University of Washington, and Children's Hospital and Medical Center, Seattle, Washington

I. Diagnosis

Children with upper and lower airway problems may present in a variety of ways: (1) with obvious symptoms denoting activity in both areas; (2) with apparent unremitting rhinitis symptoms, where part of the symptom complex is actually due to lower airway disease; and (3) with deteriorating asthma where the upper airway is silently playing a significant causative role.

The patient with allergic rhinitis may complain of a variety of problems. While nasal stuffiness and rhinorrhea are certainly the most common symptoms, cough often is another prominent one. Frequently, the cough is assumed to result from excessive secretions that cause pharyngeal irritation with little regard for the fact that a large proportion of children with allergic rhinitis have reactive airways. This may lead to ineffective courses of antihistamine and/or decongestant therapy and frustration on the part of patient, parent, and physician with the lack of response. The involvement of the lower airways is important and may take special tests to uncover. This was previously demonstrated when approximately 40% of children with allergic rhinitis, but not clinical asthma, were found to manifest exercise induced asthma as the main evidence of their airway bronchial hyperreactivity (1). Cough, in fact, may be the only presenting complaint in patients with asthma (2). Among children evaluated with methacholine challenge to rule out a diagnosis of asthma, 40% complained of cough rather than wheezing as their primary symptom (3). Given these startling figures, one cannot overlook airway reactivity as a cause for cough in patients who also have rhinitis. The same caveat applies to sinusitis. Though it is well established that cough and rhinorrhea are the most common chief complaints in children with radiographic and culture-proven sinusitis (4), this does not exclude lower airway inflammation and bronchoconstriction from the differential diagnosis of the patient's cough.

Which clues suggest that the patient with upper respiratory difficulty, rhinitis and/or sinusitis, may have clinically significant airways hyperresponsiveness (Table 1)? Typically, cough is the most prominent symptom. The history among

Table 1 Clues to Hyperresponsiveness of Lower Airways

Symptoms:	Cough
Signs:	Wheezing
	Increased expiratory phase of respiration
Diagnostic tests:	PEFR <80% predicted
	FEV_1 <80% predicted
	$FEF_{25-75\%}$ <65% predicted
	Bronchodilator inhalation to assess reversibility of above
	Bronchoprovocation tests
	Exercise
	Methacholine, histamine
	Cold air
	Distilled water (Fog)
	Hypertonic saline

patients, however, may vary. Sometimes the patient will complain of persisting cough, even after medical therapy, e.g., antihistamines, decongestants, nasal cromolyn, and/or nasal corticosteroids and antimicrobial therapy can control nasal symptoms. This is often increased during the night and early morning hours. Others will complain of increased cough following broncho-provocative stimuli such as cold air and exercise. In a smaller number of children, instead of cough, the child may experience bronchospasm with exercise and present with shortness of breath on exertion or unwillingness to participate in physical activities.

Physical examination may reveal an increased anterior-posterior chest diameter, increased expiratory phase of respiration and wheezing, obvious signs of bronchospasm. The physical examination in most cases may not, however, be very helpful. If the chest examination is unremarkable, but history is suggestive, certain diagnostic tests can be employed to make the diagnosis. Pulmonary function testing may show abnormalities in lung volumes and airflow that are not visually evident. Peak expiratory flow rate, a measure of airflow through larger airways, can be decreased from predicted normal for age in patients with reactive airways currently experiencing bronchospasm. Peak flow determinations are easily performed by children age 3 years and older who can readily be taught to exhale forcefully into a peak flow meter. Patients with intermittent symptoms can be given a portable peak flow meter to use at home. It may be valuable to have patients use these twice a day to establish a baseline and also to assess any flow changes that may occur during times of coughing.

Spirometry is more sensitive than peak flow (5). Children may have abnormalities in forced expiratory flow in one second (FEV_1) and/or forced expiratory flow in 25–75% of vital capacity (FEF_{25-75}). When the PEFR remains normal, if FEV_1 is less than 80% of normal predicted for age and sex, or $FEF_{25-75\%}$ is less than 65%, bronchodilator inhalation producing reversibility of >15% in the former or >25% in the latter confirms that reversible obstruction was present. Two actuations of a metered dose inhaler of a beta agonist such as metaproterenol, terbutaline, or albuterol with spirometry 10–30 min later is adequate for this assessment.

Patients with reactive airways and intermittent obstruction may have normal spirometry. If lower airway disease remains a likelihood, bronchoprovocation testing will be helpful. One form of this, exercise, is easily accomplished by having the patient run for 6–8 min at a rate capable of causing tachycardia to approximately 170 beats per min, fairly easily achieved in children by having them run up and down corridors or around office buildings. Factors that cannot be standardized with this technique such as air temperature and ambient pollutants may enhance the bronchoprovocative challenge. Treadmill or cycloergometer exercise allow for standardizing of the workload but are not absolutely necessary for a clinical diagnosis.

Methacholine, an acetylcholine congener with potent but short-lived bronchoconstrictive properties, is more sensitive than exercise for defining hyperreactive airways. While a methacholine challenge may be positive in asymptomatic children, selective testing of patients who have symptoms and/or physical findings favoring a diagnosis of obstructive airway disease increases the likelihood that a positive test is clinically relevant. Alternative bronchoprovocative challenges that are valuable methods for confirming lower airway disease are histamine challenge, inhalation of cold dry air (isocapneic hyperventilation), distilled water inhalation, and hypertonic water inhalation (6).

II. TREATMENT

Proper therapy for the rhinitis/sinusitis patient with reversible airways obstruction will depend on the chronicity of symptoms. If patients demonstrate intermittent daytime cough, a beta agonist by inhalation from a metered dose inhaler or orally in the case of younger children may be adequate. Two inhalations of beta agonist prior to exercise is the treatment of choice for exercise-induced asthma. More persistent problems require therapy that is longer lasting than inhaled beta agonist therapy and that addresses the problem of underlying airway inflammation, not simple smooth muscle constriction. Primary drugs for chronic therapy could be inhaled cromolyn or corticosteroids or theophylline. Beta agonists will be important additions to these on an as-needed or regular basis. Oral corticosteroids may be necessary for refractory situations and certain acute exacerbations. One of the most common problems in the child with both upper and lower airway involvement occurs when the child who is known to have asthma suffers from "upper airway neglect." Commonly, physicians will aggressively pursue a medical regimen for the patient who is hospitalized, in status asthmaticus, or has frequent emergency room visits for asthma. When the high intensity situation has resolved, the patient may be wheeze-free but have persistent rhinorrhea and congestion. Since allergic rhinitis is common in children with asthma, proper management must include attention to upper airway situations in addition to the pulmonary abnormalities.

This attention to the upper airway is not merely to provide symptomatic relief of rhinorrhea and nasal congestion. To gain a better perspective of the relationship between upper and lower airways, further discussion is necessary concerning the role of upper respiratory tract disease on the course of asthma. It is well accepted that antigen exposure of allergic individuals can heighten bronchial reactivity. For example, during pollen seasons, pollen-sensitive individuals will have more severe exercise-induced asthma than at other times (7). The issue of whether nasal antigen challenge enhances bronchial reactivity is controversial. Schumacher et al. (8), Hoehne and Reed (9), and Rosenberg et al. (10) were unable to find pulmonary function changes after nasal antigen challenge, even though nasal resistance increased. However, nasal histamine challenges of patients with perennial allergic rhinitis have shown significant changes in FEV_1 in 8 of 12 subjects, all of whom had increases in nasal resistance after challenge (11). Perhaps antigen and/or allergic mediators influence subjects with active disease differently than subjects who are challenged while in an asymptomatic state (12).

The ability of rhinosinusitis to adversely affect asthma is another controversial issue. There exists a fascinating array of historical anecdotes attesting to asthma remissions after nasal polyp removal and other surgical approaches to the sinuses.

The adult and pediatric literature contains a number of compelling reports on the effect of sinusitis on asthma that are difficult to minimize because of their poignant content and the discriminating clinical acumen of their authors. Slavin and co-workers (23) describe a group of patients with severe asthma and radiographically documented sinusitis. Most of these patients experienced marked improvement in lower respiratory disease following therapy, including aggressive use of antimicrobials or surgical intervention. An important subgroup of this sample had markedly abnormal sinus radiogrpahs but were asymptomatic aside from asthma-related problems. Nevertheless, the clearing of their sinus films correlated well with improvement in asthma. The authors warn clinicians to consider sinusitis in patients with difficult to control asthma. Friedman and co-workers (14) were similarly impressed with a group of eight children with sinusitis and asthma. Aspiration of the sinuses yielded positive bacterial cultures in five of eight *Branhamella catarrhalis, Haemophilus influenzae*, and *Streptococcus pneumoniae* being recovered. All patients were treated with antibiotics with significant improvement in pulmonary function in all subjects and improvement in the radiograph in six of the eight children.

Rachelefsky and co-workers (15) identified 48 children who had required bronchodilator therapy for at least 3 months and had markedly abnormal maxillary sinuses on radiograph: severe thickening in 10, opacity of one or both antra in 30, and air fluid level in 8. After 2–5 weeks of antibiotic therapy, 39 patients had improved radiographs, while 9 required antral lavage. Following this medical or surgical therapy, many patients achieved normal pulmonary function, became asymptomatic and were able to discontinue asthma therapy (Table 2).

Table 2 Disease Characteristics Before and After Treatment for Sinus Disease in 48 Children

	Before		After	
Characteristic	No.	%	No.	%
Cough	48	100	14	29
Wheeze	48	100	7	15
Rhinorrhea	30	63	10	21
Bronchodilator treatment	48	100	10	21
Normal pulmonary function tests	0/30	0	20/30	67
Normal sinus radiograph	0	0	38	79

Source: Rachelefsky et al. (15, p. 528).

III. SINUSITIS AND ASTHMA

These uncontrolled reports match the clinical impressions of many. Nevertheless, the relationship of sinus disease and asthma requires additional delineation before the controversy will be put to rest. There needs to be a placebo-controlled evaluation of antibiotic therapy for sinus disease with asthma. This, however, poses ethical problems relating to withholding antibiotics from children with radiographically documented sinusitis when the likelihood of bacterial disease is high (4). The ethical dilemma is compounded if one's clinical bias is that not only the sinus disease but asthma, too, will worsen if antibiotics are omitted. Further complicating the problem is the group of children with mucosal thickening who radiographically do not have bacterial infection and, therefore, do not respond to antimicrobial therapy.

In contrast with the reports above, other investigators remain unconvinced of a relationship between sinus disease and asthma. Zimmerman and associates (16) found sinus radiograph abnormalities in 43 of 138 patients with asthma compared with 0 of 50 controls. They found the same incidence of sinus abnormalities in patients with mild, moderate, and severe asthma and conclude there is no support from these data for the belief that sinusitis aggravates asthma.

While this evaluation proves that there is a high incidence of radiographically abnormal sinuses in people with asthmna, it fails to answer the question of a causal association, since it assesses disease at one moment in time. One needs to know whether asthma gets better if the patients with sinusitis are treated or, if it gets worse if the sinus disease progresses. Such a prospective investigation needs to be done with appropriate randomization and placebo controls.

Another missing element in the sinusitis-asthma debate is the absence of a proven mechanism for an association. Slavin et al. (13) postulated three possible mechanisms: (1) bacterial seeding of the lungs by sinus disease with resulting bronchospasm, (2) enhanced beta blockade due to sinus infection, and (3) vagal reflex-mediated bronchospasm. Bacterial seeding seems unlikely since asthma and not bacterial pneumonia occur. Also, asthma is reportedly worsened even when sinusitis is sterile. Recent studies involving the insertion of balloon catheters into maxillary antra of patients with antrostomies have shown that the inflation of the catheters results in increased lower airway resistance, presumably through reflex mechanisms (17).

Recent evaluations of the pathologic findings in chronic sinusitis draw striking similarities between chronic asthma and sinus disease. Harlin et al. (18) examined sinus mucosa from 26 patients with chronic sinusitis, including 13 who had asthma. There was a significant association of tissue eosinophilia and asthma as well as an association of eosinophil major basic protein with presence of asthma. As in the pulmonary tree, the presence of eosinophils and eosinophil products correlated with membrane damage and inflammation. This represents another link connecting upper and lower airway dysfunction.

Though the relationship between sinusitis and asthma awaits definitive proof, the clinician must consider this relationship in caring for patients with asthma (Table 3). During asthma exacerbations, one should consider sinusitis among possible causative factors, particulary when usual therapy for acute asthma,

Table 3 Features Suggesting Sinusitis in the Patient with Asthma Exacerbations

Symptoms:	Nasal
	Headache
	Sore throat
Signs:	Periorbital edema
	Purulent rhinorrhea
	Pharyngeal drainage
	Middle ear dysfunction
	Otitis
	Effusion
	Extremely negative pressure
Nasal cytology:	Predominance of neutrophils and bacteria

including high dose corticosteroids, fails to give a satisfactory resolution to the obstructive picture. One should ask about the coexistence of nasal congestion and rhinorrhea, since in children with sinusitis, headache, fever, and malaise are less frequent sinusitis-related complaints than are cough and rhinorrhea. Physical examination must include a global evaluation. Some children with sinusitis show marked periorbital pallor and edema, sometimes with darkness under the eyes, indistinguishable from so-called "allergic shiners." The nasal exam should assess the presence of edema, erythema (more common with infection than allergy), and the quality of nasal secretions since purulence often suggests infection. The pharynx may show purulent drainage, even when the nasal examination is benign. Middle ear disease commoly accompanies sinusitis (19). One must look for acute otitis, middle ear effusions, and abnormal tympanic membrane mobility indicative of abnormal middle ear pressure, which may be confirmed with tympanometry.

The microscopic examination of the nasal secretions can be a helpful adjunct to the physical examination. Hansel's strain will allow clear separation of neutrophils and eosinophils. If eosinophils predominate, chronic noninfectious inflammation is likely. If one sees huge numbers of neutrophils and bacteria in secretions from a patient with symptoms longer than one week in duration, the likelihood of sinusitis is high. Normal individuals will have an assortment of epithelial cells, other mononuclear cells, and neutropils.

Clear distinctions are not always possible with nasal cytology, and clinical impression should guide the physician in the decision to obtain radiographs. A Waters film, which will show maxillary antra well but ethmoid sinuses poorly, is usually sufficient for assessiing sinusitis in children. However, if the Waters view is normal and other factors suggest sinusitis, one should consider the addition of the Caldwell and lateral views. In certain situations, coronal computerized tomography of the paranasal sinuses may be worthwhile. This is certainly true if sinus surgery is being considered.

IV. SUMMARY

Treatment of the child with asthma exacerbations and sinusitis must obviously address both situations. Antimicrobial therapy must be directed to the pathogens most often isolated form sinus aspirates: *B. catarrhalis, H. influenzae*, and *S. pneumoniae* (4). While amoxicillin remains the favored drug, in many communities amoxicillin-resistant strains have led to the increased use of amoxicillin-clavulinic acid and cefaclor. Individuals with persistent or recurrent sinusitis may have anaerobic infection for which clindamycin is often effective. While the addition of agents that decrease membrane edema—antihistamines, decongestants and nasal steroids—seem reasonable as additional therapies, they have not been evaluated in sinusitis. Asthma exacerbations will require an assessment of the patient's usual therapy with an eye toward optimizing bronchodilator use and consideration of starting corticosteroid therapy or increasing maintenance therapy with a high dose burst of prednisone. Since there is concurrence of upper and lower eosinophilic inflammatory disease in some patients with chronic sinusitis and asthma, steroid therapy will serve well for both conditions.

REFERENCES

1. Kawabori I, Pierson WE, Conquest LL, Bierman CW. Incidence of exercise-induced asthma in children. J Allergy Clin Immunol 1976; 58:447–455.
2. Corrao WH, Bramen SS, Irwin RS. Chronic cough as the sole presenting manifestation of bronchial asthma. N Engl J med 1979; 300:633–637.
3. Shapiro GG, Furukawa CT, Pierson WE, Bierman CW. Methacholine bronchial challenge in children. J Allergy Clin Immunol 1987; 69:365–369
4. Wald ER, Milmore GI, Bowen AD, et al. Acute maxillary sinusitis in children. N Engl J Med 1981; 304:749–752.
5. Ferguson AC. Persisting airway obstruction in asymptomatic children with asthma with normal peak expiratory flow rates. J Allergy Clin Immunol 1988; 82:19–22.
6. Bierman CW, Shapiro GG. Clinical expression of bronchial hyperreactivity in children. Clinical Reviews in Allergy 1989; 7(3):301–320..
7. Eggleston PA. Methods of exercise challenge. J Allergy Clin Immunol 1984; 73 (suppl):666.
8. Schumacher MJ, Cota KA, Taussig LM. Pulmonary response to nasal-challenge testing of atopic subjects with stable asthma. J Allergy Clin Immunol 1986; 78:30.
9. Hoehne JH, Reed CE. Where is the allergic reaction in ragweed asthma? J Allergy Clin Immunol 1971; 48:36.
10. Rosenberg GL, Rosenthal RH, Norman PS. Inhalational challenge with ragweed pollen and ragweed-sensitive asthmatics. J Allergy Clin Immunol 1983; 71:302.
11. Yan K, Salome C. The response of the airways to nasal stimulation in asthmatics with rhinitis. Eur J Respir Dis 1983; 64(suppl 128):105.
12. McFadden ER Jr. Nasal-sinus-pulmonary reflexes and bornchial asthma. J Allergy Clin Imunol 1986; 78:1–3.
13. Slavin RG, Cannon RE, Friedman WH, et al. Sinusitis and bronchial asthma. J Allergy Clin Immunol 180; 66:250–257.
14. Friedman R, Ackerman H, Wald E, et al. Asthma and bacterial sinusitis in children. J Allergy Clin Immunol 1984; 74:185–189.
15. Rachelefsky GS, Katz RM, Siegel SC. Chronic sinus disease with associated reactive airway disease in children. Pediatrics 1984; 73:526–529.

16. Zimmerman B, Stringer D, Feanny S, et al. Prevalence of abnormalities found by sinus x-rays in childhood asthma: lack of relation to severity of asthma. J Allergy Clin Immunol 1987; 80:268–673.
17. Druce H. Personal communication.
18. Harlin SL, Ansel DG, Lane SR, et al. A clinical and pathologic study of chronic sinusitis: the role of the eosinophil. J Allergy Clin Immunol 1988; 81:867–875.
19. Shapiro GG. Sinusitis in children. J Allergy Clin Immunol 1988; 81(5) (suppl): 1025–1027.

Glossary of Abbreviations

AU	Arbitrary allergy units
BU/ml	Biological units per milliliter
CAT	Computed tomography
CBC	Complete blood cell count
CEP	Ciliated epithelial cell
CGRP	Calcitonin gene-related peptide
CS	Cromolyn sodium
CTMC	Connective tissue mast cell
Da	Dalton
DAG	1,2-Diacylglycerol
ECO	Eosinophil cationic protein
EDN	Eosinophil-derived neurotoxin
ELISA	Enzyme-linked immunosorbent assay
EPO	Eosinophil peroxidase
ER	Emergency room
FAST	Fluorescent allergosorbent test
Fc RI	High-affinity Fc receptors
Fc_{ϵ} RII	Lower-affinity Fc receptors
FDA	Food and Drug Administration
GAGs	Glycosaminoglycans
GM-CSF	Granulocyte-macrophage colony stimulating factor
GMPc	Cyclic guanosine monophosphate
HEP	Histamine equivalent prick
HEPA	High-efficiency particulate air filter
HETEs	Hydroxyeicosatetraenoic acids

HPETE	Acyclic hydroperoxyeicosatetraenoic
IgE-BFs	IgE-binding regulatory factors
IL-2	Interleukin 2
IL-3	Interleukin 3
IL-5	Interleukin 5
IU	International units
IUIS	International Union of Immunological Societies
LAST	Latex allergosorbent test
LTC4	Leukotriene C4
MAb	Monoclonal antibodies
MAG	L-Monoacylglycerol
MAST	Multiple allergosorbent test
MBP	Major basic protein
MC	Chymase
MMC	Metachromatic mucosal cell
MRI	Magnetic resonance imaging
MT	Tryptase
NANC	Nonadrenergic, noncholinergic
NAR	Nasal airway resistance
NARES	Nonallergic rhinitis with eosinophilia
NCA	Neutrophil chemotactic activity
NS	Nedocromil sodium
PAF	Platelet-activating factor
PEG	Polyethylene glycol
PGs	Prostaglandins
PI	Phosphatidylinositol
PMEE	Persistent middle ear effusion
PNU	Protein nitrogen units
PPD	Packs per day
RAST	Radioallergosorbent test
RIA	Radioimmunoassay
SNF	Sensory nerve fiber
sP	Somatostatin
TAME	Esterase tosyl arginine methyl ester
TXs	Thromboxanes
URI	Upper respiratory infection
VIP	Vasoactive intestinal peptide
WHO	World Health Organization
W/V	Weight per volume

Index

B

C

D

K

O

P

R

S

T

About the Editors

CHARLES K. NASPITZ is Professor and Chief of the Division of Allergy, Immunology, and Rheumatology in the Department of Pediatrics at the Escola Paulista de Medicine, in São Paulo, Brazil, where he has taught since 1962. From 1965 to 1967 he served as a Research and Clinical Fellow in the Division of Allergy at McGill University in Montreal, Canada. He is the author or coauthor of some 40 journal articles on immunology, pediatrics, and asthma, as well as coeditor, with David G. Tinkelman and Constantine J. Falliers, of the book *Childhood Asthma* (Marcel Dekker, Inc.). He is past president of the Brazilian Society of Allergy and Clinical Immunology. Dr. Naspitz received the M.D. degree (1959) from the Escola Paulista de Medicina and M.Sc. degree (1967) from McGill Universtiy.

DAVID G. TINKELMAN is Clinical Associate Professor of Pediatrics at the Medical College of Georgia in Augusta. He also conducts a private practice and research center at the Atlanta Allergy Clinic, P.A., and serves as editor of the *Journal of Asthma* (Marcel Dekker, Inc.). A participant in many research projects, he is the author or coauthor of over 50 journal articles, book chapters, and abstracts primarily in the field of asthma. With Constantine J. Falliers and Charles K. Naspitz, he coedited the book *Childhood Asthma* (Marcel Dekker, Inc.). From 1974 to 1976 he held a fellowship in allergy and immunology at the National Jewish Hospital and Research Center in Denver, Colorado. He is a member of the American Academy of Pediatrics, American Academy of Allergy and Immunology, and American College of Allergy. Dr. Tinkelman received the B.A. degree (1968) from Temple Univesity and M.D. degree (1972) from Hahnemann Medical College.